Frontiers in Clinical Drug Research-Alzheimer Disorders

(Volume 7)

Edited by

Atta-ur-Rahman, *FRS*
Honorary Life Fellow, Kings College, University of Cambridge, Cambridge, UK

Frontiers in Clinical Drug Research - Alzheimer Disorders

Volume # 7

Editor: Atta-ur-Rahman

ISSN (Online): 2214-5168

ISSN (Print): 2451-8743

ISBN (Online): 978-1-68108-560-9

ISBN (Print): 978-1-68108-561-6

General:

1. Any dispute or claim arising out of or in connection with this License Agreement or the Work (including non-contractual disputes or claims) will be governed by and construed in accordance with the laws of the U.A.E. as applied in the Emirate of Dubai. Each party agrees that the courts of the Emirate of Dubai shall have exclusive jurisdiction to settle any dispute or claim arising out of or in connection with this License Agreement or the Work (including non-contractual disputes or claims).
2. Your rights under this License Agreement will automatically terminate without notice and without the need for a court order if at any point you breach any terms of this License Agreement. In no event will any delay or failure by Bentham Science Publishers in enforcing your compliance with this License Agreement constitute a waiver of any of its rights.
3. You acknowledge that you have read this License Agreement, and agree to be bound by its terms and conditions. To the extent that any other terms and conditions presented on any website of Bentham Science Publishers conflict with, or are inconsistent with, the terms and conditions set out in this License Agreement, you acknowledge that the terms and conditions set out in this License Agreement shall prevail.

Bentham Science Publishers Ltd.
Executive Suite Y - 2
PO Box 7917, Saif Zone
Sharjah, U.A.E.
Email: subscriptions@benthamscience.org

BENTHAM SCIENCE

CONTENTS

PREFACE

The book series, "***Frontiers in Clinical Drug Research – Alzheimer Disorders***" presents the important recent advancements in the form of cutting edge reviews written by experts. ***Volume*** *7* of this eBook series is a compilation of seven well written chapters contributed by prominent researchers in the field. They include articles on brain stimulation, ASS234 – an Anti-Alzheimer agent, Alzheimer's drug discovery research, proteasome, Ca^{2+}/cAMP signalling interaction, non-pharmacological therapies, drug development and other related areas.

Chapter 1 by Lavano *et al.*, discusses the role of deep brain stimulation in the treatment of Alzheimer's disease (AD). In chapter 2, Romero *et al.*, summarize the neuroprotective effects of ASS234 in counteracting several steps in the pathological processes of AD. Liu *et al.* in chapter 3 focus on recent advances in Alzheimer's drug discovery research. In Chapter 4, Ding and Zhu highlight the basic information and updates on the proteasome system and related cellular complexes.

In chapter 5, Bergantin discusses the fundamental concepts and current therapies to treat AD, including therapeutic outcomes resulting from the Ca^{2+}/cAMP signalling interaction. Chapter 6 by Gottlieb *et al.*, emphasizes the role of different non-pharmacological therapies administered by a multi-professional health team to maintain the acceptable quality of life for the elderly with AD. The last chapter by Sahu *et al.*, discusses the scope and limitations of some currently marketed drugs in the management of AD.

The 7th volume of this book series represents the results of a huge amount of work by many eminent researchers. I am grateful to the authors for their excellent contributions. I would also like to express my gratitude to the editorial staff of Bentham Science Publishers, particularly Mr. Mahmood Alam (Director Publication), Mr. Shehzad Naqvi (Editorial Manager Publications) and Ms. Fariya Zulfiqar (Manager Publications) for their hard work and persistent efforts.

Atta-ur-Rahman, *FRS*
Honorary Life Fellow
Kings College
University of Cambridge
Cambridge
UK

List of Contributors

Alejandro Romero	Department of Pharmacology and Toxicology, Faculty of Veterinary Medicine, Complutense University, Madrid, Spain
Ana P. Fernández	The Neurovascular Research Group, Department of Translational Neurobiology, Cajal Institute (CSIC), Madrid, Spain
Angelo Lavano	Unit of Functional Neurosurgery, Department of Medical and Surgical Sciences, University "Magna Graecia", Catanzaro, Italy
Attilio Della Torre	Unit of Functional Neurosurgery, Department of Medical and Surgical Sciences, University "Magna Graecia", Catanzaro, Italy
A von Gunten	Department of Psychiatry, University Hospital Lausanne, Lausanne, Switzerland
Bharat Bhusan Subudhi	School of Pharmaceutical Sciences, Siksha O Anusandhan Deemed University, Bhubaneswar, Odisha, India
Brati Das	Department of Neuroscience, UConn Health, 263 Farmington Avenue, Farmington, CT, USA
BJP Lopes Filho	Graduate Program in Biomedical Gerontology (GERONBIO) of the School of Medicine, Pontifícia Universidade Católica do Rio Grande do Sul, Porto Alegre, RS, Brazil
Carmelino Angelo Stroscio	Unit of Functional Neurosurgery, Department of Medical and Surgical Sciences, University "Magna Graecia", Catanzaro, Italy
CR Oliveira	Psychology Graduate Program, Faculdade Meridional Imed., Passo Fundo, RS, Brazil
Domenico Chirchiglia	Unit of Functional Neurosurgery, Department of Medical and Surgical Sciences, University "Magna Graecia", Catanzaro, Italy
Donatella Gabriele	Unit of Functional Neurosurgery, Department of Medical and Surgical Sciences, University "Magna Graecia", Catanzaro, Italy
Eva Ramos	Department of Pharmacology and Toxicology, Faculty of Veterinary Medicine, Complutense University, Madrid, Spain
F Loureiro	Graduate Program in Biomedical Gerontology (GERONBIO) of the School of Medicine, Pontifícia Universidade Católica do Rio Grande do Sul, Porto Alegre, RS, Brazil
Giorgio Volpentesta	Unit of Functional Neurosurgery, Department of Medical and Surgical Sciences, University "Magna Graecia", Catanzaro, Italy
Giusy Guzzi	Unit of Functional Neurosurgery, Department of Medical and Surgical Sciences, University "Magna Graecia", Catanzaro, Italy
Haiyan Zhu	Department of Biological Sciences, Kent State University, East Liverpool, OH, USA
José Marco-Contelles	Laboratory of Medicinal Chemistry, Institute of General Organic Chemistry (CSIC), Madrid, Spain
Julia Serrano	The Neurovascular Research Group, Department of Translational Neurobiology, Cajal Institute (CSIC), Madrid, Spain

JP Rocha	Graduate Program in Biomedical Gerontology (GERONBIO) of the School of Medicine, Pontifícia Universidade Católica do Rio Grande do Sul, Porto Alegre, RS, Brazil
Leandro Bueno Bergantin	Department of Pharmacology, Universidade Federal de São Paulo (UNIFESP), São Paulo, Brazil
MGV Gottlieb	Graduate Program in Biomedical Gerontology (GERONBIO) of the School of Medicine, Pontifícia Universidade Católica do Rio Grande do Sul, Porto Alegre, RS, Brazil
Prashant Tiwari	School of Pharmaceutical Sciences, Siksha O Anusandhan Deemed University, Bhubaneswar, Odisha, India
Pratap Kumar Sahu	School of Pharmaceutical Sciences, Siksha O Anusandhan Deemed University, Bhubaneswar, Odisha, India
Qunxing Ding	Department of Biological Sciences, Kent State University, East Liverpool, OH, USA
Ricardo Martínez-Murillo	The Neurovascular Research Group, Department of Translational Neurobiology, Cajal Institute (CSIC), Madrid, Spain
Sathyanarayanan V Puthanveettil	Department of Neuroscience, The Scripps Research Institute, Jupiter, FL, USA
Shakti Ketan Prusty	School of Pharmaceutical Sciences, Siksha O Anusandhan Deemed University, Bhubaneswar, Odisha, India
VE Closs	Study Group on Cardiometabolic Risk, Aging And Nutrition (GERICEN) of the Institute of Geriatrics and Gerontology (IGG), Pontifícia Universidade Católica do Rio Grande do Sul., Porto Alegre, RS, Brazil
VM Junges	Integrated Center for Obesity Treatment (CINTRO), Porto Alegre, RS, Brazil
Xin-An Liu	Department of Neuroscience, The Scripps Research Institute, Jupiter, FL, USA Department of Neuroscience, Icahn School of Medicine at Mount Sinai, One Gustave L. Levy Place, NewYork, NY, USA
Xu Tian	Department of Environmental Sciences and Engineering, School of Public Health, University of North Carolina, Chapel Hill, NC, USA
Yosef Avchalumov	Department of Neuroscience, The Scripps Research Institute, Jupiter, FL, USA
Youjun Chen	Department of Neurology, School of Medicine, University of North Carolina, Chapel Hill, NC, USA
Zuxin Chen	Department of Neuroscience, Icahn School of Medicine at Mount Sinai, One Gustave L. Levy Place, New York, NY, USA
ZCL Lindôso	Federal University of Pelotas, Pelotas, RS, Brazil

CHAPTER 1

Deep Brain Stimulation in the Treatment of Alzheimer's disease

Angelo Lavano*, Giusy Guzzi, Attilio Della Torre, Domenico Chirchiglia, Carmelino Angelo Stroscio, Donatella Gabriele and **Giorgio Volpentesta**

Unit of Functional Neurosurgery, Department of Medical and Surgical Sciences, University "Magna Graecia", Catanzaro, Italy

Abstract: Alzheimer's disease (AD) is the leading neurological cause of dementia of advanced predominance worldwide. The pathogenic mechanisms may concern accumulations of beta amyloid and tau protein, inflammatory pathways, altered oxidative metabolism and responses to oxidative stress. The currently available therapeutic options for AD have limited efficacy. Deep Brain Stimulation (DBS) may represent a chance in order to ameliorate cognitive performances modifying cortical and hippocampal circuits. Fornix and Nucleus basalis of Meynert are the most promising targets in terms of delaying and reversing the cognitive impairment; other targets like entorhinal cortex/hippocampus, pedunculopontine tegmental nucleus, anterior thalamic nucleus are under investigation with some success. The mechanism of action and stimulation parameters remain unclear.

Keywords: Alzheimer's disease, Brain neuromodulation, Deep Brain Stimulation, Fornix, Hippocampus, Nucleus basalis of Meynert.

INTRODUCTION

Alzheimer's disease (AD) was diagnosed for the first time in 1901 by Dr. Alzheimer [1]. It is estimated that about 35 million people worldwide are affected by AD and its incidence may be the cause of an increase in ageing populations over the next decade, posing significant challenges for public health and allocation of health care resources [2, 3]. The medical therapy, currently used, includes acetyl cholinesterase inhibitors, NMDA (N-methyl D-aspartate) receptors blockers, vitamin E, that improve only temporarily the symptoms. The modest efficacy and the substantial adverse effects, such as restlessness, dizziness, motor slowing, of drugs led to find out alternative non-pharmacological options for AD [4]. It is already acknowledged that the pathological phases implicated in

* **Corresponding author Angelo Lavano:** Unit of Functional Neurosurgery, Department of Medical and Surgical Sciences, University Magna Graecia, Campus "S. Venuta" of Germaneto, Viale Europa, 88100 Catanzaro, Italy; Tel +3909613647389; E-mail lavano@unicz.it

Atta-ur-Rahman (Ed.)

AD produce a focal synaptic dysfunction that interrupts correlated brain regions generating disseminated interferences in the normal function of circuits and networks entailed in cognition [5]. Deep Brain Stimulation (DBS) is an established way of treatment in neurodegenerative and neuropsychological conditions such as Parkinson's disease or obsessive compulsive disorder [6 - 11]. In the last years some investigations have been published concerning the possibility that DBS of select regions of the limbic system can improve memory processing and cognitive abilities [12, 13].

DBS TARGETS USED IN PATIENTS WITH AD

Anatomically AD has implications for many structures of the brain, but the most important circuitry is the limbic system. Selection of targets of the "memory circuits" with deep electrodes in AD is a new application of DBS [14]. DBS targets analysed are fornix, nucleus basalis of Meynert (NBM), entorhinal cortex (EC), pedunculopontine tegmental nucleus (PPN), anterior thalamic nucleus (ATN) and anterior limb of internal capsule/nucleus accumbens (ALIC/NAc).

Fornix

Based on the observation both on unexpected memory improvement and spatial - verbal learning in a case of bilateral hypothalamic DBS for obesity management by Hamani [15], the first phase I trial of DBS of the fornix was published in 2010 by Laxton *et al.* [16]. Fornix is a fiber bundle conducting nearly 1.2 million axons, which constitutes the major beaming connecting various nodes within the circuit of Papez. Six patients with early AD were treated with forniceal DBS bilaterally, over 1 year, supervising both neuropsychological assessments and FDG-PET scans. The parameters of stimulation were: 130 Hz, 90 μs pulse width, voltage between 1.0 and 10 V, monopolar mode. The authors used positron emission tomography (PET) imaging to demonstrate that this therapy was effective in reversing altered glucose consumption in the temporal and parietal lobes. Clinical evaluation with the Alzheimer's disease Assessment Scale-Cognitive Subscale (ADAS-COG) and the Mini Mental State Examination (MMSE) suggested a reduction in cognitive decline rate. The follow-up PET studies after 1 year demonstrated an increasing cerebral glucose metabolism both in frontal-temporal-parietal-striatal-thalamic circuit and frontal-temporal-pariet-l-occipital-hippocampal circuit that was subsequently associated with improved cognitive status and quality of life [17]. Fontaine *et al.* [18] prove stabilization of mnesic scores and augmented metabolism in the mesial-temporal lobe after bilateral DBS of fornix in a patient with moderate AD. Bilateral low frequency stimulation of fornix (bipolar square waves of 0.2 μs duration at 5 Hz with current intensity of 8 mA/phase) has been demonstrated to enhance MMSE in 11 patients with intractable epilepsy over a period of 4 h [19].

Sankar *et al.*, observed with structural MRI bilateral hippocampal volume increases in two of six AD patients that underwent to bilateral fornix DBS. Following this treatment, in one patient hippocampal volume was maintained three years after diagnosis. Mean hippocampal atrophy was significantly slower in the DBS group compared to the AD group, correlated strongly with hippocampal metabolism and with volume change in the fornix and mammillary bodies, suggesting a circuit-wide effect of stimulation. This is the first in-human evidence that, in addition to modulating neural circuit activity, DBS may potentially change the natural course of brain atrophy in a neurodegenerative condition [20]. Lozano *et al.*, considered ON/OFF bilateral DBS of the fornix in a randomized, double-blind trial in 42 patients with mild AD. They evaluated cognitive performance and cerebral glucose metabolism up to 12 months post-implantation, showing that DBS for AD was linked to the improved cerebral glucose metabolism. There were no further variations in cognitive functions for patients in its entirety, while it is conceivable a possible deterioration in patients aged<65 years with stimulation.

Nucleus Basalis of Meynert

The first case report of DBS for dementia traces back approximately to thirty years ago and Nucleus basalis of Meynert (NBM) was targeted. In 1984 Turnbull implanted a unilateral electrode into the left NBM by frontal approach in a 74-year-old patient with moderate AD [21]. The modulation of NBM can enhance the behavioural state and boost memory, attention and perception. Patients eligible for NBM DBS trials are those who have already tested cholinesterase inhibitors before, have minimal cortical atrophy on imaging, lack of significant comorbidities and lucid intervals and capacity to consent. In one 71-year-old patient with Parkinsonian Dementia Disease, Freund *et al.* [22] performed bilateral monopolar low frequency DBS of Ch4i subsector of NBM was (1 V, 20 Hz, 120 μs) associated with bilateral STN stimulation. NBM DBS enhances substantially cognitive and memory functioning: after surgery score on Auditory Verbal Learning Test for immediate episodic memory and learning (AVLT - sum) demonstrated improvement of immediate episodic memory and score on Auditory Verbal Learning Test for long term memory (AVLT - recog) improvement of long term memory performance. Cognitive profits have been supported for 2 months during chronic stimulation (time locked). This expansion in cognitive and behavioral functions can be ascribed to the strengthening of leftover cholinergic projections in the memory circuits [23].

Entorhinal Cortex/Hippocampus

Neuropsychological details counsel that the verbal learning is a function of the left medial temporal lobe while non-verbal learning is the prerogative of the right medial temporal lobe. Starting from this examination, in 2012, Suthana *et al.* [24] observed that bilateral DBS of the hippocampus or entorhinal cortex in seven pharmacologically intractable temporal lobe epilepsy patients may enhance memory functions. Improved spatial memory was observed when the medial temporal lobe was stimulated. This finding is the proof that improvement could be registered in patients with other memory disorders like Alzheimer's disease. Fell *et al.* evaluated in a pilot study the effects of low frequency stimulation of EC and hippocampus in 11 patients with temporal lobe epilepsy. A linear relationship of stimulation on correctly remembered words was reported [25].

Pedunculopontine Tegmental Nucleus

In a small group of six Parkinsonian patients Stefani *et al.* were the first to stimulate simultaneously both the subthalamic nucleus (STN) and the pedunculopontine tegmental nucleus (PPN). PPN-ON/STN-OFF stimulation condition (bipolar contacts 0-1/4-5, 25 Hz, 1.5 to 2.4 V and 60 μs pulse width) elicited better results in both executive and attentive functions, associated with augmented glucose consumption in prefrontal and frontal bilateral cortical areas, including both lateral and more antero-medial cortices. Moreover, during PPN-ON stimulation, a more recognizable reduction of FDG (fluorodeoxyglucose) was observed in the left ventral striatum. These data would corroborate the hypothesis of a positive effect of 25 Hz PPN-DBS on Parkinsonian patients' cognitive profile, probably due to a facilitatory effect exerted by PPN on both associative and limbic circuits [26].

Anterior Thalamic Nucleus

According to Gao, bilateral anterior thalamic nucleus (ATN) stimulation in rats increased glucose utilization in the target region, the thalamus and hippocampus, and decreased glucose consumption in the cingulate cortex and frontal cortex [27]. In 2011, Oh examined the cognitive outcomes at least 12 months after bilateral DBS of the ATN for controlling epilepsy in nine patients with intractable epilepsy who were not candidates for resective surgery. Bilateral ATN DBS directly activated both the limbic and the thalamo-cortical pathway, with significant advantages in verbal memory or verbal fluency after chronic stimulation. Thus, bilateral DBS of the ATN is responsible for metabolic activation of the target area and changes in energy metabolism in remote brain regions *via* efferent or afferent fibers [28].

Anterior Limb of Internal Capsule/Nucleus Accumbens

Modulation of ventral capsule, ventral striatum and nucleus accumbens are entailed in motivation and is a part of reward circuitry. The stimulation of these neural pathways might strengthen the cognitive and behavior functions in patients with AD [29]. The initial stimulating results of the study involving bilateral DBS of anterior limb of internal capsule/nucleus accumbens (ALIC/NAc) in patients with AD are yet to be published.

DISCUSSION

AD is a neurodegenerative disorder that affects behaviour and cognition clinically and many structures in the limbic system even anatomically. Neuroimaging studies have highlighted widespread structural and metabolic aberrations, mainly in areas associated with memory functions [30]. In pathogenesis of AD accumulations of beta amyloid and tau protein, inflammatory cascades, abnormal responses to oxidative stress and alteration in oxidative metabolism are implicated [4, 8 - 10]. At molecular level, these proteins are responsible for the loss of synaptic functions, faulty metabolism, altered cell repair and cell death. These molecular alterations lead to neuronal loss and cerebral atrophy in different regions of the brain involving frontal, temporal, parietal, hippocampus and entorhinal cortex. AD also disrupts the neural connections between the cortical and subcortical areas [4, 7, 9].

Interest in the potential role of neurosurgery for patients with diagnosis of dementia has gradually increased: encapsulated cell biodelivery (ECB) implant and Deep Brain Stimulation (DBS) represent a new strategy.

Several animal studies have shown that delivery of nerve growth factor (NFG) – a neurotrophin that is involved in cholinergic synaptic remodeling in the adult CNS - in basal forebrain (anterior part of the brain, cerebral hemispheres, thalamus and hypothalamus) by ECB could arrest or even reverse the neuronal degeneration process. In 2012 Wahlberg *et al.* demonstrated the restorative role of ECB implants in patients with AD [31].

The results of DBS on the neural circuitry in diseases like Parkinson's disease, primary dystonia, Obsessive Compulsive Disorders, Major Depression and Tourette syndrome have prompted researchers to translate its potential utility to AD [32 - 36]. Several targets have been explored as potential targets to enhance memory functions in the circuit of Papez that is one of the major pathways of the limbic system and is primarily involved in the cortical control of emotions and in storing memory. In the so-called "memory circuit" the entorhinal cortex projects to the hippocampus *via* the perforant pathway that projects to the dentate gyrus, to the subiculum and to the CA3 and CA1 subfield of the hippocampus. From the hippocampus the information proceeds through the subiculum to the fimbria and the fornix. The pre-commissural branch of the fornix projects to the anterior cingulated cortex *via* the septal nuclei, the nucleus basalis of Meynert and the ventral striatum. The post-commissural branch of the fornix projects to the anterior thalamic nucleus and the mammillary bodies. Because the mammillo-thalamic tract couples the mammillary bodies and the anterior thalamic nucleus, the hippocampus can have direct as well as indirect effect on the thalamus [37].

As recent data suggest system-level defects characterized by alterations in memory circuits, it is reasonable to expect that external stimulation of subareas within the circuitry will ameliorate symptoms. Stimulation of the "memory circuit" activates hippocampus and the para-hippocampalgyrus and thus improves hippocampus-dependent memory functions. The anterior thalamic nucleus plays an important role in the Papez circuit. Previous studies in rats have shown that high current stimulation of the ATN interrupted the acquisition of contextual fear conditioning and reduced performance on a spatial alternating task; stimulation of this area also modulates regional cerebral metabolism as detected by FDG-microPET [27]. Stimulation of the nucleus basalis of Meynert (NBM) should improve or stabilize memory and cognitive performance in patients with AD. Medial temporal structures, including the hippocampus and the entorhinal cortex, have long been known to be important in memory formation and recall [24]. Previous studies in refractory epileptic patients have shown that entorhinal stimulation enhanced the memory of spatial information when applied during learning. The CA1 region of the hippocampus is another interesting target. A rodent model study showed that application of high-frequency stimulation to isolated hippocampal slices significantly increased synaptic plasticity in the CA1 region and promoted a twofold increase of non-amyloidogenic α-secretase activity.

Although we rely on a small series, the fornix is the current target most frequently chosen for treating dementia with 2.5-3.5 V, 130 Hz and 60-90 μs as stimulation parameters: DBS of this target improves memory functions and slows progression of memory loss in AD patients mainly in those affected by mild cognitive impairment [15, 16, 18]. As to other potential target, there are investigations dealing with the effects of low-frequency (20-50 Hz, 1-3 V, 120-210 μs) DBS in the NBM for treating patients with Parkinsonian Dementia Disease and Senile Dementia of Alzheimer's type, stressing results regarding memory and other cognitive functions like attention, visual processing or practical symptoms [19, 27]. NBM DBS also improves memory performance, as a result of Ach release from the NBM. The nucleus basalis of Meynert may be a promising target structure in dementia thanks to its afferent and efferent projections and its pool of

90% cholinergic neurons [23, 35]. Other potential DBS targets under evaluation in patients with dementia are the entorhinal cortex (0.5-1.5 mA, 50-130 Hz,300-450 μs as stimulation parameters) [24], the pedunculopontine tegmental nucleus (2.4 mA, 25 Hz and 60 μs) [26] and the anterior thalamic nucleus (1.5-3.1 mA, 100-185 Hz, 90-150 μs) [28], because at least in some areas of cognition such as spatial orientation, executive functions and attention, slight improvements appeared to occur in humans. Currently there are six clinical trials (ranging from March 2007 to May 2012) for DBS in AD that are listed by the National Institutes Health of Clinical Trial registry. One of these is a double-blind design (stimulation on/off), which should prove to be very informative in evaluating the effectiveness of DBS as a therapeutic technique in AD [30].

For AD patients undergoing DBS, very few adverse effects are described so far. Independently of the target structure stimulated, patients recovered quickly from surgery and only rarely experienced cognitive deterioration caused by the operation. Generally chronic stimulation was well tolerated, except for sensations of warmth, flushing and sweating.

The mechanisms underlying the effects of DBS in AD are still uncertain. Increase in neuritic arborization with restoration of functional connectivity, induction of hippocampal neurogenesis, increase of neurotrofic grown factors (NGF) release and acetylcholine release in hippocampus may be activated by fornix or NBM DBS [32, 35].

The promotion of neurogenesis has been demonstrated in animal studies involving the electrical stimulation of fornix, anterior thalamic nucleus and entorhinal cortex and stimulation-induced memory enhancement may depend on the ability of electrical neural stimulation to induce the development of functional mature hippocampal neurons.

In addition to the aforementioned potential mechanism that can be at the basis of long-term effects (arrest or slowing of cognitive decline), DBS can induce a modulation of oscillatory rhythms which may be responsible for the immediate effects of stimulation on cognition (enhancement of memory functions)by means of theta phase activity resetting in the hippocampus [24, 35].

Neuroethical aspects concerning the use of DBS in AD and/or cognitive impairments represent a challenge for clinical research. Taking into account that DBS is a surgical procedure, it requires an informed consent. The ability to express or to sign an informed consent in a patient affected by dementia or cognitive disorder may be lack and the surgical procedure is not explainable only on the basis of the clinical diagnosis [38]. Also the decision-making capacity of caregivers to give consent in difficult situations poses ethical and legal questions [39, 40].

CONCLUSION

AD is a multifactorial disease with significant financial and health-care impact. Medical therapy is of modest advantage and associated with significant side effects. In selected patients with AD, DBS of key regions of memory circuit with tailored stimulation parameters can delay cognitive decline, enhance memory functions and improve overall quality of life. Fornix and NBM are the most promising targets for DBS in terms of delaying and reversing the cognitive deterioration. Other potential targets for DBS treatment of AD have been assessed and include the nucleus basalis of Meynert, the entorhinal cortex, the pedunculopontine nucleus, ATN with encouraging results. Moreover, DBS in AD patients seems to be feasible and safe, even if the debate on the ethical issues moves clinical research to reevaluate this technique within the framework of cognitive degenerative disorders, with strict protocols and inclusion criteria. However, long-term randomized controlled trials are required to validate the efficacy of neurostimulation, to determine the most optimal target and stimulation parameters, to define mechanisms through which DBS produces therapeutic effects in AD patients, and to check for possible adverse effects in the long period.

CONSENT FOR PUBLICATION

Not applicable.

CONFLICT OF INTEREST

The author (editor) declares no conflict of interest, financial or otherwise.

ACKNOWLEDGEMENTS

Declared none.

REFERENCES

[1] Shampo MA, Kyle RA, Steensma DP. Alois Alzheimer-Alzheimer disease. Mayo Clin Proc 2013; 88(12): e155.
[http://dx.doi.org/10.1016/j.mayocp.2013.01.031] [PMID: 24290132]

[2] Ballard C, Gauthier S, Corbett A, Brayne C, Aarsland D, Jones E. Alzheimer's disease. Lancet 2011; 377(9770): 1019-31.
[http://dx.doi.org/10.1016/S0140-6736(10)61349-9] [PMID: 21371747]

[3] Winblad B, Amouyel P, Andrieu S, *et al.* Defeating Alzheimer's disease and other dementias: a priority for European science and society. Lancet Neurol 2016; 15(5): 455-532.
[http://dx.doi.org/10.1016/S1474-4422(16)00062-4] [PMID: 26987701]

[4] Zibly Z, Shaw A, Harnof S, *et al.* Modulation of mind: therapeutic neuromodulation for cognitive disability. J Clin Neurosci 2014; 21(9): 1473-7. [http://dx.doi.org/10.1016/j.jocn.2013.11.040] [PMID: 24882563]

[5] Lozano AM, Fosdick L, Chakravarty MM, *et al.* A Phase II Study of Fornix Deep Brain Stimulation in Mild Alzheimer's Disease. J Alzheimers Dis 2016; 54(2): 777-87. [http://dx.doi.org/10.3233/JAD-160017] [PMID: 27567810]

[6] Rezai RA, Sharma M. Deep brain stimulation (DBS): current and emerging applications. Japanese Journal of Neurosurgery 2014; 23: 648-60. [http://dx.doi.org/10.7887/jcns.23.648]

[7] Lyketsos CG, Targum SD, Pendergrass JC, Lozano AM. Deep brain stimulation: a novel strategy for treating Alzheimer's disease. Innov Clin Neurosci 2012; 9(11-12): 10-7. [PMID: 23346514]

[8] Rocca WA, Petersen RC, Knopman DS, *et al.* Trends in the incidence and prevalence of Alzheimer's disease, dementia, and cognitive impairment in the United States. Alzheimers Dement 2011; 7(1): 80-93. [http://dx.doi.org/10.1016/j.jalz.2010.11.002] [PMID: 21255746]

[9] Pereira JL, Downes A, Gorgulho A, Patel V, Malkasian D, De Salles A. Alzheimer's disease: The role for neurosurgery. Surg Neurol Int 2014; 5 (Suppl. 8): S385-90. [http://dx.doi.org/10.4103/2152-7806.140191] [PMID: 25289167]

[10] Watt AD, Villemagne VL, Barnham KJ. Metals, membranes, and amyloid-β oligomers: key pieces in the Alzheimer's disease puzzle? J Alzheimers Dis 2013; 33 (Suppl. 1): S283-93. [PMID: 22699851]

[11] Bronstein JM, Tagliati M, Alterman RL, *et al.* Deep brain stimulation for Parkinson disease: an expert consensus and review of key issues. Arch Neurol 2011; 68(2): 165. [http://dx.doi.org/10.1001/archneurol.2010.260] [PMID: 20937936]

[12] Damoiseaux JS, Prater KE, Miller BL, Greicius MD. Functional connectivity tracks clinical deterioration in Alzheimer's disease. Neurobiol Aging 2012; 33(4): 828.e19-30. [http://dx.doi.org/10.1016/j.neurobiolaging.2011.06.024] [PMID: 21840627]

[13] Hamani C, Stone SS, Garten A, Lozano AM, Winocur G. Memory rescue and enhanced neurogenesis following electrical stimulation of the anterior thalamus in rats treated with corticosterone. Exp Neurol 2011; 232(1): 100-4. [http://dx.doi.org/10.1016/j.expneurol.2011.08.023] [PMID: 21906593]

[14] Hescham S, Lim LW, Jahanshahi A, *et al.* Deep brain stimulation of the forniceal area enhances memory functions in experimental dementia: the role of stimulation parameters. Brain Stimul 2013; 6(1): 72-7. [http://dx.doi.org/10.1016/j.brs.2012.01.008] [PMID: 22405739]

[15] Hamani C, McAndrews MP, Cohn M, *et al.* Memory enhancement induced by hypothalamic/fornix deep brain stimulation. Ann Neurol 2008; 63(1): 119-23. [http://dx.doi.org/10.1002/ana.21295] [PMID: 18232017]

[16] Laxton AW, Tang-Wai DF, McAndrews MP, *et al.* A phase I trial of deep brain stimulation of memory circuits in Alzheimer's disease. Ann Neurol 2010; 68(4): 521-34. [http://dx.doi.org/10.1002/ana.22089] [PMID: 20687206]

[17] Smith GS, Laxton AW, Tang-Wai DF, *et al.* Increased cerebral metabolism after 1 year of deep brain stimulation in Alzheimer disease. Arch Neurol 2012; 69(9): 1141-8. [http://dx.doi.org/10.1001/archneurol.2012.590] [PMID: 22566505]

[18] Fontaine D, Deudon A, Lemaire JJ, *et al.* Symptomatic treatment of memory decline in Alzheimer's disease by deep brain stimulation: a feasibility study. J Alzheimers Dis 2013; 34(1): 315-23. [PMID: 23168448]

[19] Koubeissi MZ, Kahriman E, Syed TU, Miller J, Durand DM. Low-frequency electrical stimulation of a fiber tract in temporal lobe epilepsy. Ann Neurol 2013; 74(2): 223-31.
[PMID: 23613463]

[20] Sankar T, Chakravarty MM, Bescos A, *et al.* Deep brain stimulation influences brain structure in Alzheimer's disease. Brain Stimul 2015; 8(3): 645-54.
[http://dx.doi.org/10.1016/j.brs.2014.11.020] [PMID: 25814404]

[21] Turnbull IM, McGeer PL, Beattie L, Calne D, Pate B. Stimulation of the basal nucleus of Meynert in senile dementia of Alzheimer's type. A preliminary report. Appl Neurophysiol 1985; 48(1-6): 216-21.
[PMID: 3915647]

[22] Freund HJ, Kuhn J, Lenartz D, *et al.* Cognitive functions in a patient with Parkinson-dementia syndrome undergoing deep brain stimulation. Arch Neurol 2009; 66(6): 781-5.
[http://dx.doi.org/10.1001/archneurol.2009.102] [PMID: 19506141]

[23] Gratwicke J, Kahan J, Zrinzo L, *et al.* The nucleus basalis of Meynert: a new target for deep brain stimulation in dementia? Neurosci Biobehav Rev 2013; 37(10 Pt 2): 2676-88.
[http://dx.doi.org/10.1016/j.neubiorev.2013.09.003] [PMID: 24035740]

[24] Suthana N, Haneef Z, Stern J, *et al.* Memory enhancement and deep-brain stimulation of the entorhinal area. N Engl J Med 2012; 366(6): 502-10.
[http://dx.doi.org/10.1056/NEJMoa1107212] [PMID: 22316444]

[25] Fell J, Staresina BP, Do Lam AT, *et al.* Memory modulation by weak synchronous deep brain stimulation: a pilot study. Brain Stimul 2013; 6(3): 270-3.
[http://dx.doi.org/10.1016/j.brs.2012.08.001] [PMID: 22939277]

[26] Stefani A, Pierantozzi M, Ceravolo R, Brusa L, Galati S, Stanzione P. Deep brain stimulation of pedunculopontine tegmental nucleus (PPTg) promotes cognitive and metabolic changes: a target-specific effect or response to a low-frequency pattern of stimulation? Clin EEG Neurosci 2010; 41(2): 82-6.
[http://dx.doi.org/10.1177/155005941004100207] [PMID: 20521490]

[27] Gao F, Guo Y, Zhang H, *et al.* Anterior thalamic nucleus stimulation modulates regional cerebral metabolism: an FDG-MicroPET study in rats. Neurobiol Dis 2009; 34(3): 477-83.
[http://dx.doi.org/10.1016/j.nbd.2009.03.001] [PMID: 19303441]

[28] Oh YS, Kim HJ, Lee KJ, Kim YI, Lim SC, Shon YM. Cognitive improvement after long-term electrical stimulation of bilateral anterior thalamic nucleus in refractory epilepsy patients. Seizure 2012; 21(3): 183-7.
[http://dx.doi.org/10.1016/j.seizure.2011.12.003] [PMID: 22209542]

[29] Bichot NP, Heard MT, Desimone R. Stimulation of the nucleus accumbens as behavioral reward in awake behaving monkeys. J Neurosci Methods 2011; 199(2): 265-72.
[http://dx.doi.org/10.1016/j.jneumeth.2011.05.025] [PMID: 21704383]

[30] Barbosa Pereira JL, Downes A, Gorgulho A, Patel V, Malkasian D, De Salles A. Alzheimer's disease: the role for neurosurgery. Surg Neurol Int 2014; 5(Suppl 8): S385-90.
[http://dx.doi.org/10.4103/2152-7806.140191] [PMID: 25289167]

[31] Wahlberg LU, Lind G, Almqvist PM, *et al.* Targeted delivery of nerve growth factor *via* encapsulated cell biodelivery in Alzheimer disease: a technology platform for restorative neurosurgery. J Neurosurg 2012; 117(2): 340-7.
[http://dx.doi.org/10.3171/2012.2.JNS11714] [PMID: 22655593]

[32] Grieve SM, Williams LM, Paul RH, Clark CR, Gordon E. Cognitive aging, executive function, and fractional anisotropy: a diffusion tensor MR imaging study. AJNR Am J Neuroradiol 2007; 28(2): 226-35.
[PMID: 17296985]

[33] Bishop KM, Hofer EK, Mehta A, Ramirez A, Sun L, Tuszynski M. Therapeutic potential of CERE-

110 (AAVG-NGF): targeted, stable and sustained NGF delivery and trophic activity on rodent basal forebrain cholinergic neurons. Exp Neurol 2008; 211(2): 574-84.
[http://dx.doi.org/10.1016/j.expneurol.2008.03.004] [PMID: 18439998]

[34] Petersen RC, Jack. Jr. CR. Imaging and biomarkers in early Alzheimer's disease and mild cognitive impairment. Clin Pharmacol Ther 2009; 86(4): 438-41.
[http://dx.doi.org/10.1038/clpt.2009.166]

[35] Hardenacke K, Shubina E, Bührle CP, Zapf A, Lenartz D. Deep brain stimulation as a tool for improving cognitive functioning in Alzheimer's dementia: a systematic review. Front Psychiatry 2013; 4: 159.
[http://dx.doi.org/10.3389/fpsyt.2013.00159] [PMID: 24363647]

[36] Lavano A, Della Torre A, Volpentesta G, *et al.* Deep brain stimulation for treatment-resistant depression: review of the literature. Brain Disord Ther 2015; 4: 168-70.

[37] Hescham S, Lim LW, Jahanshahi A, Blokland A, Temel Y. Deep brain stimulation in dementia-related disorders. Neurosci Biobehav Rev 2013; 37(10 Pt 2): 2666-75.
[http://dx.doi.org/10.1016/j.neubiorev.2013.09.002] [PMID: 24060532]

[38] Siegel AM, Barrett MS, Bhati MT. Deep Brain Stimulation for Alzheimer's Disease: Ethical Challenges for Clinical Research. J Alzheimers Dis 2017; 56(2): 429-39.
[http://dx.doi.org/10.3233/JAD-160356] [PMID: 27983548]

[39] Ovadia D, Bottini G. Neuroethical implications of deep brain stimulation in degenerative disorders. Curr Opin Neurol 2015; 28(6): 598-603.
[http://dx.doi.org/10.1097/WCO.0000000000000263] [PMID: 26551238]

[40] Lavano A. Neurosurgical treatment of Alzheimer's disease: where do we stand? J Neurosurg Sci 2016; 60(2): 151-3.
[PMID: 27150540]

CHAPTER 2

ASS234: A New and Promising Anti-Alzheimer Agent

Alejandro Romero[1,*], **Eva Ramos**[1], **Ana P. Fernández**[2], **Julia Serrano**[2], **Ricardo Martínez-Murillo**[2] and **José Marco-Contelles**[3]

[1] *Department of Pharmacology and Toxicology, Faculty of Veterinary Medicine, Complutense University of Madrid, Madrid, Spain*

[2] *The Neurovascular Research Group, Department of Translational Neurobiology, Cajal Institute (CSIC), Madrid, Spain*

[3] *Laboratory of Medicinal Chemistry, Institute of General Organic Chemistry (CSIC), Madrid, Spain*

Abstract: Physiopathological events associated with the development and progression of Alzheimer's disease (AD) are complex and require new therapeutical approaches. Consequently, *N*-((5-(3-(1-benzylpiperidin-4-yl) propoxy)-1- methyl-1H-indol-2-yl) methyl)-*N*-methylprop-2-yn-1-amine (ASS234), synthesized as a new multitarget-directed molecule, has focused a great interest in this field. *In vitro*, it is able to cross the blood-brain barrier and has less toxicity than donepezil. It acts simultaneously as a reversible inhibitor of both human acetyl and butyrylcholinesterase, and as an irreversible inhibitor of human monoamine oxidase A and B. It inhibits both $A\beta_{1-42}$ and $A\beta_{1-40}$ self-aggregation and possesses antioxidant and neuroprotective properties. Recently, it was demonstrated that ASS234 is able to induce the wingless-type MMTV integration site family (Wnt) signaling pathway, which is involved in neuroprotective activities related to AD and it also promotes the induction of several key antioxidant genes that counteract oxidative stress. *In vivo* experiments, ASS234 exhibited a reduction of amyloid plaque burden and gliosis in the cortex and hippocampus and significantly decreased scopolamine-induced learning deficits in C57BL/6J mice. Herein, we summarize the neuroprotective effects of ASS234 in counteracting several steps in the pathological processes of AD.

Keywords: AChE, Alzheimer disease, ASS234, BuChE, Gene expression, MAO-A/B, Neuroprotection, Oxidative stress, Wnt signaling pathway.

* **Corresponding author Alejandro Romero:** Department of Pharmacology and Toxicology, Faculty of Veterinary Medicine, Complutense University of Madrid, Madrid, Spain; Tel: +34 91 394 39 70; E-mail: manarome@ucm.es

Atta-ur-Rahman (Ed.)

INTRODUCTION

Alzheimer's disease (AD) is the most common neurodegenerative disorder at any age worldwide, which involves progressive memory loss and dementia [1]. Initially, the extracellular deposit of *β*-amyloid (A*β*) intraneuronal and accumulations of hyperphosphorylated tau (pTau) (neurofibrillary tangles) were the main hypotheses for this disease [2 - 4]. However, both molecular manifestations do not fully explain all of the disturbances in AD development, which, in the last years, has come under sharp criticism. It is clear that AD is a multifactorial disorder and it seems to result from a complex interaction of multiple environmental and genetic factors [5]. Besides these, numerous other mechanisms, such as disturbances in the structure and functions of mitochondria [6], chronic oxidative stress (OS) [7], neuroinflammation [8], metal ion metabolism disorders [9], abnormalities of lipid metabolism [10] and/or deregulation of the Cyclin-dependent kinase 5 (Cdk5) [11] are involved.

In this complex scenario, the scientific community is exploring multiple approaches to modify the natural course of this disease. Until now, four acetylcholinesterase inhibitors (tacrine, donepezil, rivastigmine and galantamine) and one NMDA receptor antagonist (memantine) have been FDA-approved for this pathology. However, these drugs had not produced the expected results. Combination or hybridizing therapy is an alternative strategy to address the complex pathophysiology of AD through multiple pathways at several steps, offering a higher efficacy. Consequently, the design and synthesis of molecules able to interact with two or more targets, the so called multitarget-directed ligands (MTDLs), have raised a great interest in this field as a powerful drug design alternative and run parallel to drug combination for the treatment of AD [12, 13].

In this chapter, we summarize the interesting perspectives given by the studies carried out with the multipotent monoamine oxidase (MAO) A and B plus cholinesterase inhibitor *N*-((5-(3-(1-benzylpiperidin-4-yl) propoxy)-1- methyl-1- -indol-2-yl) methyl)-*N*-methylprop-2-yn-1-amine (ASS234) by several *in vitro* and *in vivo* experimental studies through enzymatic and other specific targets.

Design and Synthesis of ASS234 Strategy

Possibly, the multifactorial and complex nature of AD is the main cause that no effective drug exists in clinics, even after more than a century of the first diagnosed case of AD. Consequently, multiple new therapeutic strategies have been conceived to find the statement drug, among them, of particular interest and acceptation is the multi-target directed ligand (MTDL) [2] approach, based on the "*one molecule, multiple targets*" paradigm [14]. Thus, the idea was that a single drug acting on a specific target might not be adequate for AD therapy. Thereby, the MTDL approach has captured an increasing attention in many laboratories, which have reported a large number of ligands able to bind several biological targets simultaneously [12, 15 - 19].

Thus, based on our previous developments of monoamine oxidase inhibitors (MAOIs) to treat neurodegenerative diseases [20], our choice was to design new potential hybrids able to inhibit both MAO and cholinesterase (ChE) for AD treatment. Consequently, novel hybrids were designed combining selected pharmacophoric motifs from donepezil (**1**, Aricept®), one of the current cholinesterase inhibitor (ChEI) administered to AD patients, and *N*-[(- -benzyloxy-1-methyl-1*H*-indol-2-yl)methyl]-*N*-methylprop-2-yn-1-amine (**2**), one of the most interesting MAOIs previously investigated in our laboratory (IQOG, CSIC, Madrid, Spain). (Fig. **1**) [21]. The underlying strategy was to retain the 1-benzylpiperidine fragment of donepezil (**1**), with the 1-methyl-1*H*-indol-2-yl)methyl]-*N*-methylprop-2-yn-1-amine moiety of the compound **2** (Fig. **1**), that is the responsible key motif for MAO inhibition. Moreover, this fragment presumably interacts at the peripheral anionic site (PAS) of the AChE, which was expected to give the resulting compound a dual AChEI binding site. This conjunctive approach should result in a significant AChE inhibition power, to counteract the symptomatology of cholinergic deficit in AD. And moreover, this PAS blockade appears to mediate the A*β* proagreggating action of the AChE [22].

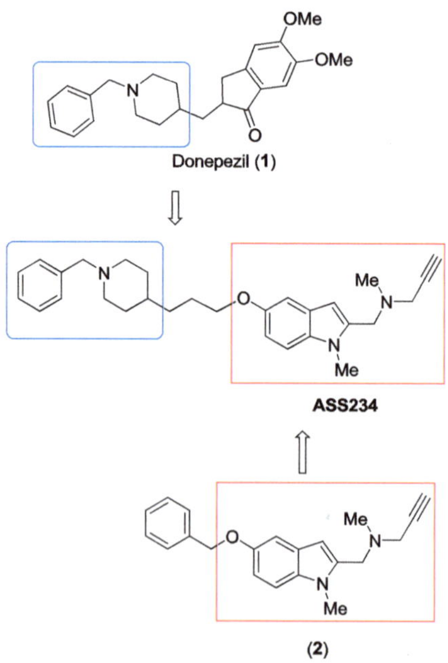

Fig. (1). ASS234, a hybrid from donepezil (1) and indole 2, as a MTDL to inhibit ChEs and MAO enzymes.

In this context, ASS234 was designed, being the most attractive hybrid identified in a research program, directed to find novel multitarget agents against AD.

The synthesis of ASS234 has been carried out as showed in Scheme (**1**), by sodium hydride/DMF promoted reaction of chloride **8**, and 1-methyl-2-{[ethyl(prop-2-yn-1-yl)amino]ethyl}-1*H*-indol-5-ol **9** [23]. Key intermediate 1-benzyl-4-(3-chloropropyl) piperidine **8** was prepared easily obtained starting from 4-pyridinecarboxaldehyde **3**, *via* the known intermediate **4** [24], which hydrogenation [25], under Pd/C and PtO_2 catalysis, in the presence of hydrochloric acid, and work-up with methanol, afforded methyl ester **5** [26]. Next, *N*-benzylation to give 1-benzylpiperidine **6**, reduction with lithium aluminium hydride to provide alcohol **7** [27], and treatment with thionyl chloride, furnished the desired chloride derivative **8** in quantitative yield.

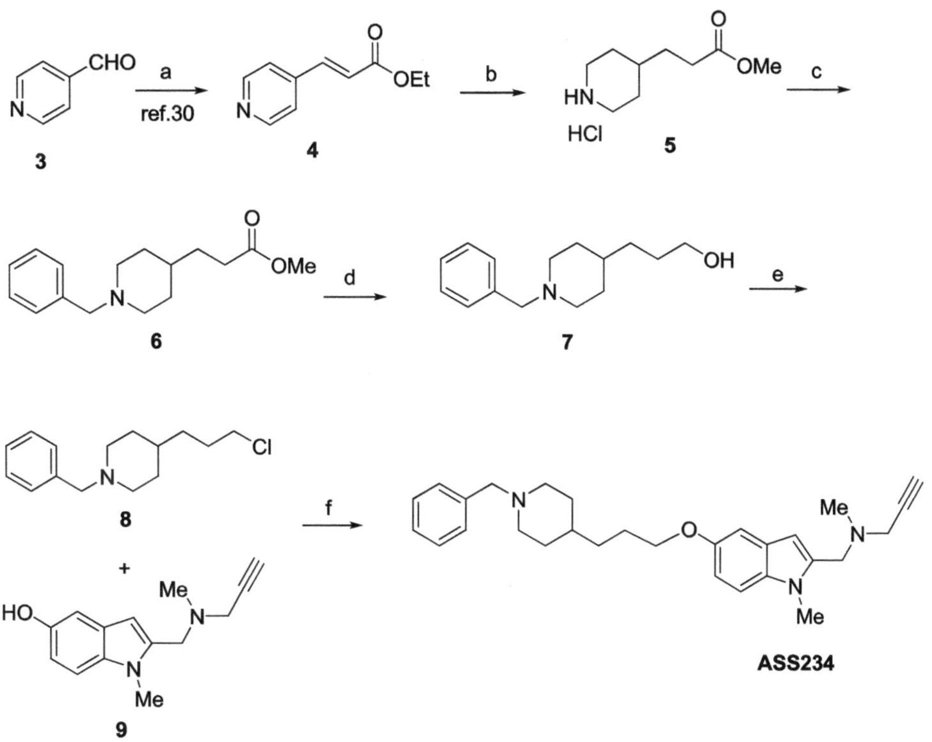

Scheme (1). (a) $(EtO)_2P(O)CH_2CO2Et$, THF, K_2CO_3, reflux (92%); (b) i. H_2, Pd/C 10%, PtO_2, 4N HCl in dioxane, EtOH, rt; ii. MeOH (90%); (c) BnBr, TEA, CH_2Cl_2 (75%); (d) $LiAlH_4$, THF, reflux (98%); (e) $SOCl_2$, CH_2Cl_2, reflux (99%); (f) NaH, DMF, rt (56%).

ASS234 was the most interesting and promising hit-compound among a new series of hybrid derivatives containing the benzyl piperidine moiety of donepezil (**1**) and the indolyl propargylamine moiety of *N*-[(5-benzyloxy-1-methyl-1*H*-

indol-2-yl)methyl]-*N*-methylprop-2-yn-1-amine (**2**). ASS234 was identified both as the most potent MAOI and AChEI. The ability of ASS234 to inhibit butyrylcholinesterase (BuChE), in the submicromolar range, was remarkable, in view of the renewed interest of ChEIs as therapeutic agents for AD [28]. Additionally, ASS234 inhibits MAO-B, which may modulate the cholinergic and the serotoninergic neurotransmission, and also inhibits MAO-A, which produces antidepressant activity [29]. Moreover, it behaves as a $A\beta$-self-induced and human AChE-dependent aggregation inhibitor, even more potent than donepezil.

To sum up, ASS234 is not only an interesting MTDL-hit with a good IMAO/IAChE profile and with a significant activity against $A\beta$ formation and aggregation, but also a potential disease-modifying agent for AD treatment.

Biological and Pharmacological Evaluation of ASS234

As noted above, ASS234 is able to inhibit AChE, BuChE and MAO (A and B), playing an interesting role modulating and enhancing cholinergic and monoaminergic neurotransmission [30]. In order to confirm the neuroprotective profile of ASS234, an *in vitro* study in SH-SY5Y neuroblastoma cells, subjected to amyloid beta peptide fragments $A\beta_{1-40}$ and $A\beta_{1-42}$, was carried out [31]. Under these experimental conditions, ASS234 inhibited the $A\beta_{1-40}$ and $A\beta_{1-42}$ self-aggregation and $A\beta_{1-40}$ and $A\beta_{1-42}$ AChE-dependent aggregation, in a micromolar range. At the same time, ASS234 significantly reduced $A\beta_{1-42}$ (40 μM for 24 h) mediated toxicity in a dose-dependent manner. The highest protection was achieved at 10 μM dose.

To evaluate the role of ASS234 as a modulator of the apoptosis process, Bolea and coworkers [31] investigated the expression of three initiator caspases (caspase-8, caspase-9 and caspase-12) and one executioner caspase (caspase-3). Preincubation with ASS234 at a dose of the 5 and 10 μM, displayed an antiapoptotic effect in SH-SY5Y cells after $A\beta_{1-42}$ (40 μM for 24 h), decreasing caspase-9 and caspase-3 activation. In this sense, the authors hypothesized that the intrinsic pathway of apoptosis could be altered by ASS234 avoiding AD-related neuronal cell death. Furthermore, and to assess the antioxidant profile of ASS234, they evaluated its free radical species scavenger capacity by Oxygen Radical Absorbance Capacity by Fluorescence (ORAC-FL) method [32] and, at the same time, its effect on two antioxidant enzymes; catalase and superoxide dismutase (SOD-1). ASS234 showed a moderate capacity to capture free radical species, with the half ORAC value (0.5 ± 0.1) than the reference compound (Trolox). Besides, pre-incubation with ASS234 (5 and 10 μM) counteracted the $A\beta_{1-42}$-induced reduction of both catalase (19.1 ± 3.0%) and SOD-1 (84.7 ± 5.4%) expression.

ASS234 showed a high effectiveness to permeate central nervous system (CNS) tissues, in the parallel artificial membrane permeation assay for the blood-brain barrier (PAMPA-BBB), with an effective permeability value of P_e = 10.3 x 10^{-6} cm/s, suggesting that ASS234 is able to penetrate into the brain [33].

MAO-A and MAO-B catalyze the oxidative deamination of several biogenic and xenobiotic amines, including monoamine neurotransmitters, such as serotonin (5-HT), noradrenaline (NA) and dopamine (DA). The increased activity of these mitochondrial enzymes enhances OS, aggravates brain homeostasis and contributes to depression and aggressiveness in AD [34, 35]. Furthermore, the activity and gene expression of MAO-A have been found up-regulated in different brain areas of AD patients [36]. Esteban *et al.* [37], performed the biochemical and structural analysis of ASS234 in human enzymes, evidencing that it acts both as a reversible AChEI/BuChEI, (IC_{50} = 0.81 ± 0.06 µM and 1.82 ± 0.14 µM respectively), as well as a potent irreversible inhibitor of MAO-A (IC_{50} = 5.44 ± 1.74 nM). Based on these data, this group evaluated the possible modulator role of ASS234 on the monoaminergic system *in vitro* (PC12 and SH-SY5Y cells) and *in vivo* in a microdialysis experimental model [38]. ASS234 at 1 µM displayed a complete inhibition of MAO-A, both in SH-SY5Y and PC12 cell lines. Furthermore, it increased the 5-HT levels in SH-SY5Y after a 24 h-incubation period, which is associated with a significant reduction in the levels of its metabolite 5-hydroxyindoleacetic acid (5-HIAA). These findings, place ASS234 as a 5-HT modulator agent *in vitro*. Indeed, in PC12 cells, ASS234 significantly decreased two DA metabolites levels: 3,4-dihydroxyphenylacetic acid (DOPAC) and homovanillic acid (HVA). Which confirms a prevention of the DA metabolism by MAO inhibition. As expected, ASS234 *in vivo* (5, 15 and 30 mg/kg), increased the levels of 5-HT and NA in the hippocampus, as well as DA and NA levels in the prefrontal cortex [38]. Based on these data, the authors concluded that ASS234 could enhance the monoaminergic system, indicating that increased monoamines in specific brain regions may improve neuronal survival in AD patients.

Based on the diverse pharmacological properties of ASS234, Stasiak *et al.* [39] tested this molecule in a permanent bilateral occlusion of the common carotid arteries (BCCAO) model with impaired cognitive functions. BCCAO rats treated with ASS234 showed less negative effects, caused by cerebral hypoperfusion, on cognitive parameters than control rats [39].

Nevertheless, the molecular and cellular mechanisms underlying ASS234 actions should be further explored and preclinical studies carried out to confirm the neurotherapeutic value of this molecule.

Signal Transduction Pathways Involved in ASS234-Induced Neuroprotection

The biochemistry of AD is characterized by a plethora of pathophysiological cascades, and every step of them is modulated through multiple pathways. Understanding this complex molecular *status quo* is mandatory in order to develop new therapeutic approaches.

The wingless-type MMTV integration site family (Wnt) signaling pathway, is an interesting target against age-related diseases, particularly in brain functioning Wnt family, is represented by the "canonical" Wnt/b-catenin pathway (Wnt1, Wnt2b, Wnt3a...), and the "noncanonical" Wnt/PCP and Wnt/ Ca^{2+} pathway (Wnt6, Wnt5a...). Wnt signaling plays an important role in the CNS throughout life, and it has emerged in the last years as a new attractive target against AD [40].

Thus, our group explored whether ASS234 at a concentration of 5 μM for 24 h modulates the expression of Wnt1, Wnt2b, Wnt3a, Wnt6 and Wnt5a in SH-SY5Y cells. Wnt2 has a critical participation in the decay of neurogenesis and synapse maintenance and its expression decreases in the aged brain. Interestingly, the reduction of Wnt5 may also have consequences at the synaptic level. It has been demonstrated that Wnt5a promotes synaptic assembly on both excitatory and inhibitory hippocampal neurons [41]. In this sense, when ASS234 (5 μM) was incubated in SH-SY5Y cells for 24h-period, both Wnt2 and Wnt5a expression were significantly increased in 6.89 and 4.80-fold change respectively [42]. These preliminary results open a new therapeutic approach, given that ASS234 may modulate Wnt regulation in the CNS.

It has been established that OS and neuronal apoptosis are important hallmarks in AD [43]. Furthermore, the presence of an extensive OS and antioxidant enzymes expression alteration are prevalent features in the AD brain. In a recent study, Ramos *et al.* [44] evaluated whether ASS234 was able to induce the expression of antioxidant enzymes in SH-SY5Y neuroblastoma cells during a 24-h period, as a mechanism of neuroprotection. After incubating with 5 μM ASS234, it was evidenced that this molecule was able to significantly induce the gene expression of catalase (CAT) (1.89-fold change), superoxide dismutase (SOD1) (1.65-fold change), glutamate-cysteine ligase catalytic subunit (GCLC) (1.97-fold change), gamma-glutamylcysteine synthetase (GCLM) (2.25-fold change), glutathione reductase (GSR) (6.22-fold change), Sequestosome 1 (SQSTM1) (4.84-fold change), thioredoxin reductase 1 (TXNRD1) (4.85-fold change) and quinone oxidoreductase 1 (NQO1) (5.43-fold change).

The increased expression of these genes mitigated the free radical generation and reduced the neuronal tissue damage caused by OS. Taken these data together, ASS234 arises as a promising and new MTLD to fight against AD.

The Proof of Concept of ASS234

Recently, promising results after ASS234 treatment has been obtained on cognition, lowering Aβ and gliosis both, in transgenic mouse model (APPswe/PS1ΔE9) of AD and in an *in vivo* rodent model of scopolamine induced cognitive impairment. Also, *in vitro* toxicology studies showed that the ASS234 is less toxic than donepezil or tacrine. Reportedly ASS234, is a multipotent AChE/BuChE/MAO A-B inhibitor and a potent Aβ aggregation inhibitor, with antioxidant and antiapoptotic properties. In view of these results, we suggest that ASS234 should be considered as a promising alternative drug to treat the cognitive decline and neurodegeneration underlying in AD.

Cholinergic deficit is a consistent and early finding, which correlates with the severity of the cognitive symptoms in AD. Therefore, AChE remains a highly viable target for the symptomatic improvement in AD [45]. In addition, neuropsychological symptoms, such as depression and anxiety, are often observed in AD patients, which suggests that the dysfunction of the dopaminergic systems might be further implicated [46, 47]. Since the mechanisms of memory loss are related to the amount of soluble Aβ oligomers [48, 49] and the MAO-B is overexpressed in AD brains [50], any compound able to show dual AChE and MAO inhibition with antioxidant and inhibitory effects on Aβ-aggregation can be suggested as a potential candidate to treat AD progression [51]. The multifactorial nature of AD makes that the treatment with ChEIs or MAOIs alone cannot provide a significant delay or stop in the disease progression. For this reason, the synthesis of new compounds capable of targeting different enzymatic systems related to AD (ChEs, and MAO A/B) are actively pursued [52]. Hence, this heterogeneity demands the development of multitarget drugs to treat the symptoms and the progression of AD. As AChE and MAO dysfunctions are involved in the neuropathological process of AD, it can be assumed that therapies focused on these two targets may be effective.

Thereby, we examined the effect of ASS234 on the cognition of healthy adult C57BL/6J mice in a scopolamine model. This study confirms that *in vivo* cholinergic properties of ASS234 are as efficacious in cognition as with donepezil treatment. It is noteworthy that clinical studies revealed that AChEIs have a small beneficial effect on amyloid plaque load. We have shown in a previous study that the potent inhibitory AChE profile of ASS234 together with the presence of the propargylamine group of a MAOI, reinforces its action against the aggregation of the most relevant Aβ isoforms [31]. These results have been confirmed *in vivo* in our laboratory, peripherally administered ASS234 to a transgenic mouse model (APPswe/PS1ΔE9) of AD enters the central nervous system and reduces pathology [53].

The generation of Aβ deposits, derived from its precursor protein APP, induces OS, which plays a critical role in the pathogenesis and development of AD, leading to a neuronal injury together with the loss, inflammation and characteristic activation of microglia and astrocytic cells [54 - 57]. As microgliosis and astrocytosis are prominent aspects of the APPswe/PS1ΔE9 transgenic mouse model and indicative of neuroinflammation [58 - 61], we studied the effect of ASS234 on neuroinflammation through the evaluation of the immunohistochemical distribution of the astrocyte marker protein GFAP and of the microglia/macrophage-specific protein iba-1. A significant reduction of GFAP and iba-1 immunostainings were observed in the cortex of treated transgenic mice compared to control mice, suggesting a beneficial effect of ASS234 on neuroinflammation [53].

CONCLUDING REMARKS

The multifactorial nature of AD leads to many possible therapeutic targets. ASS234, as a new multitarget directed propargylamine, acts on several pathophysiological targets involved in the progress and development of AD. ASS234 has a good MAO/AChE inhibitory potency profile, as well as an interesting neuroprotective and antiapoptotic activity. Furthermore, ASS234 is able to regulate different signaling pathways involved in the antioxidant capacity and in the Wnt components in brain functioning. Besides, one single chemical entity offers several advantages, such as, the simplification of dosing regimen, improving patient compliance, obviating thus, the challenge of administering multiple single-drug entities, which may have different bioavailability, pharmacokinetics, and metabolic profiles [2]. Collectively, these results suggest that ASS234 is a promising tool to fight against AD. However, additional investigations are necessary before extrapolating the obtained ASS234 data to clinical studies, to determine doses and the optimal timing of administration.

CONSENT FOR PUBLICATION

Not applicable.

CONFLICT OF INTEREST

The author (editor) declares no conflict of interest, financial or otherwise.

ACKNOWLEDGEMENTS

JMC thanks the Ministerio de Ciencia e Innovación (SAF2006-08764-C02-01), Comunidad de Madrid (S/SAL-0275-2006), Instituto de Salud Carlos III [Retic RENEVAS (RD06/0026/1002)], and COST Action D34/0003/05 (2005-2010) for financial support.

REFERENCES

[1] Fiest KM, Roberts JI, Maxwell CJ, *et al.* The prevalence and incidence of dementia due to alzheimer's disease: a systematic review and meta-analysis. Can J Neurol Sci 2016; 43 (Suppl. 1): S51-82. [http://dx.doi.org/10.1017/cjn.2016.36] [PMID: 27307128]

[2] León R, Garcia AG, Marco-Contelles J. Recent advances in the multitarget-directed ligands approach for the treatment of Alzheimer's disease. Med Res Rev 2013; 33(1): 139-89. [http://dx.doi.org/10.1002/med.20248] [PMID: 21793014]

[3] Spillantini MG, Goedert M. Tau pathology and neurodegeneration. Lancet Neurol 2013; 12(6): 609-22. [http://dx.doi.org/10.1016/S1474-4422(13)70090-5] [PMID: 23684085]

[4] Lue LF, Guerra A, Walker DG. Amyloid Beta and Tau as Alzheimer's Disease Blood Biomarkers: Promise From New Technologies. Neurol Ther 2017; 6 (Suppl. 1): 25-36. [http://dx.doi.org/10.1007/s40120-017-0074-8] [PMID: 28733956]

[5] Scheltens P, Blennow K, Breteler MM, *et al.* Alzheimer's disease. Lancet 2016; 388(10043): 505-17. [http://dx.doi.org/10.1016/S0140-6736(15)01124-1] [PMID: 26921134]

[6] Yan MH, Wang X, Zhu X. Mitochondrial defects and oxidative stress in Alzheimer disease and Parkinson disease. Free Radic Biol Med 2013; 62: 90-101. [http://dx.doi.org/10.1016/j.freeradbiomed.2012.11.014] [PMID: 23200807]

[7] Liu Z, Zhou T, Ziegler AC, Dimitrion P, Zuo L. Oxidative stress in neurodegenerative diseases: from molecular mechanisms to clinical applications. Oxid Med Cell Longev 2017; 2017: 2525967. [http://dx.doi.org/10.1155/2017/2525967] [PMID: 28785371]

[8] Bolós M, Perea JR, Avila J. Alzheimer's disease as an inflammatory disease. Biomol Concepts 2017; 8(1): 37-43. [http://dx.doi.org/10.1515/bmc-2016-0029] [PMID: 28231054]

[9] Brewer GJ. Copper-2 hypothesis for causation of the current alzheimer's disease epidemic together with dietary changes that enhance the epidemic. Chem Res Toxicol 2017; 30(3): 763-8. [http://dx.doi.org/10.1021/acs.chemrestox.6b00373] [PMID: 28161940]

[10] Wong MW, Braidy N, Poljak A, Sachdev PS. The application of lipidomics to biomarker research and pathomechanisms in Alzheimer's disease. Curr Opin Psychiatry 2017; 30(2): 136-44. [http://dx.doi.org/10.1097/YCO.0000000000000303] [PMID: 28002106]

[11] Liu SL, Wang C, Jiang T, Tan L, Xing A, Yu JT. The Role of Cdk5 in Alzheimer's Disease. Mol Neurobiol 2016; 53(7): 4328-42. [http://dx.doi.org/10.1007/s12035-015-9369-x] [PMID: 26227906]

[12] Ramos E, Egea J, de Los Ríos C, Marco-Contelles J, Romero A. Melatonin as a versatile molecule to design novel multitarget hybrids against neurodegeneration. Future Med Chem 2017; 9(8): 765-80. [http://dx.doi.org/10.4155/fmc-2017-0014] [PMID: 28498717]

[13] de Oliveira Pedrosa M, Duarte da Cruz RM, de Oliveira Viana J, *et al.* Hybrid Compounds as Direct Multitarget Ligands: A Review. Curr Top Med Chem 2017; 17(9): 1044-79. [http://dx.doi.org/10.2174/1568026616666160927160620] [PMID: 27697048]

[14] Cavalli A, Bolognesi ML, Minarini A, *et al.* Multi-target-directed ligands to combat neurodegenerative diseases. J Med Chem 2008; 51(3): 347-72. [http://dx.doi.org/10.1021/jm7009364] [PMID: 18181565]

[15] Rodríguez-Franco MI, Fernández-Bachiller MI, Pérez C, Castro A, Martínez A. Design and synthesis of N-benzylpiperidine-purine derivatives as new dual inhibitors of acetyl- and butyrylcholinesterase. Bioorg Med Chem 2005; 13(24): 6795-802.

[http://dx.doi.org/10.1016/j.bmc.2005.07.019] [PMID: 16183292]

[16] Rosini M, Antonello A, Cavalli A, *et al.* Prazosin-related compounds. Effect of transforming the piperazinylquinazoline moiety into an aminomethyltetrahydroacridine system on the affinity for alpha1-adrenoreceptors. J Med Chem 2003; 46(23): 4895-903.
[http://dx.doi.org/10.1021/jm030952q] [PMID: 14584940]

[17] Elsinghorst PW, Cieslik JS, Mohr K, Tränkle C, Gütschow M. First gallamine-tacrine hybrid: design and characterization at cholinesterases and the M2 muscarinic receptor. J Med Chem 2007; 50(23): 5685-95.
[http://dx.doi.org/10.1021/jm070859s] [PMID: 17944454]

[18] Fang L, Appenroth D, Decker M, *et al.* Synthesis and biological evaluation of NO-donor-tacrine hybrids as hepatoprotective anti-Alzheimer drug candidates. J Med Chem 2008; 51(4): 713-6.
[http://dx.doi.org/10.1021/jm701491k] [PMID: 18232655]

[19] Marco-Contelles J, León R, de Los Ríos C, *et al.* Novel multipotent tacrine-dihydropyridine hybrids with improved acetylcholinesterase inhibitory and neuroprotective activities as potential drugs for the treatment of Alzheimer's disease. J Med Chem 2006; 49(26): 7607-10.
[http://dx.doi.org/10.1021/jm061047j] [PMID: 17181144]

[20] Schäfer H, Servais P, Muyzer G. Successional changes in the genetic diversity of a marine bacterial assemblage during confinement. Arch Microbiol 2000; 173(2): 138-45.
[http://dx.doi.org/10.1007/s002039900121] [PMID: 10795685]

[21] Pérez V, Marco JL, Fernández-Alvarez E, Unzeta M. Relevance of benzyloxy group in 2-indolyl methylamines in the selective MAO-B inhibition. Br J Pharmacol 1999; 127(4): 869-76.
[http://dx.doi.org/10.1038/sj.bjp.0702600] [PMID: 10433493]

[22] Inestrosa NC, Alvarez A, Pérez CA, *et al.* Acetylcholinesterase accelerates assembly of amyloid-bet--peptides into Alzheimer's fibrils: possible role of the peripheral site of the enzyme. Neuron 1996; 16(4): 881-91.
[http://dx.doi.org/10.1016/S0896-6273(00)80108-7] [PMID: 8608006]

[23] Cruces MA, Elorriaga C, Fernández-Alvarez E. The kinetics of monoamine oxidase inhibition by three 2-indolylmethylamine derivatives. Biochem Pharmacol 1990; 40(3): 535-43.
[http://dx.doi.org/10.1016/0006-2952(90)90553-W] [PMID: 2383286]

[24] Hallinan EA, Hagen TJ, Husa RK, *et al.* N-substituted dibenzoxazepines as analgesic PGE2 antagonists. J Med Chem 1993; 36(22): 3293-9.
[http://dx.doi.org/10.1021/jm00074a010] [PMID: 7901416]

[25] Yamanaka T, Ohkubo M, Kuroda S, *et al.* Design, synthesis, and structure-activity relationships of potent GPIIb/IIIa antagonists: discovery of FK419. Bioorg Med Chem 2005; 13(13): 4343-52.
[http://dx.doi.org/10.1016/j.bmc.2005.03.056] [PMID: 15927840]

[26] Frølund B, Kristiansen U, Brehm L, Hansen AB, Krogsgaard-Larsen P, Falch E. Partial GABAA receptor agonists. Synthesis and in vitro pharmacology of a series of nonannulated analogs of 4,5,6,7-tetrahydroisoxazolo[5,4-c]pyridin-3-ol. J Med Chem 1995; 38(17): 3287-96.
[http://dx.doi.org/10.1021/jm00017a014] [PMID: 7650683]

[27] Kitbunnadaj R, Zuiderveld OP, De Esch IJ, *et al.* Synthesis and structure-activity relationships of conformationally constrained histamine H(3) receptor agonists. J Med Chem 2003; 46(25): 5445-57.
[http://dx.doi.org/10.1021/jm030905y] [PMID: 14640553]

[28] Mandelli GR, Maiorana S, Terni P, Lamperti G, Colibretti ML, Imbimbo BP. Synthesis of new cardioselective M2 muscarinic receptor antagonists. Chem Pharm Bull (Tokyo) 2000; 48(11): 1611-22.
[http://dx.doi.org/10.1248/cpb.48.1611] [PMID: 11086886]

[29] Cai Z. Monoamine oxidase inhibitors: promising therapeutic agents for Alzheimer's disease (Review). Mol Med Rep 2014; 9(5): 1533-41. [Review].

[PMID: 24626484]

[30] Bolea I, Juárez-Jiménez J, de Los Ríos C, *et al.* Synthesis, biological evaluation, and molecular modeling of donepezil and N-[(5-(benzyloxy)-1-methyl-1H-indol-2-yl)methyl]-N-methlprop-2-yn-1-amine hybrids as new multipotent cholinesterase/monoamine oxidase inhibitors for the treatment of Alzheimer's disease. J Med Chem 2011; 54(24): 8251-70. [http://dx.doi.org/10.1021/jm200853t] [PMID: 22023459]

[31] Bolea I, Gella A, Monjas L, *et al.* Multipotent, permeable drug ASS234 inhibits Aβ aggregation, possesses antioxidant properties and protects from Aβ-induced apoptosis in vitro. Curr Alzheimer Res 2013; 10(8): 797-808. [http://dx.doi.org/10.2174/15672050113109990151] [PMID: 23919774]

[32] Ou B, Hampsch-Woodill M, Prior RL. Development and validation of an improved oxygen radical absorbance capacity assay using fluorescein as the fluorescent probe. J Agric Food Chem 2001; 49(10): 4619-26. [http://dx.doi.org/10.1021/jf010586o] [PMID: 11599998]

[33] Di L, Kerns EH, Fan K, McConnell OJ, Carter GT. High throughput artificial membrane permeability assay for blood-brain barrier. Eur J Med Chem 2003; 38(3): 223-32. [http://dx.doi.org/10.1016/S0223-5234(03)00012-6] [PMID: 12667689]

[34] Finberg JP. Update on the pharmacology of selective inhibitors of MAO-A and MAO-B: focus on modulation of CNS monoamine neurotransmitter release. Pharmacol Ther 2014; 143(2): 133-52. [http://dx.doi.org/10.1016/j.pharmthera.2014.02.010] [PMID: 24607445]

[35] Vermeiren Y, Van Dam D, Aerts T, Engelborghs S, De Deyn PP. Monoaminergic neurotransmitter alterations in postmortem brain regions of depressed and aggressive patients with Alzheimer's disease. Neurobiol Aging 2014; 35(12): 2691-700. [http://dx.doi.org/10.1016/j.neurobiolaging.2014.05.031] [PMID: 24997673]

[36] Naoi M, Riederer P, Maruyama W. Modulation of monoamine oxidase (MAO) expression in neuropsychiatric disorders: genetic and environmental factors involved in type A MAO expression. J Neural Transm (Vienna) 2016; 123(2): 91-106. [http://dx.doi.org/10.1007/s00702-014-1362-4] [PMID: 25604428]

[37] Esteban G, Allan J, Samadi A, *et al.* Kinetic and structural analysis of the irreversible inhibition of human monoamine oxidases by ASS234, a multi-target compound designed for use in Alzheimer's disease. Biochim Biophys Acta 2014; 1844(6): 1104-10. [http://dx.doi.org/10.1016/j.bbapap.2014.03.006] [PMID: 24642166]

[38] Esteban G, Van Schoors J, Sun P, *et al.* In-vitro and in-vivo evaluation of the modulatory effects of the multitarget compound ASS234 on the monoaminergic system. J Pharm Pharmacol 2017; 69(3): 314-24. [http://dx.doi.org/10.1111/jphp.12697] [PMID: 28134992]

[39] Stasiak A, Mussur M, Unzeta M, Samadi A, Marco-Contelles JL, Fogel WA. Effects of novel monoamine oxidases and cholinesterases targeting compounds on brain neurotransmitters and behavior in rat model of vascular dementia. Curr Pharm Des 2014; 20(2): 161-71. [http://dx.doi.org/10.2174/13816128113199990026] [PMID: 23701539]

[40] Riise J, Plath N, Pakkenberg B, Parachikova A. Aberrant Wnt signaling pathway in medial temporal lobe structures of Alzheimer's disease. J Neural Transm (Vienna) 2015; 122(9): 1303-18. [http://dx.doi.org/10.1007/s00702-015-1375-7] [PMID: 25680440]

[41] Cuitino L, Godoy JA, Farías GG, *et al.* Wnt-5a modulates recycling of functional GABAA receptors on hippocampal neurons. J Neurosci 2010; 30(25): 8411-20. [http://dx.doi.org/10.1523/JNEUROSCI.5736-09.2010] [PMID: 20573888]

[42] del Pino J, Ramos E, Aguilera OM, Marco-Contelles J, Romero A. Wnt signaling pathway, a potential target for Alzheimer's disease treatment, is activated by a novel multitarget compound ASS234. CNS Neurosci Ther 2014; 20(6): 568-70.

[http://dx.doi.org/10.1111/cns.12269] [PMID: 24712554]

[43] Rojas-Gutierrez E, Muñoz-Arenas G, Treviño S, *et al.* Alzheimer's disease and metabolic syndrome: A link from oxidative stress and inflammation to neurodegeneration. Synapse 2017. [http://dx.doi.org/10.1002/syn.21990] [PMID: 28650104]

[44] Ramos E, Romero A, Marco-Contelles J, Del Pino J. Upregulation of Antioxidant Enzymes by ASS234, a Multitarget Directed Propargylamine for Alzheimer's Disease Therapy. CNS Neurosci Ther 2016; 22(9): 799-802. [http://dx.doi.org/10.1111/cns.12590] [PMID: 27380946]

[45] Mehta M, Adem A, Sabbagh M. New acetylcholinesterase inhibitors for Alzheimer's disease. Int J Alzheimers Dis 2012; 2012: 728983. [http://dx.doi.org/10.1155/2012/728983] [PMID: 22216416]

[46] Zhang L, Zhou FM, Dani JA. Cholinergic drugs for Alzheimer's disease enhance in vitro dopamine release. Mol Pharmacol 2004; 66(3): 538-44. [http://dx.doi.org/10.1124/mol.104.000299] [PMID: 15322245]

[47] Giménez-Llort L, Blázquez G, Cañete T, *et al.* Modeling behavioral and neuronal symptoms of Alzheimer's disease in mice: a role for intraneuronal amyloid. Neurosci Biobehav Rev 2007; 31(1): 125-47. [http://dx.doi.org/10.1016/j.neubiorev.2006.07.007] [PMID: 17055579]

[48] Broersen K, Rousseau F, Schymkowitz J. The culprit behind amyloid beta peptide related neurotoxicity in Alzheimer's disease: oligomer size or conformation? Alzheimers Res Ther 2010; 2(4): 12. [http://dx.doi.org/10.1186/alzrt36] [PMID: 20642866]

[49] O'Nuallain B, Klyubin I, Mc Donald JM, *et al.* A monoclonal antibody against synthetic Aβ dimer assemblies neutralizes brain-derived synaptic plasticity-disrupting Aβ. J Neurochem 2011; 119(1): 189-201. [http://dx.doi.org/10.1111/j.1471-4159.2011.07389.x] [PMID: 21781116]

[50] Gulyás B, Brockschnieder D, Nag S, *et al.* The norepinephrine transporter (NET) radioligand (S,S)-[18F]FMeNER-D2 shows significant decreases in NET density in the human brain in Alzheimer's disease: a post-mortem autoradiographic study. Neurochem Int 2010; 56(6-7): 789-98. [http://dx.doi.org/10.1016/j.neuint.2010.03.001] [PMID: 20211213]

[51] Zheng H, Amit T, Bar-Am O, Fridkin M, Youdim MB, Mandel SA. From anti-Parkinson's drug rasagiline to novel multitarget iron chelators with acetylcholinesterase and monoamine oxidase inhibitory and neuroprotective properties for Alzheimer's disease. J Alzheimers Dis 2012; 30(1): 1-16. [PMID: 22387411]

[52] Yáñez M, Viña D. Dual inhibitors of monoamine oxidase and cholinesterase for the treatment of Alzheimer disease. Curr Top Med Chem 2013; 13(14): 1692-706. [http://dx.doi.org/10.2174/15680266113139990120] [PMID: 23889051]

[53] Serrano MP, Herrero-Labrador R, Futch HS, *et al.* The proof-of-concept of ASS234: Peripherally administered ASS234 enters the central nervous system and reduces pathology in a male mouse model of Alzheimer disease. J Psychiatry Neurosci 2017; 42(1): 59-69. [http://dx.doi.org/10.1503/jpn.150209] [PMID: 27636528]

[54] Niranjan R. Molecular basis of etiological implications in Alzheimer's disease: focus on neuroinflammation. Mol Neurobiol 2013; 48(3): 412-28. [http://dx.doi.org/10.1007/s12035-013-8428-4] [PMID: 23420079]

[55] Perez-Nievas BG, Stein TD, Tai HC, *et al.* Dissecting phenotypic traits linked to human resilience to Alzheimer's pathology. Brain 2013; 136(Pt 8): 2510-26. [http://dx.doi.org/10.1093/brain/awt171] [PMID: 23824488]

[56] Orre M, Kamphuis W, Osborn LM, *et al.* Isolation of glia from Alzheimer's mice reveals

inflammation and dysfunction. Neurobiol Aging 2014; 35(12): 2746-60.
[http://dx.doi.org/10.1016/j.neurobiolaging.2014.06.004] [PMID: 25002035]

[57] Trujillo-Estrada L, Dávila JC, Sánchez-Mejias E, *et al.* Early neuronal loss and axonal/presynaptic damage is associated with accelerated amyloid-β accumulation in AβPP/PS1 Alzheimer's disease mice subiculum. J Alzheimers Dis 2014; 42(2): 521-41.
[PMID: 24927710]

[58] Hong HS, Hwang JY, Son SM, Kim YH, Moon M, Inhee MJ. FK506 reduces amyloid plaque burden and induces MMP-9 in AβPP/PS1 double transgenic mice. J Alzheimers Dis 2010; 22(1): 97-105.
[http://dx.doi.org/10.3233/JAD-2010-100261] [PMID: 20847451]

[59] Kamphuis W, Mamber C, Moeton M, *et al.* GFAP isoforms in adult mouse brain with a focus on neurogenic astrocytes and reactive astrogliosis in mouse models of Alzheimer disease. PLoS One 2012; 7(8): e42823.
[http://dx.doi.org/10.1371/journal.pone.0042823] [PMID: 22912745]

[60] Kook SY, Lee KM, Kim Y, *et al.* High-dose of vitamin C supplementation reduces amyloid plaque burden and ameliorates pathological changes in the brain of 5XFAD mice. Cell Death Dis 2014; 5: e1083.
[http://dx.doi.org/10.1038/cddis.2014.26] [PMID: 24577081]

[61] Wang SM, Lee YC, Ko CY, *et al.* Increase of zinc finger protein 179 in response to CCAAT/enhancer binding protein delta conferring an antiapoptotic effect in astrocytes of Alzheimer's disease. Mol Neurobiol 2015; 51(1): 370-82.
[http://dx.doi.org/10.1007/s12035-014-8714-9] [PMID: 24788683]

CHAPTER 3

Recent Advances in Alzheimer's Drug Discovery Research

Xin-An Liu[1,6,*], **Brati Das**[2], **Youjun Chen**[3], **Zuxin Chen**[4], **Yosef Avchalumov**[1], **Xu Tian**[5] and **Sathyanarayanan V. Puthanveettil**[1,*]

[1] *Department of Neuroscience, The Scripps Research Institute, Jupiter, FL33458, USA*

[2] *Department of Neuroscience, UConn Health, 263 Farmington Avenue, Farmington, CT 06030-3401, USA*

[3] *Department of Neurology, School of Medicine, University of North Carolina at Chapel Hill, NC 27599, USA*

[4] *Department of Neuroscience, Icahn School of Medicine at Mount Sinai, One Gustave L. Levy Place, New York, NY 10029-6574, USA*

[5] *Department of Environmental Sciences and Engineering, School of Public Health, University of North Carolina at Chapel Hill, NC 27599, USA*

[6] *Department of Neuroscience, Icahn School of Medicine at Mount Sinai, One Gustave L. Levy Place, NewYork, NY 10029-6574, USA*

Abstract: Alzheimer's disease (AD) is the most common cause of age-related dementia, a deleterious neurodegenerative disorder that impairs memory, where neuropathological changes develop gradually over years to affect cognitive functions. AD is one of the most important health-care problems with over 20 million people suffering worldwide and has become a critical issue to human health, especially in aging societies. Current treatments do not prevent, stop, or delay disease progression, despite the considerable advances in knowledge of the pathogenesis of AD and in medicinal chemistry over the past quarter of a century. The neuropathologic hallmarks of AD are extracellular senile plaques of aggregated β-amyloid and intracellular neurofibrillary tangles, mainly containing the hyperphosphorylated microtubule-associated protein tau. Additional changes that may also occur in the brains of AD patients include age-related brain atrophy, synaptic pathology, and neuron loss, which contribute to cognitive impairment. So far, only four cholinesterase inhibitors and memantine have been marketed as the therapeutic strategies for Alzheimer's disease. Despite advancements in prevention strategies, potential targets, effective biomarkers, clinical development methods, and the evaluation of potential treatments in clinical trials. This chapter summarizes our best understanding of the etiology, animal models

* **Corresponding authors, Xin-An Liu:** Department of Neuroscience, Icahn School of Medicine at Mount Sinai, One Gustave L. Levy Place, NewYork, NY 10029-6574, USA; Tel: 5615427758; E-mail: xinan.liu@mssm.edu;
Sathyanarayanan V. Puthanveettil: Department of Neuroscience, The Scripps Research Institute, Jupiter, FL 33458, USA; Tel: 5612282243; Fax: 5612282249; E-mail: SPuthanv@scripps.edu

Atta-ur-Rahman (Ed.)

currently under study, pharmacotherapeutic targets, and molecular pathways that curtail the progression of AD. This knowledge will help to strategize the development and clinical use of any new drugs for AD therapy in future.

Keywords: Alzheimer's Disease, Drug Development, Pharmacotherapeutic Targets, Transgenic Models.

INTRODUCTION

The Prevalence of Alzheimer's Disease from Epidemiological Studies and Public Health Impact

Alzheimer's disease is a fatal, progressive, degenerative brain disease that slowly destroys memory and thinking skills, often starting 5, 10 or even 20 years before symptoms appear. It is also the most common form of dementia worldwide and the top cause for disabilities in later life. According to 2017 Alzheimer's Statistics, nearly 44 million people have Alzheimer's or a related dementia around the world and an estimated 5.5 million Americans of all ages have Alzheimer's disease, in another words, one in 10 people age 65 and older (10 percent) has Alzheimer's dementia (Latest Facts & Figures Report from Alzheimer's Association). Alzheimer is most common in Western Europe and least prevalent in Sub-Saharan Africa (Alzheimer's Disease International).

Of the 5.5 million Americans with Alzheimer's in 2017, an estimated 5.3 million are age 65 and older and approximately 200,000 individuals are under age 65 and have younger-onset Alzheimer's (early onset Alzheimer's) (Data from 2017 Alzheimer's Disease facts and figures at alz.org). Further, AD is the sixth-leading cause of death in the United States and the fifth-leading cause of death among those aged 65 and older. Alzheimer's care has become an overwhelming burden for society and families as the global cost of Alzheimer's and dementia is estimated to be $605 billion, which is equivalent to 1% of the entire world's gross domestic product. According to the data from Alzheimer's Association, people with Alzheimer's disease are hospitalized three times more often than people without Alzheimer's, the caregivers have estimated $236 billion in additional health care costs of their own in 2016. These numbers will escalate rapidly in coming years. By 2030, it is estimated that there will be 74.7 million people with dementia, and the cost of caring these individuals could rise to some US$2 trillion [1]. By 2050, the number of people age 65 and older with Alzheimer's disease may nearly triple, barring the development of medical breakthroughs to prevent or cure the disease.

The etiology of Alzheimer disease, which is multi-faceted, other than older age and genetic susceptibility, remains unclear. In the past decade, large strides have been made towards a better understanding of the pathogenesis of AD for possible interventions to delay the course of disease. While AD is rare in young individuals, especially below age 60 years, mutations in known early-onset genes are reported to contribute to ~50% of early-onset cases [2]. Incidence of AD increases with age in all populations [3, 4] with annual incidence in US increasing from ~1% at ages 65-70 years, to 6–8% by age 85 years and up [5, 6]. Although aging is the primary risk factor for AD, there are many other risk factors that may affect the progression of AD. 1) Researches have shown that adults with Type 2 diabetes mellitus (T2D) have a higher risk of later developing Alzheimer's and neurodegeneration compared with healthy individuals [7] and T2D is associated with a progressive cognitive decline [8]. Some work has suggested that brain insulin resistance may be an early and common AD marker [9] and anti-diabetic agents are a promising therapeutic approach for AD patients [10 - 12]. 2) Chronic psychosocial stress is increasingly recognized as a risk factor for late-onset Alzheimer's disease (LOAD) and has been shown to exacerbate tau pathology, abnormal accumulation of Aβ, neurodegeneration, and cognitive performance [13]. Chronic stress primes microglia and the immune system to induce inflammatory responses in the adult brain, which contributes to synaptic dysfunction and cognitive impairment in AD [14, 15]. Other risk factors include family history and genetics, head trauma, Down syndrome history, high cholesterol, high blood pressure, alcohol, smoking and obesity. Evidence is steadily and increasingly accumulating to confirm that women are at significantly greater risk of developing Alzheimer's disease, and recent evidence has shown poorer cognitive outcomes for women than men with Alzheimer's disease at the same disease stage [16]. More strikingly, a recent study of multiomic evaluation of AD-associated virome integrating genomic, transcriptomic, proteomic, and histopathological data from human post-mortem tissue has observed the increased human herpesvirus 6A (HHV-6A) and human herpesvirus 7 (HHV-7) from subjects with AD and the regulatory relationships linking viral abundance and the modulators of APP metabolism [17].

Apart from AD, there are other causes of dementia including cerebrovascular disease, dementia with Lewy bodies (DLB), frontotemporal lobar degeneration, Parkinson's disease, as well as combined dementia such as AD and vascular dementia, AD and DLB, and the combination of these three, which make accurate diagnosis a complex task. Other forms of dementia need to be ruled out for an appropriate diagnosis of AD, including metabolic disorders (for example, thyroid disease, vitamin B12 deficiency and heavy metal poisoning), chronic infections, brain tumors, depression, and medication-induced dementia [18]. It has been established that the pathological changes of AD start with neuronal death in the entorhinal cortex, whose connections to the hippocampus, support transformation of short-term memories to long-term memories. At the early stages of AD, forgetfulness, deficits in problem solving and attention are common. The progression of the dementia to another stage lasts for around 2 to 5 years. The mild stage is recognized by memory loss, visuospatial difficulty, language dysfunction, and personality changes. In the following moderate stage, the brain damage spreads to the cerebral cortex that controls language, reasoning, sensory processing, and consciousness. Various visual functions decline in ageing and is exacerbated in AD patients, such as complex visual processes and shadow-processing [19]. Symptoms of the disease begin to become more pronounced and the patient displays behavioral problems, such as hallucinations, delusions, anger outbursts and impairments in routine tasks leading to a need for supervision. After a further 2 to 4 years, the severe stage of AD is characterized by a widespread atrophy of the cerebral cortex and the enlargement of the ventricles. The patient is incapable to recognize the family and friends and unable to swallow, control bladder or bowel, walk, and sleep. In addition to cognitive deficits, a variety of adverse behavioral symptoms such as depression, aggressive behavior, psychosis, and over activity which are "noncognitive" symptoms of AD raise the direct costs of care significantly [20].

GENETIC DETERMINANTS OF ALZHEIMER'S DISEASE

Molecular Genetic Phenotypes of Alzheimer's Disease

Over the past decades, research progress on identification of disease genes and risk loci has led to some of the greatest advances in medicine and invaluable insights into pathogenic mechanisms, therapeutic targets, and guidance for drug design. Genetic factors have been shown to be key to the etiology of neurodegenerative disorders such as AD, not only as the monogenic causes of heritable disease but also as the modifiers of susceptibility to complex, sporadic disorders. AD is a highly heritable disease with great complexity in its genetic contributors. Large-scale genetic analyses, such as genome-wide association study (GWAS) Meta-Analysis, transcriptome-wide association studies (TWAS), and competitive pathway analysis, as well as novel study designs and new methodology are rapidly expanding our understanding of the genetic architecture of Alzheimer's disease. Evidence for a genetic basis for AD was first recognized more than 60 years ago [21] and was later highlighted with results from family studies [22, 23]. Genetic linkage studies in familial AD patients have identified four genes, including β-amyloid precursor protein (APP), presenilin protein 1 (PSEN1), presenilin 2 (PSEN2), and APOE. Dominantly inherited mutations in the first three genes are known to cause the early onset AD, accounting for about 1-2% of all AD cases.

The existence of families in whom the disease is transmitted in a clear autosomal dominant pattern has clearly shown the genetic contribution to the etiology of Alzheimer's disease. Both early-onset and late-onset Alzheimer's disease have a genetic component. APOE is the major risk gene associated with AD. Apolipoprotein E (APOE) encodes a pleiotropic glycoprotein, highly expressed in the brain, liver, macrophages and monocytes [24]. Three isoforms of APOE exist that differ in two amino acids, ε2, ε3 and ε4. APOE ε3 is the most abundant allele, occurring in about 72% of the general population. APOE ε2 is the rarest isoform, with a frequency of about 11% among general population and it is thought to protect against AD [25]. APOE increases the amyloid plaque accumulation by reducing the clearance of soluble Aβ and accelerating fibril formation [26, 27]. APOE ε4 has been shown to increase the risk for Alzheimer's disease and is also associated with an earlier age of disease onset [28, 29]. APOE ε4 occurs in about 17% of the general population and is a genetic risk factor for late onset AD with homozygous APOE ε4 showing up to 15-fold increase of AD risk compared to homozygous APOE ε3 [30]. The reason for the difference of AD risk among the three isoforms is probably due to their differential interaction with Aβ and tau protein [31, 32]. APOE ε4 exhibits a faster binding activity to Aβ, that promotes the formation of Aβ fibrils [27].

APP is the precursor of Aβ. It is a transmembrane glycoprotein that is proteolytically processed to generate secreted forms. Under physiological conditions, the majority of APP is cleaved within the Aβ domain by α- and γ-secretases and the resulting sAPPα and α-C-terminal fragment are nonpathogenic. Alternatively, pathological form of Aβ is generated when APP is cleaved by β- and γ-secretases. About 14% of early-onset autosomal dominant AD cases are due to dominant mutations in APP gene [33]. More than 30 pathogenic mutations within APP have been identified so far and the majority of these mutations are located in the region close to or within the Aβ domain [33]. Some mutations influence AD pathogenesis by increasing plasma Aβ levels which seems sufficient to cause AD, such as the KM670/671NL mutation that does so by regulating β-secretase cleavage efficiency [34]. Other mutations do not cause a general increase in plasma Aβ levels but result in a shift to the preferential production of Aβ42, the more aggregation prone fragment [35]. A third type of mutations causes accelerated Aβ aggregation. The 'Arctic' mutation E693G first identified in a Swedish family enhances Aβ protofibril formation that may lead to faster insoluble Aβ buildup accompanied by reduced plasma levels of Aβ42 and Aβ40 [36]. Nevertheless, all these disease causing mutation proves one point that Aβ aggregation caused by abnormal APP processing is critically involved in AD pathogenesis.

The rare, early-onset familial form of Alzheimer's disease is associated with mutations in genes on chromosomes 21, 14, and 1. Mutations on chromosome 21 cause the formation of abnormal APP which leads to neuritic plaques in AD. A mutation on chromosome 14 and chromosome 1 causes the formation of abnormal presenilin 1 and presenilin 2 [33]. Encoded by PSEN1 and PSEN2, presenilin-1 and presenilin-2 are key components of γ-secretase catalytic subunit that is involved in APP cleavage. PSEN1 is the most commonly mutated gene in AD, with over 200 pathogenic mutations identified so far, accounting for about 80% of early-onset familial AD cases. Following the second most commonly mutated APP gene, PSEN2 mutations account for about 5% of early-onset familial AD cases, with 19 pathogenic mutations [37]. Presenilin-1 and presenilin-2 are highly homologous transmembrane proteins sharing similar structural characteristics. They are enriched in the endoplasmic reticulum and Golgi compartments of neurons and are involved in protein processing [38, 39]. Because of their involvement in γ-secretase, mutations of PSEN1 and PSEN2, leads to AD pathology by altering the ratio of Aβ42 and Aβ40 fragments [40]. Meanwhile, researchers have not found a specific gene that directly causes the late-onset form of the disease except the mutations on apolipoprotein E (APOE) gene on chromosome 19-does increase a person's risk, as discussed above.

Genome-wide association studies have identified more than 20 AD risk genes, such as ABCA7, CLU, EPHA1, and, SORL1, which have been previously linked to the amyloidogenic AD pathways. Further work has suggested that AD genes might differentially regulate AD pathologic findings across the disease stages [41]. The CD33 SNP rs3865444 was associated with inhibition of CD33 expression and reductions in amyloid β (Aβ42) level in the brain thus providing protection against AD. Therefore, CD33 inactivation mitigates Aβ pathology and CD33 inhibition could represent a novel therapy for AD [42]. Miron J and colleagues (YEAR) using performed a GWAS in patients with late-onset sporadic AD from the Quebec Founder Population and identified that CDK5RAP2 plays a key role in the regulation and accumulation of Tau pathophysiology [43].

Besides the long established loci for Alzheimer's disease, numerous efforts are under way to gather evidence for involvement of the genes proposed in GWA studies [44]. The identified AD associated loci from genomic studies are classified regarding to previously known AD pathways such as, APP (SORL1, CASS4 and FERMT2), immune response and inflammation (HLA-DRB5–DRB1, INPP5D, MEF2C,TREM2), cell migration (PTK2B), lipid transport and endocytosis (SORL1), hippocampal synaptic function (MEF2C and PTK2B), cytoskeletal function and axonal transport (CELF1, NME8, and CASS4), regulation of gene expression and post-translational modification of proteins, and microglial and myeloid cell function (INPP5D and TLR2) [45, 46]. Saad M and colleagues (2015) have conducted single marker and gene-based burden tests for common and rare variants and combined association analyses with variance component linkage analysis with reference to prior studies to identify strong gene candidates that contributes to AD pathogenesis. They found a statistically significant association with age at onset (AAO) for three genes (WRN, NTN4 and LAMC3) with common associated variants, and for four genes (SLC8A3, SLC19A3, MADD and LRRK2) with multiple rare-associated variants that have a plausible biological function related to AD [47]. Sanchez-Mut and colleagues have recently identified the association of the peptidase M20-domain-containing protein 1 (PM20D1) with AD by combining GWAS and EWAS and PM20D1 is increased in human patients with AD who are carriers of the non-risk haplotype [48].

Other genetic mutations have also been found in specific populations. Recent work has identified rare Reticulon 3 (RTN3) variants in both the early-onset and late-onset Alzheimer's disease in Han Chinese. RTN3 is a neuronally-expressed reticulon family protein that was previously shown to negatively regulate BACE1 and the generation of Aβ from amyloid precursor protein [49]. Previous work from Yan *et al.* (2015) genotyped 672 representatives of the Chinese Han population for the functional rs890293 polymorphism within CYP2J2, and characterized that CYP2J2 rs890293 is a predisposing genetic factor for progression of LOAD [50]. In another Asian population, the KIBRA rs17070145C allele was demonstrated to increase the risk of AD in young Japanese with synergism with the APOE genotype [51]. Besides APOE, nine other genomic loci were identified by GWAS for LOAD, mainly in European individuals [46, 52, 53]. Shuai P *et al.* (2015) performed a meta-analysis and found that CLU SNP rs9331888 might be associated with an increased AD risk in Caucasian populations, but not in Asian populations [54]. However, on the other hand, several studies demonstrate that some of these loci show similar effects across populations, such as SORL1 loci which was reported to be associated with AD in Japanese and Koreans, was replicated also in a large European American cohort [55].

The Role of ncRNAs in AD

There is a rising recognition that noncoding (nc)RNAs are involved in both the onset and pathogenesis of AD, including microRNAs (miRNAs), long noncoding RNAs (lncRNAs), and circular RNAs (circRNAs) that regulate gene expressions, such as APOE4, APP, secretases and tau at the transcriptional and posttranscriptional levels and can serve as biomarkers and potential therapeutic targets. Recent studies have indicated that miRNAs are involved in virtually all physiological states, including development, proliferation, differentiation, and signal transduction *etc.*, with the evidence that miRNAs are highly expressed in neurons in the brain, it is not surprising that miRNA have a profound impact on cognitive functions and the dysfunction of miRNA are involved in the etiology of several neurological disorders, including AD [56, 57].

One of the pioneer studies showing miRNA regulation of APP mRNA was that of Niwa R *et al.* (2008) demonstrating the APP homolog of C. elegans, APL-1, is developmentally regulated by miRNA let-7 [58]. It is also reported by Patel N *et al.*(2008) that miRNAs hsa-mir-106a and hsa-mir-520c bind to human APP 3'UTR and negatively regulate gene expression [59] and the regulation of miRNAs belonging to the miR-20a family (that is, miR-20a, miR-17-5p and miR-106b) on APP expression was also reported *in vitro* [60]. One of the members of the miR-29 family, miR-29c, which is downregulated in AD brains, was shown to regulate the expression of BACE1 directly by targeting its 3'-UTR both in human and mouse cell lines [61, 62]. Expression of microRNA miR-107 decreases early in Alzheimer's disease and may accelerate disease progression through regulation of BACE1 [63]. miR-132 is one of the most severely down-regulated miRNAs at the intermediate and late stages of AD [64], making it a potential biomarker and therapeutic target. On the other hand, the miRNA regulations on Tau mRNA expression and metabolism have been established: It has been reported that miR-132/212 deficiency increased tau expression, phosphorylation, and aggregation, and promotes pathological aggregation in mouse models [65] and the dysregulation of miR-132/-212 expression could contribute to signaling mechanisms that are involved in an array of cognitive disorders [66]. The role of miR-132 in AD has also been validated in patients [67]. Other candidates include miR-219, miR-124, miR-9, miR-132, and miR-137, miR-15a, miR-922, which regulate tau splicing and tauopathy [68 - 71]. Another notable miRNA is miR-146a which is upregulated in AD brains and was found to be upregulated in the CSF of AD patients, another potential biomarker for AD [72, 73].

BEHAVIORAL AND ELECTROPHYSIOLOGICAL STUDIES IN TRANSGENIC MODELS OF ALZHEIMER'S DISEASE

The etiology of AD is unknown, and most of the animal models are based on genetic mutations associated with familial AD (fAD). Although, these models are invaluable in determining the molecular mechanisms of AD progression and testing potential therapeutics, no single mouse model can possibly elucidate all the aspects of AD.

Aβ plaques present in AD transgenic mice are structurally similar to those found in the human brain [74]. Transgenic mice with APP overproduction develop pathophysiology as observed in humans; they too exhibit an age dependent progression in Aβ accumulation. Notably, plaque formation is accelerated when the longer Aβ42 is preferentially cleaved from APP, as this peptide is more prone to aggregation than Aβ40 and leads to earlier an onset and more severe cognitive decline [75].

The second prominent feature for pathology of human AD is the intracellular aggregates of hyperphosphorylated tau otherwise known as neurofibrillary tangles (NFTs). Unlike human AD, these mouse models do not develop NFTs, yet many show increased tau hyperphosphorylation [76]. This could be because (A) human Aβ accumulation is not sufficient to cause NFT formation; (B) rodent tau has a different structure and sequence that may not be prone to aggregate formation; (C) the life span of mice is not prolonged enough to allow for enough hyperphosphorylation/aggregation as these pathologies develop over decades in humans; or (D) a combination of these. So, whereas Aβ accumulation in APP overexpressing mice does not lead to NFT formation, these animals still exhibit robust cognitive decline. To model the NFTs seen in human AD it has been necessary to develop transgenic mice that express further gene alterations in addition to mutated APP such as mutated human tau [77, 78] or removal of nitric oxide synthase 2 [79]. These multigenic AD transgenic models do develop NFTs similar to humans and have thus aided the explication of the relationship between Aβ and tau [80] with Aβ pathology which seem to precede the onset of tau pathology. Some of the strongest data supporting tau pathology as a downstream event of Aβ accumulation have come from the study of these mice [78].

Most AD transgenic models exhibit memory impairments, with the cognitive deficits appearing to occur earlier than the appearance of extracellular plaques. Research shifted to identifying the precursors to plaque formation and identifying how aggregation of Aβ was crucial to its toxicity. This led to the focus on soluble oligomeric Aβ species—low-molecular-weight aggregates up to ~150 kDa consisting of two to 30 Aβ peptides. As in AD transgenic mice, cognitive decline in humans is not proportional to Aβ plaque load [81].

Some of the mouse models have also been developed to target specific therapeutic approach to treat or slow the progression of AD such studying the biology of BACE1 and for investigating compounds that target β-secretase. These models are relevant for analyzing long term effect of inhibition of BACE1 on many downstream events like synaptic transmission [82], motor coordination [83], for axon guidance and many more critical functions [82].

Many of the cognitive impairments stem from disruption of synaptic transmission and plasticity. Mounting evidence suggests in various animal model of AD, Aβ as the underlying factor that causes changes in synaptic function. Other reports have demonstrated the role of NFTs in synaptic dysfunction. Modeling both tangles and plaques in AD-relevant brain regions in mouse models of AD enables one to establish the critical link between proteinaceous structures to learning and memory, synaptic plasticity and transmission. Synaptic loss occurs early in AD and accompanies Aβ accumulation [84]. It has been shown that the severity of dementia in AD patients correlates better with the extent of synaptic dysfunction rather than the loss of neurons [81, 85]. Synaptic loss is likely represent a morphological changes in dendritic spine morphology and structure that begins early in the disease [86 - 90]. It is believed that remodeling of the excitatory spine synapses contribute for the increased of functional plasticity, which in turn underlie the mechanism of learning and memory [91]. Researchers have turned their attention on LTP changes in the hippocampus as a measure of synaptic dysfunction and cognitive function in transgenic animal models. The precise mechanism underlying the interaction between amyloid and tangles pathologies in AD remains to be elucidated, and the development of mouse models of AD will help us to understand how synaptic plasticity and transmission has evolve in this disorder [92].

Some animal model with extensive studies in synaptic function and behavior assessments have been described here in Table (**1**).

Table 1. Summary of behavioral and electrophysiological properties of transgenic models of AD.

Mouse Model	Behavior Changes	Electrophysiological Changes
3xTg-AD	Cognitive impairment is observed ~ 4 months. Impairments first manifest as a retention/retrieval deficit and not as a learning deficit and occur prior to plaques and tangles. Deficits are observed in both spatial and contextual based paradigms. ~ 6.5 months, mice display learning and memory deficits in the Barnes maze, but performed better than wild-type mice in the Y maze and fear conditioning tasks. These mice are viable, fertile, and display no initial gross physical or behavioral abnormalities [93].	Synaptic dysfunction, with LTP deficits occur. High density of GFAP positive astrocytes and IBA-1 positive microglia are observed when compared to WT mice at around 7 months of age [94].

(Table 1) cont.....

Mouse Model	Behavior Changes	Electrophysiological Changes
5xFAD	High neuronal loss and deficits correspond with spatial learning deficits by 4 to 5 months [95]. Also observed is impaired stress-related memory, specifically very low levels of contextual freezing at 6 months [96].	Altered synaptic structure and function is observed at around 4 months. LTP is normal in young animals but becomes gradually impaired around 6 months [96]. In hippocampal slices the Input/output (I/O) responses at Schaffer collateral-CA1 synapses at 6 months shows severe deficits compared to WT littermates [95].
APP23	Deficits in spatial memory are observed in the Morris water maze at three months and become more severe with age [97, 98]. APP23 mice exhibit both early behavioral impairment in the large Morris maze as well as impairments in passive avoidance and small pool performance that are marked only in old age. Memory deficits in passive avoidance were observed in 25-month-old mice, but not at younger ages [98].	Basic synaptic function in the hippocampus was reduced in hemizygous APP23 mice compared with their WT littermates at 12 and 18 months of age, whereas, it was unaltered within the prefrontal cortex. LTP in the hippocampus and prefrontal cortex is normal at all ages studied: 3, 6, 9, 12, 18 and 24 months [99].
APP23 x PS1-R278I	Short-term memory deficits around 3 to 4 months as measured by the Y maze [100].	Unknown
APP751SL/PS1 KI	Age-dependent impairments in working memory as measured by the Y maze and T-maze continuous alternation task. No deficit at 2 months, but deficits at 6 and 12 months compared to PS1KI littermates [101].	~6 months a large reduction of LTP and disrupted paired pulse facilitation observed. No deficit at 4 months [102].
APP-C99 (tg13592)	Hypoactivity. The acquisition of place learning in the Morris water maze task was impaired [103].	Unknown
APP E693Δ-Tg (Osaka)	By 8 months mice exhibited memory impairment in the Morris water maze compared to mice expressing equivalent levels of WT human APP [104].	~ 8 months, transgenic mice exhibit reduced short term plasticity as shown by paired-pulse facilitation along with reduced LTP [105].
APP NL-G-F Knock-in	Memory impairment in homozygous mice by 6 months of age as measured by the Y maze [106].	Unknown

(Table 1) cont.....

Mouse Model	Behavior Changes	Electrophysiological Changes
ADanPP	Animals are tested at 6 months and 18-20 months. Mice 18-20 months of age exhibited both motor and spatial learning defects in the Morris water maze, and increased anxiety in the open field test. No impairments at 6 month-observed [107].	Unknown
APPPS1	Cognitive deficits in spatial learning and memory in the Morris water maze reported at 7 months [108]. Impaired reversal learning of a food-rewarded four-arm spatial maze task observed at 8 months [109].	Hippocampal CA1 LTP normal at 4.5 months of age, but impaired at 8 and at 15 months of age [110].
$APP^{sw/0}$; $Pdgfr\beta^{+/-}$	~9 months, $APP^{sw/0}$;$Pdgfr^{\beta+/-}$ mice perform poorly on several hippocampal-dependent behavioral tests including burrowing, nest construction, and novel object recognition, compared with age-matched $APP^{sw/0}$;$Pdgfr\beta^{+/+}$ littermates [111].	Unknown
APPSwDI x NOS2 Knock-out	Impairments in spatial memory by 52-56 weeks as measured by the radial arm maze and the Barnes maze. Bigenic mice more impaired than APPSwDI [79].	Unknown
APPSwe/PSEN1(A246E)	Age-associated cognitive impairment, as measured by the Morris water maze, was observed in 11 to 12-month-old males. Both acquisition and retention were impaired. No impairment at 3-4 months of age. At both time points mice performed normally on a position discrimination task in the T-maze [112].	Unknown
APPswe/PSEN1dE9	Impairment in the Morris water maze ~12 months, specifically during acquisition of the hidden platform sub-task and the probe trial, but not in the visible platform test [113]. ~ 13 months the mice commit more errors in the Morris water maze, but not ~7 months [114].	Transient long-term potentiation (t-LTP) is reduced ~3 months. The degree of impairment is not related to age from 3 to 12 months [114].
APP(V642I)KI	Impairments at the water finding task at age 27-29 months, a test of long-term memory. No differences in the open field test of the elevated plus maze indicating no difference in general behavioral patterns, activity level, or emotional state [115].	Unknown

(Table 1) cont.....

Mouse Model	Behavior Changes	Electrophysiological Changes
APP(V717I)	~ 6 months, spatial and non-spatial orientation and memory deficits by Morris water maze and other tests. Also deficits in associative learning has been observed [116, 117].	Significant deficit in LTP in CA1 region of the hippocampus at 6 months [117].
APP(V717I) x PS1(A246E)	~5 months, spatial and non-spatial orientation and memory deficits observed by Morris Water Maze are observed. Impaired associative learning, hyperactivity, anxiety, and aggression [118].	Significant deficit in LTP in CA1 region of the hippocampus ~ 6 months [118].
Arc48 (APPSw/Ind/Arc)	At 3-4 months the Arc48 mouse was able to learn a task involving escape to a cued platform in the Morris water maze, but were impaired in the ability to use extramaze cues to navigate to the hidden platform [119].	Unknown
ArcAβ	Cognitive impairment measured from the age ~ 6 months in the Morris water maze and Y-maze, as well as in active avoidance behavior [120].	LTP is severely impaired in slices~3.5 and ~7.5 month old mice. LTP and basal synaptic transmission were normal in slices from 1 month old mice [120].
ARTE10	Mice exhibit age-associated cognitive deficits, mainly in episodic memory. Depending on the paradigm used, deficits were observed in an object-recognition task and in the Morris water maze at 12 months of age, but not ~4 and ~8 months [121].	Hippocampal neurons exhibit substantial changes in electrophysiological properties by 10-14 months of age, including hyperexcitability in the form of increased firing of action potentials and a more efficient transition from solitary firing to bursting [122].
BACE1 Knock-out	Decrease neuronal activity and suppress LTP, resulting in memory deficits as assessed by novel object recognition and Y maze spontaneous alternation [123].	BACE1 KO display reduced presynaptic function with an increase in paired-pulse facilitation ratio. Mossy fiber LTP, normally expressed *via* an increase in presynaptic release, is eliminated in the Kos [123, 124].
BCAE1 Conditional Knock out (CKO)	Decreased neuronal activity like tradition Knock out [125].	BACE1 deletion in the adult decreases LTP and level remains like genetic Knock out [125].

(Table 1) cont.....

Mouse Model	Behavior Changes	Electrophysiological Changes
htau	Abnormal spatial learning ~6 month compared with control mice [126]. Normal object recognition and spatial learning and memory by MWM at four months, but deficits by 12 months [127]. Impaired burrowing relative to control mice occurs by four months [128].	In hippocampal slices, LTP induced by high frequency stimulation (HFS) was normal at four months but abolished by 12 months. LTP induced by theta burst stimulation (TBS) was normal at both ages. Paired-pulse ratio (PPR) was unaffected at four months, but increased at 12 months compared with controls, suggesting a decrease in probability of transmitter release [127].
hTau-A152T	In the Morris water maze, performance was impaired after 17 months of age. Nest building was impaired at 10-14 months. Social interaction, anxiety, exploratory behavior, and motor functions were unaltered [129].	No Changes
J20 (PDGF-APPSw,Ind)	Deficits in spatial memory and learning with age ~4 months, demonstrate spatial reference memory deficits as measured by the radial arm maze [130] and Morris water maze [131]	Between ~3 and ~6 months show deficits in basal synaptic transmission. Field EPSPs at the SC to CA1 synapse in acute slices have smaller amplitude than WT. Also exhibit deficits in LTP at the SC–CA1 synapse [132].
mThy-1 3R Tau (line 13)	~ 6-8 months' memory impairment is evident as a failure to habituate to a novel environment. At ~8-10 months, transgenics also took longer than WT mice to find the hidden platform in the Morris water maze [133].	Unknown
mThy1-hAPP751 (TASD41)	Cognitive impairment observed by ~6 months by Morris Water Maze [134]. Some sex-specific differences have been observed in open field exploration and thigmotaxis, the tendency to remain close to walls when exploring a new environment [135].	Unknown

(Table 1) cont.....

Mouse Model	Behavior Changes	Electrophysiological Changes
PDAPP(line109)	This model exhibits cognitive deficits in many tasks, including spatial working memory at ~4 months *via* Morris water maze [136]. Deficits in recognition memory follow at approximately ~6 months of age, as assessed by novel object recognition [137].	The show decreased synaptic and dendritic density [135]. Alterations in LTP induced by theta burst stimulation (TBS) at ~4-5 months which is prior to plaque formation is seen. Also PPF is enhanced. Responses to high frequency stimulation bursts were distorted [138].
PLB1-triple (hAPP/hTau/hPS1)	Social recognition memory impaired by ~5 months and further worsens ~12 months. Spatial learning impairments seen ~12 months deficits in spatial acquisition learning were seen in the open field water maze [139, 140].	Impairments in LTP and STP plasticity observed at hippocampus. Basic synaptic transmission intact ~6 months but severely affected at ~12 months. PPF is reduced at both 6 and 12 months [140, 141].
PLB4 (hBACE1)	Impaired spatial representation in a habituation task ~3 months. By ~6 months, impaired learning and memory as observed from Y-maze, Morris water maze, and a test of the social transmission of food preference [142, 143].	Unknown
PS1 conditional Knock-out	Mild impairment of spatial learning and memory in the Morris water maze ~ 5 month [144].	Mice ~3-6 months exhibit normal PPF, LTP, and LTD in the SC-CA1 pathway of hippocampus [144].
PS2APP (PS2(N141I) x APPswe)	Mice develop age-associated cognitive impairment from ~8 months with impaired acquisition of spatial learning in the water maze [145].	No difference in LTP in the dentate gyrus at 3 and 10 months compared to WT mice [145].
PS/APP	Mice exhibit progressive, age-related impairments in cognitive tasks, including acquisition in the water maze and radial arm water maze working memory. Performance in these tasks deteriorates by ~15-17 months compared with performance at ~5–7 months when neuropathology is minimal [146, 147]	Unknown
PS cDKO	Deficits in the Morris water maze and contextual fear conditioning are mild at ~2 months, but are more severe with age [148].	Reduction in synaptophysin immunoreactivity in hippocampal CA1 pyramidal neurons ~6 months. Reduction in dendritic spines ~9 months [148].

(Table 1) cont.....

Mouse Model	Behavior Changes	Electrophysiological Changes
TAS10 (thy1-APPswe)	Deficits in spatial learning present by 6 months of age as measured by the Morris water maze. No difference from non-Tg at 2 months of age. Deficits in Y maze at 12 months. No deficit in fear conditioning up to 24 months of age [145].	~12 to 14 months of age, deficits in basal synaptic transmission have been observed in the CA1 region, but short- and long-term synaptic plasticity are relatively normal [145].
Tau4RTg2652	Deficits in spatial learning and memory as indicated by performance in the Barnes maze at multiple time points-3,6 and 11 months [149].	Unknown
Tau609 (Tau 10 + 16)	Deficits in spatial reference memory by 6 months of age as measured by the Morris water maze. No difference from non-Tg littermates at 4 months of age [150].	Some changes in basal synaptic transmission and significant impairment of LTP evident by 6 months [150].
TauC3 (Transgenic caspase-cleaved tau)	Learning and memory impairments as early as 1.3 months in several behavioral tests including the Y-maze, passive avoidance, and novel object recognition [151].	Unknown
TauΔK280 ("Proaggregation mutant")	Cognitive deficits in Morris water maze and in passive-avoidance paradigms reported~16 months. Deficits were seen in paradigms that test spatial learning/memory as well as contextual learning. Grip strength, Rotarod performance, and overall activity levels are normal [152].	Synapse loss. Significant reduction in pre- and postsynaptic proteins, along with fewer dendritic spines [152]. Impaired hippocampal LTP in the CA1 and CA3 areas
Tau P301L	Age-associated deficit in the passive avoidance task (significant deficit starting at 5 months) and a novel object recognition task (significant deficit at 9 months) [153]. However, at young ages (8 to 10 weeks), Tau P301L mice actually outperform WT littermates in object recognition memory [154]. The mice also develop progressive motor impairment and inactivity, accompanied by increased clasping of hind and then forelimbs around seven months [155].	Deficit in LTP in CA1 region of the hippocampus at 6 months, but enhanced LTP in the dentate gyrus at a young age (8-10 weeks) are observed [153].

(Table 1) cont.....

Mouse Model	Behavior Changes	Electrophysiological Changes
Tau P301S (Line PS19)	Impairments in spatial learning and memory ability in the Morris water maze in ~6-month-old animals [156]. Impaired memory in assays of contextual fear conditioning is also observed [157].	Impaired synaptic function is seen. Reduced LTP in the CA1 region at ~6 months is observed, as well as altered basal synaptic transmission (smaller fiber volley amplitude, fEPSP slopes, and amplitudes) [158]. Impaired LTP as measured in freely moving mice [157].
Tg2576	Exhibit age-associated cognitive deficits. impaired spatial learning and deficits in working memory and contextual fear conditioning at less than 6 months of age reported. Other studies have reported normal cognition at this age with progressive impairment at 12 months [111].	Dendritic spine reported by ~4.5 months in the CA1 region [159]. ~5 months, there is a decline in LTP in the dentate gyrus after perforant path stimulation compared to WT [160]; Both the CA1 and dentate gyrus of aged mice (>15 months) are impaired [161].
Tg4-42	Mice show an age-dependent spatial learning deficit by the Morris water maze. This deficit is not observed at ~3 months, but develops by ~8 months in homozygous animals and by ~12 months in heterozygous animals [162].	Unknown
TgCRND8	Early impairment in acquisition and learning reversal in the reference memory version of the Morris water maze, present by ~3 months [163].	In hippocampal slices from 6- to 12-month-old mice basal excitatory synaptic transmission and LTP at CA1 are reduced [164].
Tg-SwDI (APP-Swedish,Dutch,Iowa)	Learning and memory deficits seen in homozygotes at 3, 9, and 12 months in the Barnes maze task. At ~3 months, homozygotes took longer than WT C57BL/6 mice to find the escape hole. No differences in mobility, strength or coordination are reported [54].	Unknown

(Table 1) cont.....

Mouse Model	Behavior Changes	Electrophysiological Changes
THY-Tau22	Mice display learning and memory difficulties, including deficits in spatial, social, and contextual learning. The mice do not exhibit changes in overall motor activity and do not have gross motor deficits [165]. Non-spatial memory is affected as early as ~6 months, whereas spatial is impaired later, after 9 months [166]. Impaired appetitive responding has also been observed [167].	LTP is intact, but deficits in basal synaptic transmission in the hippocampus have been observed [165]. At ~9-10 months' heterozygous mice exhibit altered PPF. They also have impaired maintenance of LTD [166].

CELLULAR AND PHYSIOLOGICAL MECHANISMS OF ALZHEIMER'S DISEASE AND PHARMACOTHERAPEUTIC TARGETS

Amyloid-β Aggregation

The neuropathological hallmarks of AD include neuritic extracellular plaques in brain that consist of beta amyloid-Aβ and intraneuronal neurofibrillary tangle accumulation which comprises hyperphosphorylated tau proteins. AD can be categorized into two clinical subtypes, familial AD (fAD) and sporadic AD (sAD). Although the initiating factors for the neurodegenerative process are completely different, fAD and sAD develop similar pathological phenotypes, including not only plaques and tangles, but also the accompanying synaptic and neuronal loss, neuroinflammation and active gliosis [168].

As the dominant component of amyloid plaques and vascular deposits, Aβ is produced from mature amyloid precursor protein (APP) after its cleavage by two competing pathways *via* α-secretase (non-amyloidogenic) and β-secretase (BACE1, amyloidogenic) pathways. In the amyloidogenic pathway, it results in production of substrate for the sequential cleavage by γ-secretase leading the production of Aβ1-40/42. Aβ peptides could vary in size, from 38 to 43 amino acids and exist as monomers, dimers or oligomers by auto-aggregate; which in turn can generate fibrils that have β-sheet structure, and could deposit to form extracellular plaques (neuritic plaques) [169, 170]. In normal brains, during synaptic activity, Aβ presents at physiological levels and is involved in neuronal growth, synaptogenesis [171], cell adhesion and memory formation [172]. It can also maintain the structural integrity of blood brain barrier at picomolar level [98] and has the ability to function as a chelator and antioxidant molecule [173]. Under normal physiological conditions, the production and clearance of Aβ are balanced, but in pathological states, Aβ peptides are produced at higher amounts which causes neurotoxicity and cell death. The β-site APP cleaving enzyme is abundant in neurons and is one of the primary targets for drugs development in AD [174].

The γ-secretase complex, comprising presenilin 1 (PS1), Pen-2, Aph-1, and Nicastrin, controls a number of important cellular functions through substrate cleavage, and it also has complex regulation, through its essential subunits and other associated proteins, providing other targets for AD drugs [175].

The traditional "amyloid cascade hypothesis" asserts that the aggregation of Aβ into fibrils that deposit into the amyloid plaques initiates the pathogenesis of AD [81, 176, 177]. The accumulation of Aβ into long, unbranched fibrils is a hallmark of AD, as is the loss of neurons due to cell death in parallel with the Aβ aggregation process. Further study has suggested that oligomeric Aβ contributes the most damage to neuronal cells based on the evidence that soluble Aβ can bind to numerous extracellular molecules, including metals, cell surface receptors and cellular membranes. The oligomeric Aβ binds to a variety of Aβ receptors, such as the Aβ-binding p75 neurotrophin receptor (P75NRT), cellular prion protein (PrPc), metabotropic glutamate receptors (mGluR5), α7 nicotinic acetylcholine receptor (α7nAChR), N-methyl-D-aspartic acid receptor (NMDAR) and β-adrenergic receptor (β-AR) *et al.*, to generate neurotoxic signals into neurons, triggering cytotoxicity such as mitochondrial dysfunction and the ER stress response [178].

The proteolysis is mediated by a β-site APP cleaving enzyme 1 (BACE1) enzyme, which leads to generation of a 40–43 long amino acid sequences. These sequences form hydrophobic aggregates which constitute the senile plaques in AD [179]. The level of BACE directly co-relates with Aβ induced pathology in AD brains [180, 181]. Neurons strongly express BACE1, especially at presynaptic terminals [182 - 184]. Although BACE1 KO animals exhibit no significant morphological or functional changes from their wild type littermates they do however, display specific synaptic dysfunctions in the CA1 and CA3 regions of the hippocampus [82, 158, 184, 185]. The BACE1 KO studies have shown that inhibition of BACE1 is a good target for checking amyloid production. However BACE1 inhibition is also associated with memory impairment, subtle behavioral changes, exhibiting timid, anxious and less exploratory behavior compared to their wild type littermates in mice, evaluated *via* behavior and electrophysiology assays, suggests that only partial inhibition of BACE1 may be ideally desired [186, 187].

Tauopathies and Neurofibrillary Tangles (NFTs)

Abnormal accumulation of tau protein inside neurons forms neurofibrillary tangles, one histopathological hallmark of AD.

Tau is a microtubule binding protein that normally binds to and stabilizes microtubules by promoting microtubule polymerization and suppressing depolymerization [188 - 190]. Since NFTs are mainly composed of hyperphosphorylated tau, the function of phosphorylation has been extensively studied in Tau pathology [191]. Binding to microtubules is highly regulated by phosphorylation, with hypophosphorylated tau showing a high affinity to microtubules and hyperphosphorylation exhibiting a reduced microtubule binding capacity [192 - 194]. Tau hyperphosphorylation induces apoptotic escape and triggers neurodegeneration in Alzheimer's disease [195 - 198].

In addition to phosphorylation, other post-translational modifications (PTMs) of tau have been explored and are involved in tau pathology, including arginine mono-methylation, lysine acetylation, lysine monomethylation, lysine demethylation, lysine ubiquitination and serine O-linked N-acetylaglucosamine modification [199]. Among these PTMs, acetylation has recently been shown to contribute to tau aggregation [200]. A few tau acetylation sites have been identified, including Lys163, Lys280, Lys281 and Lys389, among which acetylation of Lys280 has been found to be prominently associated with tau aggregations in tauopathies brains, including AD and corticobasal degeneration [200]. Elevated tau acetylation is also detected in the frontal cortex of patients at early and moderate Braak stages of tauopathy [201].

Although Aβ plaques and NFTs are two distinct histopathological hallmarks of AD, tau is involved in Aβ-induced neurotoxicity. Reduction of tau in a mouse model of AD suppressed behavioral abnormalities caused by Aβ and the life span of mice [202]. Additionally, deleting tau in APP/PS1 mice that overexpress mutant forms of human APP and presenilin-1 and causes Aβ plaque accumulation, not only protects the mice from memory loss, but also suppresses synapse loss and neuronal death [203]. On the other hand, Aβ has also been shown to promote tau aggregation. Injection of synthetic Aβ fibrils substantially increased tangle formation in a mouse model that overexpressed a human tau carrying P301L mutation [204]. Mice that overexpress both tau-P301L and Aβ causing mutant APP also show an accelerated tangle formation compared with tau-P301L alone without altering plaque formation [77].

Since drugs targeting Aβ for AD have not been proven very successful clinically, there is a growing interest targeting tau as a potential therapeutic strategy [205]. A few drug candidates that potentially alters tau-mediated toxicity are being explored, including anti-tau vaccines, tau aggregation blockers, microtubule stabilizers, molecules interfering with tau hyperphosphorylation and acetylation [206, 207].

Molecular Pathways of Neurodegeneration in Alzheimer's Disease

Although the mechanism behind AD pathogenesis is largely unknown, there is a plethora of evidence implicating pathways where metabolites from Aβ monomers may lead to neurodegeneration and synaptic damage. Some of the potential mechanisms have been discussed below.

- *Formation of pore-like structures on cell membranes*: Aβ 41-42 can increase Ca^{2+} uptake which then can induce neuritic abnormality in a dose and time-dependent fashion. Mutant amyloid proteins can also form morphologically indistinguishable annular protofibrils which can lead to membrane permeabilization and thus might be the cause of cell dysfunction and even cell death [208].
- *Alterations in glutamate receptors and excitotoxicity*: Physiological concentrations of naturally secreted Aβ dimers and trimers, induce progressive loss of hippocampal synapses. Aβ-mediated spine loss requires activity of NMDA-type glutamate receptors (NMDARs) and occurs through a pathway involving cofilin and calcineurin. Furthermore, NMDAR-mediated Ca^{2+} influx into active spines is reduced by Abeta oligomers [209]. Aβ oligomers also facilitate electrically evoked LTD in the CA1 region. Aβ-enhanced LTD is mediated by mGluR or NMDAR activity. Synaptic glutamate uptake is significantly decreased by soluble Aβ. Therefore, soluble Aβ oligomers perturb synaptic plasticity by altering glutamate recycling at the synapse and promoting synapse depression [200].
- *Mitochondrial Dysfunction*: In addition to forming extra-cellular aggregates, Aβ, or its precursor APP, has complicated intracellular effects involving a variety of subcellular organelles, including mitochondria. Within AD brain samples, levels of mitochondrial APP are found to be higher in more affected brain areas and in subjects with more advanced disease. Several groups have found that Aβ interacts with mitochondria, impairing mitochondrial function and increasing free radical generation [7]. Generation of excessive nitric oxide (NO), in due to oligomers of Aβ protein or overactivity of the NMDA-subtype of glutamate receptor, can enhance mitochondrial fission. The mitochondrial fragmentation can lead to bioenergetic failure, synaptic damage, and eventually neuronal apoptosis [210].
- *Lysosomal Failure*: With the initial cathepsin findings in AD brain samples, many lysosomal system pathologies in mouse models of AD, including both amyloidosis and tauopathy models have been elucidated. Involving more than just degenerating neurons in AD brain, lysosome proliferation has been noted in nearly all neurons within vulnerable brain regions, including regions affected only at very late stages of AD. These findings suggest that lysosomal system mobilization precedes neurodegeneration. Mobilization of the lysosomal system in AD has now been traced to heightened activity and eventual dysfunction of its two main branches, the autophagic and endocytic pathways, involved either in survival of neurons, in addition to protein turnover. The autophagic and endocytic pathways, which are also known to be sites of Aβ production, begin to

fail at the earliest stages of AD [211].

Some of the signaling pathways related to synaptic plasticity, neuronal cell death and neurogenesis and involved in AD are discussed below.

Roles of Glycogen Synthase Kinase 3 (GSK-3) in AD

GSK-3 could play a critical role in Aβ production *via* enhancing β-secretase activity, modulating APP process of Aβ generation, interfering with APP cleavage at the γ-secretase complex. On the other hands, Aβ leads to GSK3β activation. Soluble Aβ binds to the insulin receptor and interfere with the functions of GSK3β. An impaired PI3K/Akt/GSK3β axis contributes to the hyperphosphorylation of Tau.

Roles of Cyclin-Dependent Kinase 5–p25

Misregulated p25/Cdk5 activity can lead to aberrant APP processing and intracellular Aβ accumulation *in vivo* with a significant increase in endogenous mouse and mutant human Aβ levels in CK–p25 and CK–p25/PD-APP Tg mouse models. Aberrant APP processing, tau pathology, and neuronal loss, can all develop from p25/Cdk5 deregulation [212]. Expression of the p25/Cdk5 complex in cultured primary neurons induces cytoskeletal disruption, morphological degeneration and apoptosis. Thus, accumulation of p25, may be involved in the pathogenesis of cytoskeletal abnormalities and neuronal death in neurodegenerative diseases [213, 214].

Roles of MAPK and ERK Kinases

The secreted form of the Aβ precursor protein (beta-APP) stimulates mitogen-activated protein (MAP) kinases [215]. All MAPK pathways, *i.e.*, the extracellular signal-regulated kinase (ERK), c-Jun N-terminal kinase (JNK) and p38 pathways, are activated in vulnerable neurons in patients with AD suggesting that MAPK pathways are involved in the pathophysiology and pathogenesis of AD [216]. Activation of ERK in astroglial cells in the white matter is accompanied by intense astrogliosis. In contrast, in patients with more advanced AD, pERK immunoreactivity was associated with neuronal cell bodies and dystrophic neurites around plaques. Levels of astroglial pERK immunoreactivity in the white matter were strongly correlated with scores of cognitive performance (Blessed, Mini-Mental Status Examination, and Clinical Dementia Rating) and with the severity of AD neuropathology (Braak stage). These findings suggest that astroglial ERK activation may be an important early response to the onset of AD pathology. Identification of cell signaling events unique to early AD may provide therapeutic targets for the prevention or delay of dementia [217], therefore ERK pathway is dysregulated in AD and also indicate an active role for this pathway in disease pathogenesis [218].

Roles of Fyn Kinase

Soluble Fyn levels are directly correlated with the cognitive scores and levels of synaptophysin immunoreactivity, and inversely correlated with neurofibrillary tangle counts in the frontal cortex. In AD cases, Fyn levels are decreased in the synapses and increased in the neuronal cell bodies where it is colocalized with neurofibrillary tangles [41]. In cells incubated with aged Aβ 1-42, the amount of immunoprecipitable FAK-Fyn complex increases up to 280%. Therefore aberrant Fyn activity due to the Aβ evoked association with FAK could play a role in neuronal degeneration and also cause anomalies in synaptic plasticity [219].

Roles of p21-Activated Kinase

p21-activated kinases (PAKs) regulate actin filaments and morphogenesis of dendritic spines regulated by the Rho family GTPases Rac and Cdc42. Active PAK is markedly reduced in AD, accompanied by downstream loss of the spine actin-regulatory protein Drebrin. Aβ oligomer is implicated in PAK defects. PAK is aberrantly activated and translocated from cytosol to membrane in AD brain and in 22-month-old Tg2576 transgenic mice with AD. The active PAK coimmunoprecipitates with the small GTPase Rac and both translocated to granules. Aβ 42 oligomer treatment of cultured hippocampal neurons induces similar effects, which is accompanied by reduction of dendrites. Therefore, PAK is involved in Aβ oligomer-induced signaling and synaptic deficits in AD.

Roles of JNK Kinases

c-Jun N-terminal kinase/Stress activated protein kinase (JNK/SAPK), a major cellular stress response protein induced by oxidative stress, plays an important role in AD. JNK2/SAPK-alpha and JNK3/SAPK-beta are related to neurofibrillary pathology and JNK1/SAP-Kgamma is related to Hirano bodies in cases of AD. Hippocampal and cortical regions of individuals with severe AD, the activated phospho-JNK/SAPK is localized exclusively in association with neurofibrillar alterations including neurofibrillary tangles, senile plaque neurites, neuropil threads and granulovacuolar degeneration structures (GVD), completely overlapping with tau-positive neurofibrillary pathology, though virtually absent in age matched controls. These findings suggest that JNK/SAPK dysregulation, probably resulting from oxidative stress, plays an important role in the increased phosphorylation of cytoskeletal proteins found in AD [200].

Inflammation and Immune Response

Recent evidence has brought up neuroinflammation as an important player in the pathogenesis of AD. Genome wide association studies identified polymorphisms of genes involved in inflammation and immune response including TREM2 and CD33 in AD [42, 220 - 222]. Cerebrospinal fluid and plaques from AD patients contain cytokines, chemokines and other molecules that are pro-inflammatory [223].

Microglia and astrocytes are the main cellular players involved in neuroinflammation in AD [224]. Microglia are the CNS resident phagocytes that survey for pathogens and cellular debris and are responsible for their clearance [225]. In AD, binding of Aβ to the receptors on the cell surface of microglia leads to microglia activation, which engulf Aβ fibrils by phagocytosis and attempt to degrade Aβ fibrils through the endolysosomal pathway [226]. Inefficient Aβ clearance due to increased cytokine concentrations leads to pathogenesis in sporadic AD [227, 228].

Astrocytes are the most abundant cells in adult brain that regulate synaptic activity as well as neurogenesis [229]. Normal adult astrocytes are able to clear exogenously added Aβ or Aβ deposits from human APP overexpressing mice [230, 231]. Astrocyte atrophy is observed in the early stage to pathogenesis in AD animal models [232]. Additionally, release of pro-inflammatory cytokines by astrocytes as a result of Aβ exposure further augments inflammatory response [224].

In addition to Aβ accumulation, recently, neuroinflammation has been shown as a trigger for tau pathology [233]. Exposure of neurons to neuroinflammatory stress leads to tau re-localization in neuritic foci and the accumulated tau in those structures are mostly hypo-phosphorylated and acetylated. Histone deacetylase HDAC6 plays a substantial role in this neuroinflammation induced tau aggregation, since deletion of HDAC6 suppressed the abnormal tau accumulation within neurons as well as in mouse brains.

Drugs targeting neuroinflammation may thus represent a new promising direction in development therapeutic strategies for AD and other neurodegenerative tauopathies. More efforts will be required in this line of research and drug development.

Apoptosis and Aberrant Cell Cycle Regulation

One prominent pathological feature of AD is brain atrophy caused by neuronal loss, mainly in hippocampus and cerebral cortex. Accumulating evidence suggests that apoptosis plays a key role in neuronal loss in AD. Impaired regulation of apoptosis leads to devastating neurodegenerative diseases including AD.

The first line of evidence of neuronal apoptosis came from histological analysis of AD brains. Detection of DNA fragmentation by the Apop Tag system showed that numerous neuronal nuclei in AD brains exhibited distinct apoptotic morphology, suggesting that apoptosis may contribute to neuronal loss in AD brains [234]. TUNEL staining of hippocampal sections from AD and non-AD brains revealed that more cells in AD hippocampus were undergoing apoptosis than that of non-AD brains [235]. Cytoplasmic immunoreactivity of activated caspase-3, the central effector enzyme of the apoptotic cascade, was also present in neurons with apoptotic morphology in AD brain while no positive staining was observed in control brains [236].

Although the exact cause of neuronal loss in AD is still elusive, several factors have been shown to contribute to this process and various hypotheses have been proposed, One such hypothesis is that neuronal loss may be due to Aβ induced neurotoxicity [237]. Arguments for this hypothesis are that extracellular Aβ deposition is the major component of amyloid plaques and it occurs before neuronal loss or NFT formation [238, 239]. Aβ deposition may cause direct toxicity to adjacent neurons. It has been shown that application of Aβ peptides to cultured neurons induces neuronal death [240, 241]. Histological studies have not been able to found a positive correlation between neuronal loss and the severity of Aβ plaque [237]. This leads to an alternative theory that Aβ -generating abnormal protein processing may disrupt the normal functional of neurons which ultimately leads to neuronal death [237].

Oxidative stress is another possible cause of neuronal loss [242]. Several studies have suggested the presence of increased oxidative stress levels in AD patients. AD patients consume more oxygen and exhibit higher levels of free radicals and activation of intracellular signals leading to free radical production [243 - 245]. Additionally, application of vitamin E, which suppresses oxidative stress, protects neurons from Aβ induced toxicity *in vitro*. However, no consistent results have been obtained in the use of antioxidants being beneficial in ameliorating AD symptoms clinically. Additionally, other stimulants such as neuroinflammation and cholesterol burden have also been proposed to induce neurotoxicity in AD [246].

One potential cellular mechanism for neuronal death in AD is abnormal cell cycle regulation. Cell cycle dysregulation in postmitotic neurons is one of the earliest neuronal abnormalities in AD. Cell cycle proteins such cyclin D, cdk4, and proliferating cell nuclear antigen are ectopically expressed in various regions of

AD cases [247]. Aberrant cell cycle entry has been observed in cells that are not normally cycling in AD brains [248]. Cell cycle markers Cyclin B and cyclin E are detected in neurons in the hippocampi of AD patients and the expression pattern suggests that cell cycle is arrested and that these neurons are unable to undergo re-differentiation [248]. Recently, functions of microRNA have emerged in the pathogenesis of AD such as miR-26b [167]. Expression of miR-26b is significantly elevated in pathological regions of AD brains. Overexpression of miR-26b in postmitotic neurons leads to aberrant cell cycle entry and increases tau-phosphorylation. Targeting this particular microRNA may represent a therapeutic strategy for AD in the future.

However, so far, no one theory explains all the etiology and pathology of AD. AD is indeed a highly heterogeneous disorder resulting from multiple genetic and environmental stimuli and all leads to similar behavioral and histological abnormalities.

Recent Drug Development in Alzheimer's Disease

The lack of an effective treatment for AD, an increasing prevalence and severe neurodegenerative pathology has spurred scientists and doctors to look for new drugs for several decades. So far the acethylcholinesterase (AChE) inhibitors and glutamate antagonist have been approved for the palliative treatment of AD.

Acetylcholinesterase (AChE) Inhibitors to Treat Dementia Associated with Alzheimer's Disease

The cholinergic hypothesis which has a prominent role in guiding research in AD and in the associated cognitive impairment, was initially presented over 30 years ago [249]. The decline in the integrity of basal forebrain cholinergic neurons that innervate widespread areas of the fontal and temporal cortices are selectively vulnerable early in the disease process, and the loss of cholinergic neurons contributes to memory and attention deficits. The loss of cholinergic neurons and the consequent impairment in dopaminergic transmission are reported to be responsible for the AD-related psychiatric symptoms such as apathy and depression [250]. The cholinergic synapses are particularly sensitive to the neurotoxicity by Aβ oligomers at early stage [251] and the synaptic loss of hippocampal and nucleus basalis cholinergic neurons correlates with memory deficit and neuropathology severity observed in AD patients [252 - 254]. Strong AchE expression pattern around Aβ plaques at the neocortex and hippocampus was reported in aged Tg2576 mice. The choline uptake and the expressions of cholinergic receptors were reduced in the hippocampus of these animals [255].

Based on these observations and other clinical evidences, four cholinesterase inhibitors (donepezil, galantamine, rivastigmine, and tacrine) were approved by U.S. Food and Drug Administration as the pharmacologic therapies for Alzheimer disease, although in clinical practice the drugs are also prescribed for other dementias [256]. These treatments have achieved relative success for AD with statistically significant but clinically marginal amelioration of cognitive symptoms [257, 258]. Meanwhile, the role of cholinesterase inhibitors on the treatment of AD can only be effective on for a certain period of time, which is less than three years, and cannot alter disease progression [259]. Howard R *et al.*(year) have shown that continued treatment with donepezil was associated with cognitive benefits with significant benefits over 12 months in patients with moderate or severe AD [260]. The effect of long-term treatment with galantamine that significantly reduced mortality and the decline in cognition and daily living activities in mild to moderate AD patients has been confirmed in a 2-year, randomized, placebo-controlled study [261]. Rivastigmine, which is available as a transdermal patch for its ease of use and generally favorable tolerability profile, was suggested to be an effective treatment option for AD patients [262].

Besides cholinesterase inhibitors, other drugs targeting the cholinergic system might also produce promising results, such as M1 acetylcholine receptor agonists. It was shown that M1 muscarinic receptors coupling to G-proteins are impaired in the neocortex of AD patients and M1/G-protein uncoupling is correlated with the severity of cognitive symptoms [263]. M1 acetylcholine receptor agonists such as AF267B and selective allosteric activator of the M1 are considered as a potential therapeutic based on its effects on the decrease of tau hyperphosphorylation and Aβ42, as well as reversing the deficits in cognition [264, 265]. Further, M2 antagonists, such as SCH-57790 and SC-72788 have shown to block the M2-mediated inhibition of presynaptic release of Ach, and ameliorate cognitive impairment in AD [266 - 268], despite its effect on the increase in Aβ production was also observed, which might explain the observed deterioration of AD patients after initial improvements [269]. Novel carbamates are also being employed as orally active novel AChE inhibitors which improved scopolamine-induce cognition impairment in *Swiss* male mice [270]. Moreover, other recent strategy such as hybrid compounds, that fuse two or more pharmacophores to create a single molecule with multiple mechanisms of actions, have also been designed for the treatment of neurodegenerative diseases, especially AD. The strategy was designed for optimization of the therapeutic activity through structural modifications of the prototype molecules for developing the Structure Activity Relationship (SAR). They mainly act as acetylcholinesterase inhibitors, and can target the amyloid β-protein deposition as well [271, 272].

Inhibition of Amyloid-β Aggregation

The amyloid hypothesis proposes Aβ as the main cause of AD and suggests that misfolded extracellular Aβ protein are accumulated in senile plaques [273] and the intracellular deposition of misfolded tau protein in neurofibrillary tangles cause memory loss and confusion. The Aβ peptides are cleaved from the much larger precursor APP by the aspartyl proteases BACE1 or β-secretase and γ-secretase [187]. BACE1 cleaves at the N-terminus of the APP. This leads to the generation and extracellular release of beta-cleaved soluble APP and a corresponding cell-associated C-terminal fragment which is later released by γ-secretase [274].

Advances in the Identification of β-Secretase Inhibitors/BACE Inhibitors

Therapeutic research is focused on development of amyloid-lowering strategies for the treatment of AD, with BACE1 inhibition being one of the most attractive approaches. Germline deletion of BACE1 reduces Aβ production and resolves amyloid plaques and cognitive/behavioral deficiencies observed in transgenic mice overexpressing human APP with familial AD mutations [275]. This data is further strengthened by the observation that a rare human mutation at the BACE1 cleavage site of APP results in a 40% decrease in Aβ production *in vitro*, with a much reduced propensity of Aβ to aggregate, a five- to sevenfold reduced risk of developing AD, and improved cognitive function in elderly subjects without AD [276]. Efforts are underway to design and develop selective, cell-permeable, orally bioavailable, brain-penetrant BACE1 inhibitors. BACE1 has its highest expression in neurons, whereas its homolog BACE2 (64% amino acid sequence homology) is sparingly expressed in the brain, with lower APP cleaving activity [277]. BACE1 containing vesicles have also been identified near active zones, which indicates a role in synaptic communication or neurotransmission [278]. BACE1 is found to be concentrated in presynaptic dystrophic neurites that surrounds amyloid plaques [278], where it potentially increases Aβ generation and plaque growth.

Many BACE1 inhibitors have been developed with different strategies [279] and some are already in clinical trials [280]. Some of the pharmaceutical companies working on BACE1 inhibitors for AD, include Merck; Novartis; Eli Lilly and Astra Zeneca, Biogen and Eisai; a subsidiary of Johnson and Johnson; and Shionogi. Many studies are now focused on BACE inhibitors with high efficacy, and reduced or no side effects. Some of the drugs are discussed below.

- CTS-21,166 (CoMentis Inc.): This was the first BACE1 inhibitor to be brought to clinical trials. Phase 1 clinical trials suggested the drug could penetrate the brain and reduce plasma Aβ levels. Nevertheless, no further studies were conducted [281].

- LY2811376 (Eli Lilly): Is an orally available non-peptidic small-molecule BACE1 inhibitor. It was later discontinued due to toxic side effects but still provided feasibility for further development of small molecule BACE1 inhibitors to reduce brain Aβ production.
- LY2886721 (Eli Lilly): LY2886721 was the first BACE inhibitor to reach Phase II clinical research. This had sufficient brain penetrance, exposure, or other key pharmacological characteristics. However, in mid-2013 the Phase II trial was halted due to liver abnormalities.
- Verubecestat / MK-8931-(Merck & Co.): MK-8931 is a small-molecule inhibitor of BACE1 and BACE2. It is the first BACE1 inhibitor to reach phase III clinical trials. However in March 2017, news came that Merck & Co. had halted the trial of verubecestat in mild-to-moderate Alzheimer disease (AD) due to futility [282] with "virtually no chance of finding a positive clinical effect" Merck formally published the findings from the discontinued Phase 3 EPOCH trial of the BACE inhibitor verubecestat in mild to moderate AD in May 2018. The treatment showed a slight decline in plaque load as measured by amyloid PET, with the SUVR falling by 0.02 to 0.04. They also lost slightly more hippocampal volume and total brain volume than controls. The paper adds data on cerebrospinal tau levels, reporting no difference between drug and placebo in either total tau or phosphorylated tau. As expected from the drug's mechanism of action, levels of Aβ40, Aβ42, and sAPPβ in CSF fell sharply, by up to 80 percent in the high-dose group.
- AZD3839 (AstraZeneca): AZD3839 is a potent and selective BACE1 whose phase I study was completed in November 2011, and AZD3839 was not brought forward into any further clinical studies.
- AZD3293/ LY3314814 (AstraZeneca & Eli Lilly): AZD3293 is a BACE1/2 inhibitor. AZD3293 is the only BACE1 inhibitor for which prolonged suppression of plasma Aβ with a QW dosing schedule has been reported. In September 2014, AstraZeneca and Elli Lilly jointly launched phase II/III trials to develop AZD3293 in mild cognitive impairment (MCI) and mild AD patients. This critical phase II/III clinical trial of AZD3293 started in late 2014 and is expected to end in May 2019.
- E2609 or Elenbecestat (Eisai): E2609 is an orally bioavailable small-molecule BACE1 inhibitor. Phase III clinical studies aiming to assess the efficacy and safety of elenbecestat for treatment of early AD, including mild cognitive impairment due to AD and a subset of very mild AD is undergoing.
- PF-05297909 (Pfizer): Pfizer researchers have also conducted Phase I safety evaluation of the spirocyclic lactam BACE1 inhibitor PF-05297909Clinical development of PF-05297909 was halted in light of these phase I results.
- CNP520 (Amgen, Inc., Novartis Pharmaceuticals Corporation): CNP520 is an

oral, small-molecule inhibitor BACE designed to reduce Aβ production to prevent or treat AD.

- JNJ-54861911 (Janssen Research and Development): This is a potent oral BACE inhibitor used in in people with early AD.
- VTP 37948/ BI 1181181 (Boehringer Ingelheim, Vitae Pharmaceuticals): This inhibitor is targeted to the catalytic site of the enzymes BACE1 and BACE2. This compound lowers brain Aβ levels in animal models and can be given orally.

Advances in the Identification of γ-Secretase Inhibitors

The putative γ-secretase is an enzyme that cleaves the C-terminal fragment of APP following cleavage by either α or β-secretase to release the APP cytoplasmic domain. Potent, orally bioavailable γ-secretase inhibitors (GSIs) have been developed and tested in humans with Alzheimer's disease (AD) and cancer. However, due to inherent mechanism based-toxicity of non-selective inhibition of γ-secretase, clinical development of GSIs will require empirical testing with careful evaluation of benefit *versus* risk. In addition to GSIs, compounds referred to as γ-secretase modulators (GSMs) remain in development as AD therapeutics. GSMs do not inhibit γ-secretase, but modulate γ-secretase processivity and thereby shift the profile of the secreted amyloid β peptides (Aβ) peptides produced. γ-Secretase is a highly tractable therapeutic target and numerous orally-bioavailable, brain penetrant GSIs have been developed [283].

- DAPT (Elan and Eli Lilly) The first reported *in vivo* testing of a -secretase inhibitor involved the dipeptidic compound DAPT, developed by Elan and Eli Lilly [284], where high single oral doses (100 mg/kg) were needed to observe 50% Aβ lowering in the brains of young APP transgenic mice.
- BMS-299897 (Bristol-Myers Squibb (BMS)): BMS-299897 is purported to be selective for inhibiting the processing of APP over Notch [285, 286]. Also for BMS708163, another compound from the same company, an increased incidence of skin cancer was reported, most likely due to concomitant Notch inhibition. Development of Bristol-Myers-Squibb's avagacestat (BMS708163) was halted in November 2012 after Phase II trials, due to lack of positive effect on cognition, worsening cognition and increased risk of skin cancer [287].
- Benzodiazepine analog LY-411575 and benzolactam LY-450139 (Eli Lilly): These are highly potent γ-secretase inhibitors that have been tested extensively *in vivo* [288 - 290]. LY-411575 is one of the most potent -secretase inhibitors yet reported. LY-411575 also lowered brain, CSF, and plasma Aβ in an APP transgenic mouse model. The related compound, benzolactam LY-450139, is two orders of magnitude less potent however, this compound moved into clinical trials.

- Begacestat (GSI-953): Demonstrated lowered Aβ levels in the CSF during Phase I trial but development was discontinued in late 2010 (https:// clinicaltrials.gov/ ct2/ show/ NCT00959881).
- Tarenflurbil: showed positive results on cognition in Phase II but was terminated after Phase III trials due to poor results (https:// clinicaltrials.gov/ ct2/ show/ NCT00322036.) [291].
- CHF-5074 (Chiesi's): Chiesi's γ-secretase modulator CHF-5074 reached Phase II trials but was halted for undisclosed reasons www.clinicaltrials.gov/ ct2/ show/ NCT01303744.
- NIC5–15: A γ-secretase modulator, is in trials. Despite the poor results with earlier drugs hope still remains around this modulatory approach.

Advances in Immunotherapy Against Amyloid

In addition to prevention of amyloid aggregation, immunotherapy against Aß is also attracting considerable interest as it offers the possibility to reach the target with highly specific drugs. However, active and passive immunotherapy agents against Aβ lead to the clearance of deposits in humans and transgenic mice expressing human Aβ but have failed to improve memory loss [292]. Clinical trials have established immunotherapy against Aβ is able to clear plaques from the brains of AD patients but they are not without consequence as exhibited by increased immune activation within the CNS, leading to neuroinflammation and vasogenic oedema [293]. Several active and passive anti-Aβ vaccines are under clinical investigation Table (**2**).

Table 2. Summary of amyloid specific antibodies in clinical trials.

Antibody	A-type Target	Company	Clinical Trial Status
GSK933776A	Pre-fibrillary aggregates	GSK	Phase 1 - completed
SAR228810	Pre-fibrillary aggregates	Sanofi	Phase 1 - completed
BAN2401	Soluble proto-fibrils	Eisai/BioArctic Neuroscience	Phase 2- ongoing
Solanezumab	Circulating and soluble Aβ	Eli Lilly	Phase 3 (for mild AD) - terminated
Gantenerumab	Fibrillary form	Roche	Phase 3 (for mild AD) - ongoing
Crenezumab	Soluble-oligomeric, fibrillary and plaque	Genentech/Roche	CREAD study phase 3 (for mild AD)—ongoing
Bapineuzumab	Soluble and aggregated	Elan/Pfizer and Johnson&Johnson	Phase 2 trial—terminated
Aducanumab	Aggregated forms (insoluble fibrils and soluble oligomers)	Biogen	Phase 3 ENGAGE—ongoing

(Table 2) cont.....

Antibody	A-type Target	Company	Clinical Trial Status
Ponezumab	Soluble and aggregated forms	Pfizer Inc.	Phase 3 trial for older individuals who may be at risk of memory loss-ongoing

Advances in Tau-based Drug Discovery

Neuronal inclusions are comprised of the microtubule-associated protein tau — misfolded tau is a key pathological agent in AD. The huge failure of amyloid--targeted therapeutics in Phase III clinical trials suggests that it is prudent to consider alternative drug discovery strategies for AD. Transgenic animal models of tauopathies typically show an age-dependent formation of intraneuronal hyperphosphorylated tau inclusions that mimic many aspects of the NFTs observed in human tauopathies, including neuritic pathology and axonal degeneration [294].

Several strategies have been raised up on tau-focused drug discovery for AD:

Inhibition of Tau Hyperphosphorylation

Considering the evidence that tau mutations and hyperphosphorylation affect microtubule binding, a number of hyperphosphorylation sites are well characterized, most of which flank the microtubule-binding domains, except ser262 and ser356 that are within the regions. Phosphorylation at ser262, thr231 and ser235 was reported to enhance tau fibrillization and reduce tau binding to microtubules, while phosphorylation at ser214 and ser262 prevent tau aggregation [295 - 297]. The effect of kinases on phosphorylating tau *in vitro* has been well documented, including proline-directed kinases such as mitogen-activated protein kinase 1 (MAPK1), glycogen synthase kinase 3 (GSK3) and cyclin dependent kinase 5 (CDK5), specifically CDK5 and GSK3 are most relevant kinases in tauopathies [191, 298, 299]. Inhibitors of the key kinases that are implicated in tau phosphorylation have been developed with concerns on target-related side effects. The treatment with the reasonably specific GSK3 inhibitor AR-A014418 leads to a reduction of insoluble tau in AD transgenic mice which is comparable to that observed with GSK3 inhibitor Licl [300], which have also shown an anti-depression effect [301, 302]. Manipulation of tau O-linked glycosylation has also shown to modify tau phosphorylation. Certain serine and threonine residues of tau are post-translationally modified through the addition of β-N-acetylglucosamine (O-GlcNAc), and increased levels of tau O-GlcNAc results in decreased phosphorylation [303]. In this case, modulating tau phosphorylation through inhibition of O-GlcNAcase was considered as another potential approach for tau-based therapy for AD, although the potential side effects of chronic inhibition of this enzyme shall be considered regarding the fact of the broad intracellular modification by O-GlcNAc [304].

Inhibition of Tau Oligomer and Fibril Assembly

The conversion of soluble tau into oligomeric and fibrillar species could result in tau toxicities. Therefore, inhibiting tau assembly into multimeric structures could prevent the formation of toxic species and increase the levels of monomeric tau which contribute to microtubule stabilization. The first compound that was reported 20 years ago to inhibit tau-tau interactions as a tau aggregation inhibitor (TAI) was the dye methylthioninium chloride (methylene blue), which alters the structure of existing PHFs that were isolated from the brains of patients with AD [305]. Methylene blue was investigated in a Phase II clinical trial in 321 patients with mild to moderate AD for 24-weeks that failed to show significant positive effects in mild AD patients. TRx 0237 (LMTX™), a second-generation tau protein aggregation inhibitor, has shown clinical benefit on activities of daily living as measured by the modified ADCS-CGIC Alzheimer's scale and the revised Addenbrooke's Cognitive Examination (ACE-R) in the third Phase 3 trial as reported at the 2016 ICFTD conference. Several other distinct classes of small-molecule compounds that have been identified to prevent tau fibrillization include rhodanines, quinoxalines, phenylamines, exifone *et al.* Although they have shown to disaggregate fibrils or block tau aggregates, their chemical or biological properties make them unsuitable for use *in vivo* that increase the potential for off-target effects.

Enhancing Intracellular Tau Degradation.

Ubiquitination and autophagy are impaired to induce neuronal degeneration and death in AD brains [306 - 308]. Upregulation of one or both of these catabolic systems may therefore lead to a reduction of pathological tau in AD since hyperphosphorylated and misfolded tau can undergo degradation through these pathways. On the other hand, the autophagic clearance system has been implicated in the removal of larger tau oligomers and fibrils which are not be able to be reduced through the UPS, and the addition of the autophagy inhibitor 3-methyladenine indeed led to enhanced tau accumulation and aggregation [309]. Therefore, an upregulation of the autophagy–lysosomal system with drugs such as rapamycin or Licl might be a potential strategy for the treatment of tauopathies [310].

Emerging Cognitive Enhancing Drugs

There is an acute need for new drugs and therapeutic approaches for treating neurodegenerative diseases such as AD, that affect higher order thinking. Since cognitive aging and mild cognitive impairment are not considered diseases, even though older individual are clearly impaired with respect to a much younger cohort, there is no FDA-approved disease targets for cognition pharmacology.

Several cognitive enhancing drugs have been developed to combat the cognitive decline and improve the cognition impairment in AD. Early studies on AD patient's brains revealed a substantial loss of presynaptic cholinergic neurons which is thought to contribute to the cognitive decline in AD [311, 312]. Thus, restore of the cholinergic activity in the brain may improve cognitive function in AD. Base on this so-called "cholinergic hypothesis", medications have been developed for treatment of AD.

Cholinesterase inhibitors (ChEI) which can increase the level and duration of acetylcholine by inhibiting the major enzyme that breaks down acetylcholine, have been approved by FDA for AD treatment. Tacrine was the first one of this kind and it was also the first drug approved for AD treatment by FDA. Studies found that Tacrine had beneficial effect on cognitive improvement [313, 314], although it was discontinued in 2013 due to liver side effects. Donepezil is a piperidine based reversible acetylcholinesterase inhibitor that currently available for AD treatment.

A multinational placebo-controlled, double-blind trial showed that daily dose of 5 or 10mg of donepezil significantly improved cognitive and global function in mild to moderately severe AD patients [315]. These findings were consistent with a similar study conducted by a USA group [316].Compared to Tacrine, Donepezil has much longer half-life and shows no liver toxicity. Galantamine, a reversible and competitive acetylcholinesterase inhibitor, has been used for AD treatment more than 20 years. In addition of its acetylcholinesterase inhibition effect, Galantamine also can sensitize nicotinic acetylcholine receptors and enhance cholinergic transmission [317]. Two independent randomized, double blind and placebo controlled trials have been designed to evaluate the efficacy of Galantamine in patients with mild to moderate AD [318, 319]. Wilcock *et al.* showed that 4 weeks of Galantamine 24 or 32 mg/day significantly slowed the decline of functional ability and cognition [319]. Tariot et reported that Galantamine 16 or 24 mg/day for 8 weeks significantly improved the cognitive and functional symptoms of AD as compared with placebo [318]. Rivastigmine, a carbonate-based compound, is a dual inhibitor for both acetylcholinesterase and butyrylcholinesterase, the major enzymes that hydrolyse acetylcholine [320]. Rivastigmine transdermal patch was approved for AD treatment in 2007 [321] and now it has been approved for use in 60 countries globally. A recent systemic review included 13 independent randomized, double-blind, controlled trials reported that rivastigmine (6 to 12mg daily orally or 9.5mg daily transdermally) shows beneficial effects for patients with mild to moderate AD, with improvement of cognitive function and activities of daily living [322]. In conclusion, cholinesterase inhibitors provide a standard therapy for improvement of cognition function in AD. In preclinical studies, the potent neurotrophic drug J147 has been recently developed and found to be effective targeting a set of molecular changes associated with aging and AD [323 - 325].

Glutamate Excitotoxicity and New Anti-Excitotoxicity Strategies in Alzheimer's Disease

Autopsy studies on brains from Alzheimer's patients show that the neurodegeneration begins from the hippocampus then spreads to cortex as the disease progress [326]. Damages of these areas are responsible for the cognitive impairment and memory loss in the AD patients. Thus, understanding the molecular mechanism of neurodegeneration is a key to prevent and intervention for Alzheimer's disease. Excitotoxicity, which is a common mechanism for neurodegeneration, has been implicated in the pathogenesis in Alzheimer`s disease for many years [327]. Excitotoxicity was first discovered about 40 years ago that acute glutamate administration cause degeneration lesion in the mouse and monkey brain [328]. Now we know that this glutamate-induced cell death process is triggered by overstimulation of AMPA and NMDA receptors which results in excess of Ca^{2+} influx into the neurons. Overloading of free cytoplasmic Ca^{2+} in turn activates proteases and induce oxidative stress that result in cell death [329].

Glutamate Transporter Deficiency and Glutamate Excitotoxicity in AD

In the central nervous system, extracellular glutamate is tightly controlled by active glutamate transporters to avoid glutamate excitotoxicity. Failing to clear extracellular glutamate may lead to excitotoxicity and neurodegeneration caused by excessive glutamate levels. Several studies reported that glutamate transporter activity and the protein levels of glutamate transporter are decreased in the cortex of AD patients. An autopsy study from AD patients described that glutamate transporter activity was decreased in the cortex, which was associated with increased excitotoxicity and neurodegeneration [330]. A more recent study showed that the protein levels of vesicular glutamate transporter VGLUT1 and VGLUT2 were decreased in AD with the reduction of VGLUT1 highly correlated with the degree of cognitive impairment [331]. The down-regulation of vesicular glutamate transporters was observed in the mildly affected brain region suggested it might occur in the early stage of the disease [332]. EAAT1 (excitatory amino acid transporter 1) and EAAT2 (excitatory amino acid transporter 2), the two major glutamate transporters in astrocytes, were also found decreased or alterations in the AD brains [22, 333 - 335]. Immunohistochemistry with EAAT antibodies revealed that lack of EAAT expression in the vicinity of amyloid plaques [334]. Importantly, restored expression of glial EATT2 in an AD mouse model significantly improved cognitive function and reduced amyloid plaques [336]. Taken together, these studies suggest that glutamate transporter deficiency may contribute to pathogenesis in AD by triggering glutamate excitotoxicity.

Amyloid β-peptide and Glutamate Excitotoxicity in AD

Amyloid β-peptide (Aβ), is the major component of amyloid plaques which is a histological hallmark of AD [273]. Aβ derives from the amyloid precursor protein (APP), which mutations have direct links to Alzheimer's disease [337, 338]. Aβ has been implicated in glutamate excitotoxicity. First, aggregated Aβ injection into CNS or addition to cell cultures can induce neuronal death [339, 340]. It was found that Aβ can elevate resting levels of Ca^{2+} and potentiate the excitotoxicity effect of excitatory amino acid in human cerebral cortical cell cultures [327]. *in vivo* multiphoton imaging study from APP mutant mice found that resting Ca^{2+} was elevated in the neurites with cortical plaques [341]. Although it is not clear how Aβ raises cytoplasmic Ca^{2+}, but one explanation is that Aβ can insert in the cell membrane and form pore-like channels that can conduct calcium ions [342]. Moreover, Aβ can induce glutamate release from astrocytes which in turn activated extrasynaptic NMDA receptors which caused spine damage consequently [343]. The Aβ neurotoxicity effect can be enhanced by releasing glutamate from reactive microglia [344]. Aβ not only affects release glutamate but also affects clearance of glutamate from synaptic cleft. It was reported that Aβ prolonged extracellular glutamate lifetime which was accompanied with reduction of glutamate transporter 1(GLT-1) in mouse astrocytes [345]. A more recent study found that soluble forms of Aβ can also decreased expression of EAAT1 and EATT2 in human astrocytes [346]. Taken together, the combined effects of Aβ impaired glutamate clearance and enhanced release likely contribute to glutamate excitotoxicity cell death.

Anti-Glutamatergic Strategies for AD

Targeting the glutamatergic system to prevent or reduce glutamate excitotoxicity offers a novel approach to treatment of AD. This can be achieved by blocking glutamate receptors or preventing glutamate building up in the synaptic cleft. Memantine, a low affinity uncompetitive antagonist for NMDA receptors, has been approved in Europe and US to treat moderate to severe AD. Memantine acts as an open-channel blocker to inhibit prolong Ca^{2+} from NMDA receptors [347, 348]. Recent study demonstrated that Memantine preferentially inhibited the GluN2B-containing extrasynaptic NMDA receptors without affecting the normal synaptic activity [349]. Moreover, memantine can also inhibited Aβ production by blocking these calcium ions conducting NMDA receptors [350]. Interestingly, memantine treatment indeed leads to decreased levels of secreted APP and Aβ in the human neuroblastoma cells [351].

KYNA is a metabolite in the kynurenine pathway, produced from tryptophan degradation. It is a broad-spectrum antagonist for inotropic glutamate receptors including AMPA, NMDA and kainite subtypes with with highest affinity for the NMDA receptor. Several studies demonstrated that KYNA had neuroprotective properties in some neurodegenerative disorders including Huntington's disease [352], Parkinson's disease [353] and multiple sclerosis [354]. In AD, KYNA levels were found significantly decreased in the plasma [355, 356]. Chronic administration of an inhibitor of kynurenine 3-monoxygenase (KMO), which resulted in higher levels of plasma KYNA, prevented memory deficits and synaptic damage in an AD mouse model [357].The neuroprotective effect of KYNA is mainly by blocking NMDA receptors which prevents glutamate excitotoxicity [358, 359].

Glutamate dehydrogenase (GDH) is an enzyme that catalyzes the reversible interconversion of glutamate to a-ketogluatarate. In the brain, intensive neuron firing and synaptic transmission are ATP consuming process, at this energy demanding condition, GDH converts glutamate to a-ketogluatarate to produce more energy which results in reduced glutamate levels [360 - 362]. This glutamate reducing effect of GDH may prevent the cells from glutamate excitotoxicity. Deficit of GDH may contribute to neurodegeneration disorders. Interestingly, post-mortem study of cerebellum from AD found that glutamate dehydrogenase was decreased [363]. Although how GDH affects AD is still unknown, but in some other neurodegeneration disorders like ischemia, excess of GDH was correlated with reduced brain damage [364].

Overall, multiple evidences demonstrated that glutamate excitotoxicity plays an important role in the development of AD. Anti-glutamatergic strategies like blocking glutamate receptors or reducing extracellular glutamate levels are promising directions for treatment of AD.

Epigenetic Therapeutics for AD

It is known that epigenetics and the ageing process are strikingly linked with each other, and epigenetic patterns in individuals undergo changes during lifetime [365, 366]. Consider the complex pathophysiology of AD, the epigenetics allows the identification of key pathological targets in AD that could not be simply explained by conventional genetics. Major epigenetic changes in AD include alterations in DNA methylation, histone modifications, chromatin remodeling and non-coding RNA dysregulation. Alterations on the epigenomic machinery cause transcriptional gene changes that are involved in the pathogenesis of AD, such as APP. The level of the AD-associated DNA hypermethylation was positively correlated with typical AD hallmark lesions, *i.e.* β amyloid plaques and tau composed neurofibrillary tangles and the hypermethylated DNA were predominantly located in neurons [367]. PSD95 as a key player in memory and a potential therapy to treat AD, has been suggested to be a target for epigenetic editing [368]. Epigenetic modifications further trigger synaptic dysfunction and cognitive decline [369, 370].

Several studies focused on the alterations in gene-specific DNA methylation profiles, the increased methylation of SORBS3 promoter and the decreased methylation of S100A2 promoter in CpG islands of the genes associated with CNS development were screened out in AD compared with healthy controls [366], pyrosequencing analysis of post-mortem brains by Iwata *et al.* revealed the aberrant CpG methylation in APP, MAPT and GSK3β genes of the brain of sporadic AD [371]. By using neuron-specific DNA methylome analysis on the postmortem brain samples from AD patients, the etiological candidates in sporadic AD, such as the differentially hypomethylated region of BRCA1 as well as its tau-related dysfunction have been revealed [372]. Investigation on patient plasma samples for levels of vitamin B9 (folate), vitamin B12, vitamin B6, and several other metabolites related to methylation has been designed and initiated in a clinical trial of discovery of novel biomarkers for early detection of AD (NCT03136679). Many literatures have reviewed a series of DNA methyltransferase inhibitors that were proposed as candidates for therapeutic intervention in AD including epigenetic drugs and organic compounds, however earlier clinical study has shown no beneficial effect of high-dose B vitamin supplements [373] or omega-3 fatty acids [270] on cognition in individuals with mild to moderate AD.

The critical role of histone acetylation in cognition has been well studied. Preclinical data have suggested that epigenetic drugs that increase histone acetylation by inhibiting histone deacetylase (HDAC inhibitors) such as nicotinamide [374], valproic acid [375] could be a useful strategy for AD treatment [369, 376 - 378]. the HDACi suberoylanilide hydroxamic acid (SAHA, vorinostat, Zolinza) displays promising avenue for treating the cognitive deficits associated with early stage AD in APPswe/PS1dE9 mouse model [379] and a phase 1 clinical study of vorinostat in patients with mild Alzheimer Disease has been initiated in 2017.

FUTURE DIRECTIONS AND NEW TRENDS IN THE DESIGN OF DRUGS AGAINST ALZHEIMER'S DISEASE

Current drug treatment for AD patients is based on three cholinesterase inhibitors (rivastigmine, donepezil and galantamine) and memantine, which acts on the glutamatergic system. These drugs do not represent a cure, as they do not stop the progress of dementia, however, it's found that in about 60 percent of patients these drugs could delay the symptoms by about six months to a year. There is an increasing understanding towards Alzheimer disease as the most prevalent cause of dementia at any age worldwide with varied and complex underlying mechanisms, a diverse portfolio of drug targets are maintained on the novel therapeutic approaches, including small molecules, biologics, and gene therapies targeting at various pathways contributing to AD. Hung and Fu have a review of selected anti-Alzheimer's disease drugs in clinical trials (updated in June 2017) [1]. Because of the complex etiology, numerous possible drug targets have been pursued and novel targets have also emerged. However, the major class of drugs used for AD till now has been the cholinesterase inhibitors for many years. In this review, we have summarized the current anti-AD drugs which are in clinical trials targeting the various neuropathologies, including Aβ clearance, BACE inhibitor, Tau stabilization, Tau aggregation inhibitor, p-Tau clearance, and α7nAChR agonist (Table **3**).

Table 3. Summary of the developing drugs for AD in current clinical trials (Phase 1-3).

Agent	Mechanism Class	Mechanism of Action	ClinicalTrials.gov Identifier
Aducanumab	Anti-amyloid	Monoclonal antibody	NCT02484547
			NCT02477800
			NCT01561053
ALZT-OP1a + ALZT-OP1b	Anti-amyloid, anti-inflammatory	Anti-amyloid combination, inhibits neuroinflammatory response	NCT02547818
AZD3293 (LY3314814)	Anti-amyloid	BACE1 inhibitor	NCT02245737
CAD106	Anti-amyloid	Amyloid vaccine	NCT02565511
			NCT02670083
E2609	Anti-amyloid	BACE inhibitor	NCT02956486
Gantenerumab	Anti-amyloid	Monoclonal antibody	NCT02051608
			NCT01224106
			NCT01760005

(Table 3) cont.....

Agent	Mechanism Class	Mechanism of Action	ClinicalTrials.gov Identifier
Sodium Oligo-mannurarate (GV-971)	Anti-amyloid	Anti-amyloid agent	NCT02293915
Solanezumab	Anti-amyloid	Monoclonal antibody	NCT01760005
			NCT02008357
			NCT01127633
			NCT01900665
			NCT02760602
TTP488 (azeliragon)	Anti-amyloid, anti-inflammatory	Anti-amyloid RAGE antagonist	NCT02080364
			NCT02916056
Atomoxetine	Anti-amyloid	Adrenergic uptake inhibitor, SNRI	NCT02756858
			NCT01522404
			NCT02534038
AZD0530 (saracatinib)	Anti-amyloid	Kinase inhibitor	NCT02167256
			NCT02886494
			NCT02467413
Crenezumab	Anti-amyloid	Monoclonal antibody	NCT02434666
			NCT02860065
			NCT01998841
JNJ-54861911	Anti-amyloid	BACE inhibitor	NCT02503501
			NCT02406027
			NCT02002819
LY3202626	Anti-amyloid	BACE Inhibitor	NCT01843075
			NCT02129348
			NCT02791191
Valacyclovir	Anti-amyloid, Anti-tau	Antiviral agent	NCT02085265
			NCT02551809
			NCT02997982
PF-06751979	Anti-amyloid	Undisclosed mechanism	NCT02793232
Aducanumab	Anti-amyloid	Monoclonal antibody	NCT01677572
			NCT02434718
			NCT02782975

(Table 3) cont.....

Agent	Mechanism Class	Mechanism of Action	ClinicalTrials.gov Identifier
Crenezumab	Anti-amyloid	Monoclonal antibody	NCT02353598
E2609	Anti-amyloid	BACE Inhibitor	NCT02859207
KHK6640	Anti-amyloid	Amyloid aggregation inhibitor	NCT02127476
Lu AF20513	Anti-amyloid	Polyclonal antibody	NCT02388152
LY2599666 + solanezumab	Anti-amyloid	Monoclonal antibody combination	NCT02614131
LY3002813	Anti-amyloid	Monoclonal antibody	NCT01837641
			NCT02624778
LY3303560	Anti-amyloid	Monoclonal antibody	NCT02754830
MK-8931 (verubecestat)	Anti-amyloid	BACE Inhibitor	NCT02910739
NGP 555	Anti-amyloid	Gamma-secretase modulator	NCT02537938
Sargramostim (GM-CSF)	Anti-amyloid	Granulocyte colony stimulator; amyloid removal	NCT01409915
			NCT02667496
			NCT01439555
AADvac1	Anti-tau	Monoclonal antibody	NCT02579252
ABBV-8E12	Anti-tau	Monoclonal antibody	NCT02880956
			NCT02279511
			NCT02912169
Methylene blue	Anti-tau	Tau inhibitor; neuronal stimulant	NCT02380573
			NCT01300728
			NCT02720445
Nilotinib	Anti-tau	Tyrosine kinase inhibitor	NCT02947893
			NCT02471196
			NCT02035553
AADvac1	Anti-tau	Monoclonal antibody directed at Tau epitope	NCT02031198
RO7105705	Anti-tau	Anti-tau antibody	NCT02820896
TPI-287	Anti-tau	Microtubule protein modulator	NCT01966666
AC-1204	Metabolic	Ketogenic agent	NCT01741194
Pioglitazone	Metabolic	PPAR-gamma agonist, anti-amyloid effect	NCT02284906

(Table 3) cont.....

Agent	Mechanism Class	Mechanism of Action	ClinicalTrials.gov Identifier
Benfotiamine	Metabolic	Antioxidant	NCT01767311
			NCT02292238
			NCT02240693
Insulin detemir (intranasal)	Metabolic	Increases insulin signaling in the brain	NCT02672306
			NCT02833792
			NCT01595646
Insulin Aspart Intranasal	Metabolic	Increases insulin signaling in the brain	NCT02462161
Oxaloacetate (OAA)	Metabolic	Mitochondrial enhancer	NCT02593318
Aripiprazole	Neurotransmitter based	Atypical anti-psychotic (dopamine partial agonist)	NCT02168920
			NCT02442765
			NCT02446132
Brexpiprazole (OPC-34712)	Neurotransmitter based	Atypical anti-psychotic (dopamine partial agonist)	NCT02783573
			NCT02972658
			NCT01862640
Idalopirdine (Lu AE58054)	Neurotransmitter based	5-HT6 antagonist	NCT02079246
			NCT02006654
			NCT01767909
ITI-007	Neurotransmitter based	5-HT2A antagonist, dopamine receptor modulator	NCT02817906
			NCT02569398
			NCT02346201
MK-4305 (suvorexant)	Neurotransmitter based	Dual orexin receptor antagonist	NCT02750306
			NCT02351882
			NCT02017340
RVT-101 (intepirdine)	Neurotransmitter based	5-HT6 antagonist	NCT01931566
			NCT02585934
			NCT02586909

(Table 3) cont.....

Agent	Mechanism Class	Mechanism of Action	ClinicalTrials.gov Identifier
DAOIB	Neurotransmitter based	NMDA enhancer	NCT02907567
			NCT02103673
			NCT02239003
Piromelatine	Neurotransmitter based	Melatonin receptor agonist; 5-HT 1A and 1D receptor agonist	NCT02992132
			NCT02615002
			NCT02925650
SUVN-502	Neurotransmitter based	5-HT6 antagonist	NCT01255046
			NCT02580305
			NCT02079909
BI409306	Neurotransmitter based	Phosphodiesterase 9A inhibitor	NCT02392468
Bisnorcymserine (BNC)	Neurotransmitter based	Butyrylcholinesterase inhibitor	NCT01747213
HTL0009936	Neurotransmitter based	Muscarinic M1 receptor agonist	NCT02546310
TAK-071	Neurotransmitter based	Muscarinic M1 receptor modulator	NCT02769065
ANAVEX 2-73	Neuroprotective	Sigma-1 receptor agonist	NCT02244541
Candesartan	Neuroprotective, anti-inflammatory	Angiotensin receptor blocker	NCT02337907
			NCT02431468
			NCT02646982
Formoterol	Neuroprotective, anti-inflammatory	β-2 adrenergic receptor agonist	NCT02792257
Rasagiline	Neuroprotective	Monoamine oxidase B inhibitor	NCT02389413
			NCT02707458
			NCT02359552
Riluzole	Neuroprotective	Glutamate receptor antagonist; glutamate release inhibitor	NCT01703117
			NCT02910102
			NCT02626572

(Table 3) cont.....

Agent	Mechanism Class	Mechanism of Action	ClinicalTrials.gov Identifier
VX-745	Neuroprotective, anti-inflammatory	P38 mitogen-activated protein kinase inhibitor	NCT02423200
			NCT02423122
			NCT02727699
BPN14770	Neuroprotective	Negative allosteric modulator of phosphodiesterase 4D	NCT02840279
			NCT02648672
Telmisartan	Neuroprotective, anti-inflammatory	Angiotensin II receptor blocker, PPAR-gamma agonist	NCT02471833
CB-AC-02 (Placenta derived-MSCs)	Regenerative	Stem cell therapy	NCT02899091
			NCT02491268
			NCT02549196
hUCB-MSCs	Regenerative	Stem cell therapy	NCT02054208
			NCT01547689
			NCT02513706
Allopregnanolone injection	Regenerative	GABA receptor modulator	NCT02221622
hMSCs	Regenerative	Stem cell therapy	NCT02600130
RGN1016	Undisclosed	Undisclosed mechanism	NCT02820155
Vorinostat	HDACi	Undisclosed mechanism	NCT03056495

Especially, clinical trials have largely been aimed at removing insoluble beta amyloid in senile plaques but no effective treatment consistently reduced the load. The novel therapeutic approaches such as Intravenous immunoglobulin (IVIG) in AD treatment are based on the fact that IVIG can direct against Aβ. Other new therapeutic paradigms emerged for AD, supposedly the activation of the adaptive immune system directly against the self-peptide Aβ to lower its accumulation in the brain. They so far have failed to show sufficient efficacy [380 - 382]. Failure to improve cognition has also frequently been attributed to the failure of the amyloid hypothesis in the AD brain. Neuroscientists tried to understand why Alzheimer trials failed and the failure analysis of clinical trials to test the amyloid hypothesis have been carried out [383, 384]. The pharmaceutical giant, Pfizer has announced plans to end its research efforts to discover new drugs for AD in January 2018 (https: //www. reuters. com/ article/ us- pfizer- alzheimers/ pfizer-ends- research- for-new-alzheimers-parkinsons-drugs-idUSKBN1EW0TN). The example of Aβ story might indicate the incorrect direction we went for AD therapy and raise the need to bring new drugs to market, even new targets or therapeutic approaches in other mechanisms. This has in turn led to a search for imaging markers that can be used as outcomes in drug discovery and trials. Reliable biomarkers that are able to predict clinical benefit in phase III clinical trials may be helpful on the optimization of the drug development.

Biomarker research for Alzheimer's disease (AD) including CSF and blood-based biomarkers has been growing rapidly over the past years. To identify biomarkers for diagnosis and early prevention, as well as the response to therapeutic treatment, single biomarker assays are challenging to establish, instead multiplex biomarker tests are required such as mass spectrometry-based proteomics. A number of potential candidates that are associated with disease severity and disease progression have been identified in cerebrospinal fluid (CSF) and other body fluids [385]. Amyloid-beta peptide 1-42, total tau protein and hyperphosphorylated tau at threonine 181 in human CSF are regarded as the molecular biomarkers for AD, other potential candidates are being identified as well, although no molecular biomarkers have been established or translated into clinical tools so far. Many functional differences between ApoE3 and ApoE4 have been proposed to explain the increased risk of dementia due to AD associated with APOEε4 genotype, low plasma ApoE concentration predicting AD dementia was suggested by recent population-based studies [386, 387], high CSF ApoE concentrations may be especially detrimental because of their association with (p)Tau [388]. However some other groups did not confirm the conclusion or even found the opposite [389, 390] and meta-analyses shown CSF ApoE did not differ between controls and patients with AD dementia [385].

Neuroimaging and functional activity measures has played a variety of roles in the study of AD drug discovery including electroencephalography (EEG), magnetic resonance imaging (MRI), positron emission tomography (PET), single-photon emission computed tomography (SPECT) [391]. Imaging has been increasingly incorporated into trial designs to measure the effects of a therapy on fibrillary amyloid (with amyloid imaging) on atrophy (with MRI) and on metabolism (PET and fMRI) [392]. Brain imaging can also be helpful on detecting potential adverse effects of biologically active therapies. The challenge for the future will be to find the ideal imaging biomarkers that correlate most efficiently with disease stages, which can be combined for the development of effective disease-modifying therapies.

Another noted issue for drug discovery for Alzheimer's disease is the effective drug delivery strategy that the systemically administered compound can pass through the capillary endothelium of the blood-brain barrier (BBB). However,

>99% of the AD drug development enterprise were devoted to CNS drug discovery, and <1% of the effort was focused on CNS drug delivery. Although the existence of the assumption on the disruption of the BBB in AD [393], earlier PET study [394] as well as CT and MRI studies [395, 396] have failed to show any increase in permeability in AD. It is key to notice the importance of highlighting the applied science of BBB drug delivery technology in AD drug discovery, especially when a novel drug comes to the investigation on its actual work in clinical trials.

CONSENT FOR PUBLICATION

Not applicable.

CONFLICT OF INTEREST

The authors declare no conflict of interest, financial or otherwise.

ACKNOWLEDGEMENTS

We thank Dr. Alexandra G. DiFeliceantonio (Department of Psychiatry, Yale University School of Medicine, New Haven, CT 06519, USA; Max-Planc--Institute for Metabolism Research, 50931 Cologne, Germany) for editing the manuscript.

REFERENCES

[1] Hung SY, Fu WM. Drug candidates in clinical trials for Alzheimer's disease. J Biomed Sci 2017; 24(1): 47.
[http://dx.doi.org/10.1186/s12929-017-0355-7] [PMID: 28720101]

[2] Finckh U, Kuschel C, Anagnostouli M, *et al.* Novel mutations and repeated findings of mutations in familial Alzheimer disease. Neurogenetics 2005; 6(2): 85-9.
[http://dx.doi.org/10.1007/s10048-005-0211-x] [PMID: 15776278]

[3] Sosa-Ortiz AL, Acosta-Castillo I, Prince MJ. Epidemiology of dementias and Alzheimer's disease. Arch Med Res 2012; 43(8): 600-8.
[http://dx.doi.org/10.1016/j.arcmed.2012.11.003] [PMID: 23159715]

[4] Hebert LE, Scherr PA, Bienias JL, Bennett DA, Evans DA. Alzheimer disease in the US population: prevalence estimates using the 2000 census. Arch Neurol 2003; 60(8): 1119-22.
[http://dx.doi.org/10.1001/archneur.60.8.1119] [PMID: 12925369]

[5] Mayeux R. Epidemiology of neurodegeneration. Annu Rev Neurosci 2003; 26: 81-104.
[http://dx.doi.org/10.1146/annurev.neuro.26.043002.094919] [PMID: 12574495]

[6] Tanner CM, Goldman SM, Ross GW, Grate SJ. The disease intersection of susceptibility and exposure: chemical exposures and neurodegenerative disease risk. Alzheimers Dement 2014; 10(3) (Suppl.): S213-25.
[http://dx.doi.org/10.1016/j.jalz.2014.04.014] [PMID: 24924672]

[7] Biessels GJ, Staekenborg S, Brunner E, Brayne C, Scheltens P. Risk of dementia in diabetes mellitus: a systematic review. Lancet Neurol 2006; 5(1): 64-74.
[http://dx.doi.org/10.1016/S1474-4422(05)70284-2] [PMID: 16361024]

[8] de Nazareth AM. Type 2 diabetes mellitus in the pathophysiology of Alzheimer's disease. Dement Neuropsychol 2017; 11(2): 105-13.
[http://dx.doi.org/10.1590/1980-57642016dn11-020002] [PMID: 29213501]

[9] Talbot K, Wang HY, Kazi H, *et al.* Demonstrated brain insulin resistance in Alzheimer's disease patients is associated with IGF-1 resistance, IRS-1 dysregulation, and cognitive decline. J Clin Invest 2012; 122(4): 1316-38.
[http://dx.doi.org/10.1172/JCI59903] [PMID: 22476197]

[10] Benedict C, Frey WH II, Schiöth HB, Schultes B, Born J, Hallschmid M. Intranasal insulin as a therapeutic option in the treatment of cognitive impairments. Exp Gerontol 2011; 46(2-3): 112-5.
[http://dx.doi.org/10.1016/j.exger.2010.08.026] [PMID: 20849944]

[11] McNay EC, Ong CT, McCrimmon RJ, Cresswell J, Bogan JS, Sherwin RS. Hippocampal memory processes are modulated by insulin and high-fat-induced insulin resistance. Neurobiol Learn Mem 2010; 93(4): 546-53.
[http://dx.doi.org/10.1016/j.nlm.2010.02.002] [PMID: 20176121]

[12] Watson GS, Cholerton BA, Reger MA, *et al.* Preserved cognition in patients with early Alzheimer disease and amnestic mild cognitive impairment during treatment with rosiglitazone: a preliminary study. Am J Geriatr Psychiatry 2005; 13(11): 950-8.
[PMID: 16286438]

[13] Carroll JC, Iba M, Bangasser DA, *et al.* Chronic stress exacerbates tau pathology, neurodegeneration, and cognitive performance through a corticotropin-releasing factor receptor-dependent mechanism in a transgenic mouse model of tauopathy. J Neurosci 2011; 31(40): 14436-49.
[http://dx.doi.org/10.1523/JNEUROSCI.3836-11.2011] [PMID: 21976528]

[14] Piirainen S, Youssef A, Song C, *et al.* Psychosocial stress on neuroinflammation and cognitive dysfunctions in Alzheimer's disease: the emerging role for microglia? Neurosci Biobehav Rev 2017; 77: 148-64.
[http://dx.doi.org/10.1016/j.neubiorev.2017.01.046] [PMID: 28185874]

[15] Cohen S, Janicki-Deverts D, Doyle WJ, *et al.* Chronic stress, glucocorticoid receptor resistance, inflammation, and disease risk. Proc Natl Acad Sci USA 2012; 109(16): 5995-9.
[http://dx.doi.org/10.1073/pnas.1118355109] [PMID: 22474371]

[16] Laws KR, Irvine K, Gale TM. Sex differences in Alzheimer's disease. Curr Opin Psychiatry 2018; 31(2): 133-9.
[PMID: 29324460]

[17] Readhead B, Haure-Mirande JV, Funk CC, *et al.* Multiscale Analysis of Independent Alzheimer's Cohorts Finds Disruption of Molecular, Genetic, and Clinical Networks by Human Herpesvirus. Neuron 2018; 99(1): 64-82.e7.
[http://dx.doi.org/10.1016/j.neuron.2018.05.023] [PMID: 29937276]

[18] McKhann GM, Knopman DS, Chertkow H, *et al.* The diagnosis of dementia due to Alzheimer's disease: recommendations from the National Institute on Aging-Alzheimer's Association workgroups on diagnostic guidelines for Alzheimer's disease. Alzheimers Dement 2011; 7(3): 263-9.
[http://dx.doi.org/10.1016/j.jalz.2011.03.005] [PMID: 21514250]

[19] Porter G, Leonards U, Troscianko T, Haworth J, Bayer A, Tales A. Dealing with illumination in visual scenes: effects of ageing and Alzheimer's disease. PLoS One 2012; 7(9): e45104.
[http://dx.doi.org/10.1371/journal.pone.0045104] [PMID: 23028786]

[20] Eustace A, Coen R, Walsh C, *et al.* A longitudinal evaluation of behavioural and psychological symptoms of probable Alzheimer's disease. Int J Geriatr Psychiatry 2002; 17(10): 968-73.
[http://dx.doi.org/10.1002/gps.736] [PMID: 12325059]

[21] Sjogren T, Sjogren H, Lindgren AG. Morbus Alzheimer and morbus Pick; a genetic, clinical and patho-anatomical study. Acta Psychiatr Neurol Scand, Suppl 1952; 82: 1-152.

[PMID: 13171126]

[22] Gatz M, Pedersen NL, Berg S, *et al.* Heritability for Alzheimer's disease: the study of dementia in Swedish twins. J Gerontol A Biol Sci Med Sci 1997; 52(2): M117-25. [http://dx.doi.org/10.1093/gerona/52A.2.M117] [PMID: 9060980]

[23] van Duijn CM, Clayton D, Chandra V, *et al.* Familial aggregation of Alzheimer's disease and related disorders: a collaborative re-analysis of case-control studies. Int J Epidemiol 1991; 20 (Suppl. 2): S13-20. [http://dx.doi.org/10.1093/ije/20.Supplement_2.S13] [PMID: 1833349]

[24] Siest G, Pillot T, Régis-Bailly A, *et al.* Apolipoprotein E: an important gene and protein to follow in laboratory medicine. Clin Chem 1995; 41(8 Pt 1): 1068-86. [PMID: 7628082]

[25] Corder EH, Saunders AM, Risch NJ, *et al.* Protective effect of apolipoprotein E type 2 allele for late onset Alzheimer disease. Nat Genet 1994; 7(2): 180-4. [http://dx.doi.org/10.1038/ng0694-180] [PMID: 7920638]

[26] Castellano JM, Kim J, Stewart FR, *et al.* Human apoE isoforms differentially regulate brain amyloid-β peptide clearance. Sci Transl Med 2011; 3(89): 89ra57. [http://dx.doi.org/10.1126/scitranslmed.3002156] [PMID: 21715678]

[27] Sanan DA, Weisgraber KH, Russell SJ, *et al.* Apolipoprotein E associates with beta amyloid peptide of Alzheimer's disease to form novel monofibrils. Isoform apoE4 associates more efficiently than apoE3. J Clin Invest 1994; 94(2): 860-9. [http://dx.doi.org/10.1172/JCI117407] [PMID: 8040342]

[28] Bertram L, Lange C, Mullin K, *et al.* Genome-wide association analysis reveals putative Alzheimer's disease susceptibility loci in addition to APOE. Am J Hum Genet 2008; 83(5): 623-32. [http://dx.doi.org/10.1016/j.ajhg.2008.10.008] [PMID: 18976728]

[29] Corder EH, Saunders AM, Strittmatter WJ, *et al.* Gene dose of apolipoprotein E type 4 allele and the risk of Alzheimer's disease in late onset families. Science 1993; 261(5123): 921-3. [http://dx.doi.org/10.1126/science.8346443] [PMID: 8346443]

[30] Ashford JW. APOE genotype effects on Alzheimer's disease onset and epidemiology. J Mol Neurosci 2004; 23(3): 157-65. [http://dx.doi.org/10.1385/JMN:23:3:157] [PMID: 15181244]

[31] Strittmatter WJ, Weisgraber KH, Goedert M, *et al.* Hypothesis: microtubule instability and paired helical filament formation in the Alzheimer disease brain are related to apolipoprotein E genotype. Exp Neurol 1994; 125(2): 163-71. [http://dx.doi.org/10.1006/exnr.1994.1019] [PMID: 8313935]

[32] Strittmatter WJ, Weisgraber KH, Huang DY, *et al.* Binding of human apolipoprotein E to synthetic amyloid beta peptide: isoform-specific effects and implications for late-onset Alzheimer disease. Proc Natl Acad Sci USA 1993; 90(17): 8098-102. [http://dx.doi.org/10.1073/pnas.90.17.8098] [PMID: 8367470]

[33] Guerreiro RJ, Gustafson DR, Hardy J. The genetic architecture of Alzheimer's disease: beyond APP, PSENs and APOE. Neurobiol Aging 2012; 33(3): 437-56. [http://dx.doi.org/10.1016/j.neurobiolaging.2010.03.025] [PMID: 20594621]

[34] Mullan M, Crawford F, Axelman K, *et al.* A pathogenic mutation for probable Alzheimer's disease in the APP gene at the N-terminus of beta-amyloid. Nat Genet 1992; 1(5): 345-7. [http://dx.doi.org/10.1038/ng0892-345] [PMID: 1302033]

[35] Bergmans BA, De Strooper B. gamma-secretases: from cell biology to therapeutic strategies. Lancet Neurol 2010; 9(2): 215-26. [http://dx.doi.org/10.1016/S1474-4422(09)70332-1] [PMID: 20129170]

[36] Nilsberth C, Westlind-Danielsson A, Eckman CB, *et al.* The 'Arctic' APP mutation (E693G) causes

Alzheimer's disease by enhanced Abeta protofibril formation. Nat Neurosci 2001; 4(9): 887-93. [http://dx.doi.org/10.1038/nn0901-887] [PMID: 11528419]

[37] Lanoiselée HM, Nicolas G, Wallon D, *et al.* APP, PSEN1, and PSEN2 mutations in early-onset Alzheimer disease: A genetic screening study of familial and sporadic cases. PLoS Med 2017; 14(3): e1002270.
[http://dx.doi.org/10.1371/journal.pmed.1002270] [PMID: 28350801]

[38] Rogaev EI, Sherrington R, Rogaeva EA, *et al.* Familial Alzheimer's disease in kindreds with missense mutations in a gene on chromosome 1 related to the Alzheimer's disease type 3 gene. Nature 1995; 376(6543): 775-8.
[http://dx.doi.org/10.1038/376775a0] [PMID: 7651536]

[39] Kovacs DM, Fausett HJ, Page KJ, *et al.* Alzheimer-associated presenilins 1 and 2: neuronal expression in brain and localization to intracellular membranes in mammalian cells. Nat Med 1996; 2(2): 224-9. [http://dx.doi.org/10.1038/nm0296-224] [PMID: 8574969]

[40] Chávez-Gutiérrez L, Bammens L, Benilova I, *et al.* The mechanism of γ-Secretase dysfunction in familial Alzheimer disease. EMBO J 2012; 31(10): 2261-74.
[http://dx.doi.org/10.1038/emboj.2012.79] [PMID: 22505025]

[41] Apostolova LG, Risacher SL, Duran T, *et al.* Associations of the Top 20 Alzheimer Disease Risk Variants With Brain Amyloidosis JAMA Neurol 2018.

[42] Griciuc A, Serrano-Pozo A, Parrado AR, *et al.* Alzheimer's disease risk gene CD33 inhibits microglial uptake of amyloid beta. Neuron 2013; 78(4): 631-43.
[http://dx.doi.org/10.1016/j.neuron.2013.04.014] [PMID: 23623698]

[43] Miron J, Picard C, Nilsson N, *et al.* CDK5RAP2 gene and tau pathophysiology in late-onset sporadic Alzheimer's disease. Alzheimers Dement 2018; 14(6): 787-96.
[http://dx.doi.org/10.1016/j.jalz.2017.12.004] [PMID: 29360470]

[44] Holton P, Ryten M, Nalls M, *et al.* Initial assessment of the pathogenic mechanisms of the recently identified Alzheimer risk Loci. Ann Hum Genet 2013; 77(2): 85-105.
[http://dx.doi.org/10.1111/ahg.12000] [PMID: 23360175]

[45] Marei HE, Althani A, Suhonen J, *et al.* Common and Rare Genetic Variants Associated With Alzheimer's Disease. J Cell Physiol 2016; 231(7): 1432-7.
[http://dx.doi.org/10.1002/jcp.25225] [PMID: 26496533]

[46] Lambert JC, Ibrahim-Verbaas CA, Harold D, *et al.* Meta-analysis of 74,046 individuals identifies 11 new susceptibility loci for Alzheimer's disease. Nat Genet 2013; 45(12): 1452-8.
[http://dx.doi.org/10.1038/ng.2802] [PMID: 24162737]

[47] Saad M, Brkanac Z, Wijsman EM. Family-based genome scan for age at onset of late-onset Alzheimer's disease in whole exome sequencing data. Genes Brain Behav 2015; 14(8): 607-17. [http://dx.doi.org/10.1111/gbb.12250] [PMID: 26394601]

[48] Sanchez-Mut JV, Heyn H, Silva BA, *et al.* PM20D1 is a quantitative trait locus associated with Alzheimer's disease. Nat Med 2018; 24(5): 598-603.
[http://dx.doi.org/10.1038/s41591-018-0013-y] [PMID: 29736028]

[49] Zou Y, He W, Wang K, *et al.* Identification of rare RTN3 variants in Alzheimer's disease in Han Chinese. Hum Genet 2018; 137(2): 141-50.
[http://dx.doi.org/10.1007/s00439-018-1868-1] [PMID: 29356939]

[50] Yan H, Kong Y, He B, *et al.* CYP2J2 rs890293 polymorphism is associated with susceptibility to Alzheimer's disease in the Chinese Han population. Neurosci Lett 2015; 593: 56-60.
[http://dx.doi.org/10.1016/j.neulet.2015.03.024] [PMID: 25796175]

[51] Kawai E, Shibata N, Nagata T, *et al.* Genetic Association Between KIBRA Polymorphism and Alzheimer's Disease with in a Japanese Population. Neuromolecular Med 2015; 17(2): 170-7.
[http://dx.doi.org/10.1007/s12017-015-8348-8] [PMID: 25800888]

[52] Harold D, Abraham R, Hollingworth P, *et al.* Genome-wide association study identifies variants at CLU and PICALM associated with Alzheimer's disease. Nat Genet 2009; 41(10): 1088-93. [http://dx.doi.org/10.1038/ng.440] [PMID: 19734902]

[53] Hollingworth P, Harold D, Sims R, *et al.* Common variants at ABCA7, MS4A6A/MS4A4E, EPHA1, CD33 and CD2AP are associated with Alzheimer's disease. Nat Genet 2011; 43(5): 429-35. [http://dx.doi.org/10.1038/ng.803] [PMID: 21460840]

[54] Shuai P, Liu Y, Lu W, Liu Q, Li T, Gong B. Genetic associations of CLU rs9331888 polymorphism with Alzheimer's disease: A meta-analysis. Neurosci Lett 2015; 591: 160-5. [http://dx.doi.org/10.1016/j.neulet.2015.02.040] [PMID: 25703218]

[55] Miyashita A, Koike A, Jun G, *et al.* SORL1 is genetically associated with late-onset Alzheimer's disease in Japanese, Koreans and Caucasians. PLoS One 2013; 8(4): e58618. [http://dx.doi.org/10.1371/journal.pone.0058618] [PMID: 23565137]

[56] Goodall EF, Heath PR, Bandmann O, Kirby J, Shaw PJ. Neuronal dark matter: the emerging role of microRNAs in neurodegeneration. Front Cell Neurosci 2013; 7: 178. [http://dx.doi.org/10.3389/fncel.2013.00178] [PMID: 24133413]

[57] Maoz R, Garfinkel BP, Soreq H. Alzheimer's Disease and ncRNAs. Adv Exp Med Biol 2017; 978: 337-61. [http://dx.doi.org/10.1007/978-3-319-53889-1_18] [PMID: 28523555]

[58] Niwa R, Zhou F, Li C, Slack FJ. The expression of the Alzheimer's amyloid precursor protein-like gene is regulated by developmental timing microRNAs and their targets in Caenorhabditis elegans. Dev Biol 2008; 315(2): 418-25. [http://dx.doi.org/10.1016/j.ydbio.2007.12.044] [PMID: 18262516]

[59] Patel N, Hoang D, Miller N, *et al.* MicroRNAs can regulate human APP levels. Mol Neurodegener 2008; 3: 10. [http://dx.doi.org/10.1186/1750-1326-3-10] [PMID: 18684319]

[60] Hébert SS, Horré K, Nicolaï L, *et al.* MicroRNA regulation of Alzheimer's Amyloid precursor protein expression. Neurobiol Dis 2009; 33(3): 422-8. [http://dx.doi.org/10.1016/j.nbd.2008.11.009] [PMID: 19110058]

[61] Zong Y, Wang H, Dong W, *et al.* miR-29c regulates BACE1 protein expression. Brain Res 2011; 1395: 108-15. [http://dx.doi.org/10.1016/j.brainres.2011.04.035] [PMID: 21565331]

[62] Lei X, Lei L, Zhang Z, Zhang Z, Cheng Y. Downregulated miR-29c correlates with increased BACE1 expression in sporadic Alzheimer's disease. Int J Clin Exp Pathol 2015; 8(2): 1565-74. [PMID: 25973041]

[63] Wang WX, Rajeev BW, Stromberg AJ, *et al.* The expression of microRNA miR-107 decreases early in Alzheimer's disease and may accelerate disease progression through regulation of beta-site amyloid precursor protein-cleaving enzyme 1. J Neurosci 2008; 28(5): 1213-23. [http://dx.doi.org/10.1523/JNEUROSCI.5065-07.2008] [PMID: 18234899]

[64] Salta E, De Strooper B. microRNA-132: a key noncoding RNA operating in the cellular phase of Alzheimer's disease. FASEB J 2017; 31(2): 424-33. [http://dx.doi.org/10.1096/fj.201601308] [PMID: 28148775]

[65] Smith PY, Hernandez-Rapp J, Jolivette F, *et al.* miR-132/212 deficiency impairs tau metabolism and promotes pathological aggregation *in vivo*. Hum Mol Genet 2015; 24(23): 6721-35. [http://dx.doi.org/10.1093/hmg/ddv377] [PMID: 26362250]

[66] Hansen KF, Sakamoto K, Aten S, *et al.* Targeted deletion of miR-132/-212 impairs memory and alters the hippocampal transcriptome. Learn Mem 2016; 23(2): 61-71. [http://dx.doi.org/10.1101/lm.039578.115] [PMID: 26773099]

[67] Lau P, Bossers K, Janky R, *et al.* Alteration of the microRNA network during the progression of Alzheimer's disease. EMBO Mol Med 2013; 5(10): 1613-34. [http://dx.doi.org/10.1002/emmm.201201974] [PMID: 24014289]

[68] Santa-Maria I, Alaniz ME, Renwick N, *et al.* Dysregulation of microRNA-219 promotes neurodegeneration through post-transcriptional regulation of tau. J Clin Invest 2015; 125(2): 681-6. [http://dx.doi.org/10.1172/JCI78421] [PMID: 25574843]

[69] Smith P, Al Hashimi A, Girard J, Delay C, Hébert SS. *in vivo* regulation of amyloid precursor protein neuronal splicing by microRNAs. J Neurochem 2011; 116(2): 240-7. [http://dx.doi.org/10.1111/j.1471-4159.2010.07097.x] [PMID: 21062284]

[70] Hébert SS, Papadopoulou AS, Smith P, *et al.* Genetic ablation of Dicer in adult forebrain neurons results in abnormal tau hyperphosphorylation and neurodegeneration. Hum Mol Genet 2010; 19(20): 3959-69. [http://dx.doi.org/10.1093/hmg/ddq311] [PMID: 20660113]

[71] Zhao ZB, Wu L, Xiong R, *et al.* MicroRNA-922 promotes tau phosphorylation by downregulating ubiquitin carboxy-terminal hydrolase L1 (UCHL1) expression in the pathogenesis of Alzheimer's disease. Neuroscience 2014; 275: 232-7. [http://dx.doi.org/10.1016/j.neuroscience.2014.06.013] [PMID: 24950120]

[72] Denk J, Boelmans K, Siegismund C, Lassner D, Arlt S, Jahn H. MicroRNA Profiling of CSF Reveals Potential Biomarkers to Detect Alzheimer's Disease. PLoS One 2015; 10(5): e0126423. [http://dx.doi.org/10.1371/journal.pone.0126423] [PMID: 25992776]

[73] Alexandrov PN, Dua P, Lukiw WJ. Up-Regulation of miRNA-146a in Progressive, Age-Related Inflammatory Neurodegenerative Disorders of the Human CNS. Front Neurol 2014; 5: 181. [http://dx.doi.org/10.3389/fneur.2014.00181] [PMID: 25324823]

[74] Yang F, Uéda K, Chen P, Ashe KH, Cole GM. Plaque-associated alpha-synuclein (NACP) pathology in aged transgenic mice expressing amyloid precursor protein. Brain Res 2000; 853(2): 381-3. [http://dx.doi.org/10.1016/S0006-8993(99)02207-6] [PMID: 10640638]

[75] Findeis MA. The role of amyloid beta peptide 42 in Alzheimer's disease. Pharmacol Ther 2007; 116(2): 266-86. [http://dx.doi.org/10.1016/j.pharmthera.2007.06.006] [PMID: 17716740]

[76] Götz J, Deters N, Doldissen A, *et al.* A decade of tau transgenic animal models and beyond. Brain Pathol 2007; 17(1): 91-103. [http://dx.doi.org/10.1111/j.1750-3639.2007.00051.x] [PMID: 17493043]

[77] Lewis J, Dickson DW, Lin WL, *et al.* Enhanced neurofibrillary degeneration in transgenic mice expressing mutant tau and APP. Science 2001; 293(5534): 1487-91. [http://dx.doi.org/10.1126/science.1058189] [PMID: 11520987]

[78] Oddo S, Caccamo A, Kitazawa M, Tseng BP, LaFerla FM. Amyloid deposition precedes tangle formation in a triple transgenic model of Alzheimer's disease. Neurobiol Aging 2003; 24(8): 1063-70. [http://dx.doi.org/10.1016/j.neurobiolaging.2003.08.012] [PMID: 14643377]

[79] Wilcock DM, Lewis MR, Van Nostrand WE, *et al.* Progression of amyloid pathology to Alzheimer's disease pathology in an amyloid precursor protein transgenic mouse model by removal of nitric oxide synthase 2. J Neurosci 2008; 28(7): 1537-45. [http://dx.doi.org/10.1523/JNEUROSCI.5066-07.2008] [PMID: 18272675]

[80] Blurton-Jones M, Laferla FM. Pathways by which Abeta facilitates tau pathology. Curr Alzheimer Res 2006; 3(5): 437-48. [http://dx.doi.org/10.2174/156720506779025242] [PMID: 17168643]

[81] Terry RD, Masliah E, Salmon DP, *et al.* Physical basis of cognitive alterations in Alzheimer's disease: synapse loss is the major correlate of cognitive impairment. Ann Neurol 1991; 30(4): 572-80. [http://dx.doi.org/10.1002/ana.410300410] [PMID: 1789684]

[82] Das B, Yan R. Role of BACE1 in Alzheimer's synaptic function. Transl Neurodegener 2017; 6: 23. [http://dx.doi.org/10.1186/s40035-017-0093-5] [PMID: 28855981]

[83] Pettersson AF, Olsson E, Wahlund LO. Motor function in subjects with mild cognitive impairment and early Alzheimer's disease. Dement Geriatr Cogn Disord 2005; 19(5-6): 299-304. [http://dx.doi.org/10.1159/000084555] [PMID: 15785030]

[84] Pozueta J, Lefort R, Shelanski ML. Synaptic changes in Alzheimer's disease and its models. Neuroscience 2013; 251: 51-65. [http://dx.doi.org/10.1016/j.neuroscience.2012.05.050] [PMID: 22687952]

[85] Delaère P, Duyckaerts C, Brion JP, Poulain V, Hauw JJ. Tau, paired helical filaments and amyloid in the neocortex: a morphometric study of 15 cases with graded intellectual status in aging and senile dementia of Alzheimer type. Acta Neuropathol 1989; 77(6): 645-53. [http://dx.doi.org/10.1007/BF00687893] [PMID: 2501966]

[86] Calabrese B, Shaked GM, Tabarean IV, Braga J, Koo EH, Halpain S. Rapid, concurrent alterations in pre- and postsynaptic structure induced by naturally-secreted amyloid-beta protein. Mol Cell Neurosci 2007; 35(2): 183-93. [http://dx.doi.org/10.1016/j.mcn.2007.02.006] [PMID: 17368908]

[87] Hsieh H, Boehm J, Sato C, *et al.* AMPAR removal underlies Abeta-induced synaptic depression and dendritic spine loss. Neuron 2006; 52(5): 831-43. [http://dx.doi.org/10.1016/j.neuron.2006.10.035] [PMID: 17145504]

[88] Wei W, Nguyen LN, Kessels HW, Hagiwara H, Sisodia S, Malinow R. Amyloid beta from axons and dendrites reduces local spine number and plasticity. Nat Neurosci 2010; 13(2): 190-6. [http://dx.doi.org/10.1038/nn.2476] [PMID: 20037574]

[89] Malenka RC, Bear MF. LTP and LTD: an embarrassment of riches. Neuron 2004; 44(1): 5-21. [http://dx.doi.org/10.1016/j.neuron.2004.09.012] [PMID: 15450156]

[90] Malenka RC, Nicoll RA. Long-term potentiation--a decade of progress? Science 1999; 285(5435): 1870-4. [http://dx.doi.org/10.1126/science.285.5435.1870] [PMID: 10489359]

[91] Whitlock JR, Heynen AJ, Shuler MG, Bear MF. Learning induces long-term potentiation in the hippocampus. Science 2006; 313(5790): 1093-7. [http://dx.doi.org/10.1126/science.1128134] [PMID: 16931756]

[92] Gilbert BJ. The role of amyloid β in the pathogenesis of Alzheimer's disease. J Clin Pathol 2013; 66(5): 362-6. [http://dx.doi.org/10.1136/jclinpath-2013-201515] [PMID: 23526599]

[93] Stover KR, Campbell MA, Van Winssen CM, Brown RE. Early detection of cognitive deficits in the 3xTg-AD mouse model of Alzheimer's disease. Behav Brain Res 2015; 289: 29-38. [http://dx.doi.org/10.1016/j.bbr.2015.04.012] [PMID: 25896362]

[94] Caruso D, Barron AM, Brown MA, *et al.* Age-related changes in neuroactive steroid levels in 3xTg-AD mice. Neurobiol Aging 2013; 34(4): 1080-9. [http://dx.doi.org/10.1016/j.neurobiolaging.2012.10.007] [PMID: 23122920]

[95] Oakley H, Cole SL, Logan S, *et al.* Intraneuronal beta-amyloid aggregates, neurodegeneration, and neuron loss in transgenic mice with five familial Alzheimer's disease mutations: potential factors in amyloid plaque formation. J Neurosci 2006; 26(40): 10129-40. [http://dx.doi.org/10.1523/JNEUROSCI.1202-06.2006] [PMID: 17021169]

[96] Kimura R, Ohno M. Impairments in remote memory stabilization precede hippocampal synaptic and cognitive failures in 5XFAD Alzheimer mouse model. Neurobiol Dis 2009; 33(2): 229-35. [http://dx.doi.org/10.1016/j.nbd.2008.10.006] [PMID: 19026746]

[97] Van Dam D, D'Hooge R, Staufenbiel M, Van Ginneken C, Van Meir F, De Deyn PP. Age-dependent

cognitive decline in the APP23 model precedes amyloid deposition. Eur J Neurosci 2003; 17(2): 388-96.
[http://dx.doi.org/10.1046/j.1460-9568.2003.02444.x] [PMID: 12542676]

[98] Cirrito JR, May PC, O'Dell MA, *et al. in vivo* assessment of brain interstitial fluid with microdialysis reveals plaque-associated changes in amyloid-beta metabolism and half-life. J Neurosci 2003; 23(26): 8844-53.
[http://dx.doi.org/10.1523/JNEUROSCI.23-26-08844.2003] [PMID: 14523085]

[99] Roder S, Danober L, Pozza MF, Lingenhoehl K, Wiederhold KH, Olpe HR. Electrophysiological studies on the hippocampus and prefrontal cortex assessing the effects of amyloidosis in amyloid precursor protein 23 transgenic mice. Neuroscience 2003; 120(3): 705-20.
[http://dx.doi.org/10.1016/S0306-4522(03)00381-6] [PMID: 12895511]

[100] Saito T, Suemoto T, Brouwers N, *et al.* Potent amyloidogenicity and pathogenicity of Aβ43. Nat Neurosci 2011; 14(8): 1023-32.
[http://dx.doi.org/10.1038/nn.2858] [PMID: 21725313]

[101] Wirths O, Breyhan H, Schäfer S, Roth C, Bayer TA. Deficits in working memory and motor performance in the APP/PS1ki mouse model for Alzheimer's disease. Neurobiol Aging 2008; 29(6): 891-901.
[http://dx.doi.org/10.1016/j.neurobiolaging.2006.12.004] [PMID: 17215062]

[102] Breyhan H, Wirths O, Duan K, Marcello A, Rettig J, Bayer TA. APP/PS1KI bigenic mice develop early synaptic deficits and hippocampus atrophy. Acta Neuropathol 2009; 117(6): 677-85.
[http://dx.doi.org/10.1007/s00401-009-0539-7] [PMID: 19387667]

[103] Lalonde R, Dumont M, Fukuchi K, Strazielle C. Transgenic mice expressing the human C99 terminal fragment of betaAPP: effects on spatial learning, exploration, anxiety, and motor coordination. Exp Gerontol 2002; 37(12): 1401-12.
[http://dx.doi.org/10.1016/S0531-5565(02)00123-7] [PMID: 12559409]

[104] Umeda T, Maekawa S, Kimura T, Takashima A, Tomiyama T, Mori H. Neurofibrillary tangle formation by introducing wild-type human tau into APP transgenic mice. Acta Neuropathol 2014; 127(5): 685-98.
[http://dx.doi.org/10.1007/s00401-014-1259-1] [PMID: 24531886]

[105] Tomiyama T, Matsuyama S, Iso H, *et al.* A mouse model of amyloid beta oligomers: their contribution to synaptic alteration, abnormal tau phosphorylation, glial activation, and neuronal loss *in vivo.* J Neurosci 2010; 30(14): 4845-56.
[http://dx.doi.org/10.1523/JNEUROSCI.5825-09.2010] [PMID: 20371804]

[106] Saito T, Matsuba Y, Mihira N, *et al.* Single App knock-in mouse models of Alzheimer's disease. Nat Neurosci 2014; 17(5): 661-3.
[http://dx.doi.org/10.1038/nn.3697] [PMID: 24728269]

[107] Coomaraswamy J, Kilger E, Wölfing H, *et al.* Modeling familial Danish dementia in mice supports the concept of the amyloid hypothesis of Alzheimer's disease. Proc Natl Acad Sci USA 2010; 107(17): 7969-74.
[http://dx.doi.org/10.1073/pnas.1001056107] [PMID: 20385796]

[108] Serneels L, Van Biervliet J, Craessaerts K, *et al.* gamma-Secretase heterogeneity in the Aph1 subunit: relevance for Alzheimer's disease. Science 2009; 324(5927): 639-42.
[http://dx.doi.org/10.1126/science.1171176] [PMID: 19299585]

[109] Radde R, Bolmont T, Kaeser SA, *et al.* Abeta42-driven cerebral amyloidosis in transgenic mice reveals early and robust pathology. EMBO Rep 2006; 7(9): 940-6.
[http://dx.doi.org/10.1038/sj.embor.7400784] [PMID: 16906128]

[110] Gengler S, Hamilton A, Hölscher C. Synaptic plasticity in the hippocampus of a APP/PS1 mouse model of Alzheimer's disease is impaired in old but not young mice. PLoS One 2010; 5(3): e9764.
[http://dx.doi.org/10.1371/journal.pone.0009764] [PMID: 20339537]

[111] Hsiao K, Chapman P, Nilsen S, *et al.* Correlative memory deficits, Abeta elevation, and amyloid plaques in transgenic mice. Science 1996; 274(5284): 99-102. [http://dx.doi.org/10.1126/science.274.5284.99] [PMID: 8810256]

[112] Puoliväli J, Wang J, Heikkinen T, *et al.* Hippocampal A beta 42 levels correlate with spatial memory deficit in APP and PS1 double transgenic mice. Neurobiol Dis 2002; 9(3): 339-47. [http://dx.doi.org/10.1006/nbdi.2002.0481] [PMID: 11950278]

[113] Lalonde R, Kim HD, Maxwell JA, Fukuchi K. Exploratory activity and spatial learning in 12-mont--old APP(695)SWE/co+PS1/DeltaE9 mice with amyloid plaques. Neurosci Lett 2005; 390(2): 87-92. [http://dx.doi.org/10.1016/j.neulet.2005.08.028] [PMID: 16169151]

[114] Volianskis A, Køstner R, Mølgaard M, Hass S, Jensen MS. Episodic memory deficits are not related to altered glutamatergic synaptic transmission and plasticity in the CA1 hippocampus of the APPswe/PS1δE9-deleted transgenic mice model of ß-amyloidosis. Neurobiol Aging 2010; 31(7): 1173-87. [http://dx.doi.org/10.1016/j.neurobiolaging.2008.08.005] [PMID: 18790549]

[115] Abe Y, Kouyama K, Tomita T, *et al.* Analysis of neurons created from wild-type and Alzheimer's mutation knock-in embryonic stem cells by a highly efficient differentiation protocol. J Neurosci 2003; 23(24): 8513-25. [http://dx.doi.org/10.1523/JNEUROSCI.23-24-08513.2003] [PMID: 13679420]

[116] Moechars D, Dewachter I, Lorent K, *et al.* Early phenotypic changes in transgenic mice that overexpress different mutants of amyloid precursor protein in brain. J Biol Chem 1999; 274(10): 6483-92. [http://dx.doi.org/10.1074/jbc.274.10.6483] [PMID: 10037741]

[117] Schneider I, Reverse D, Dewachter I, *et al.* Mutant presenilins disturb neuronal calcium homeostasis in the brain of transgenic mice, decreasing the threshold for excitotoxicity and facilitating long-term potentiation. J Biol Chem 2001; 276(15): 11539-44. [http://dx.doi.org/10.1074/jbc.M010977200] [PMID: 11278803]

[118] Dewachter I, Van Dorpe J, Smeijers L, *et al.* Aging increased amyloid peptide and caused amyloid plaques in brain of old APP/V717I transgenic mice by a different mechanism than mutant presenilin1. J Neurosci 2000; 20(17): 6452-8. [http://dx.doi.org/10.1523/JNEUROSCI.20-17-06452.2000] [PMID: 10964951]

[119] Cheng IH, Palop JJ, Esposito LA, Bien-Ly N, Yan F, Mucke L. Aggressive amyloidosis in mice expressing human amyloid peptides with the Arctic mutation. Nat Med 2004; 10(11): 1190-2. [http://dx.doi.org/10.1038/nm1123] [PMID: 15502844]

[120] Knobloch M, Konietzko U, Krebs DC, Nitsch RM. Intracellular Abeta and cognitive deficits precede beta-amyloid deposition in transgenic arcAbeta mice. Neurobiol Aging 2007; 28(9): 1297-306. [http://dx.doi.org/10.1016/j.neurobiolaging.2006.06.019] [PMID: 16876915]

[121] Willuweit A, Velden J, Godemann R, *et al.* Early-onset and robust amyloid pathology in a new homozygous mouse model of Alzheimer's disease. PLoS One 2009; 4(11): e7931. [http://dx.doi.org/10.1371/journal.pone.0007931] [PMID: 19936202]

[122] Šišková Z, Justus D, Kaneko H, *et al.* Dendritic structural degeneration is functionally linked to cellular hyperexcitability in a mouse model of Alzheimer's disease. Neuron 2014; 84(5): 1023-33. [http://dx.doi.org/10.1016/j.neuron.2014.10.024] [PMID: 25456500]

[123] Filser S, Ovsepian SV, Masana M, *et al.* Pharmacological inhibition of BACE1 impairs synaptic plasticity and cognitive functions. Biol Psychiatry 2015; 77(8): 729-39. [http://dx.doi.org/10.1016/j.biopsych.2014.10.013] [PMID: 25599931]

[124] Wang H, Song L, Laird F, Wong PC, Lee HK. BACE1 knock-outs display deficits in activity-dependent potentiation of synaptic transmission at mossy fiber to CA3 synapses in the hippocampus. J Neurosci 2008; 28(35): 8677-81.

[http://dx.doi.org/10.1523/JNEUROSCI.2440-08.2008] [PMID: 18753368]

[125] Hu X, Das B, Hou H, He W, Yan R. BACE1 deletion in the adult mouse reverses preformed amyloid deposition and improves cognitive functions. J Exp Med 2018; 215(3): 927-40. [http://dx.doi.org/10.1084/jem.20171831] [PMID: 29444819]

[126] Phillips M, Boman E, Osterman H, Willhite D, Laska M. Olfactory and visuospatial learning and memory performance in two strains of Alzheimer's disease model mice--a longitudinal study. PLoS One 2011; 6(5): e19567. [http://dx.doi.org/10.1371/journal.pone.0019567] [PMID: 21573167]

[127] Polydoro M, Acker CM, Duff K, Castillo PE, Davies P. Age-dependent impairment of cognitive and synaptic function in the htau mouse model of tau pathology. J Neurosci 2009; 29(34): 10741-9. [http://dx.doi.org/10.1523/JNEUROSCI.1065-09.2009] [PMID: 19710325]

[128] Geiszler PC, Barron MR, Pardon MC. Impaired burrowing is the most prominent behavioral deficit of aging htau mice. Neuroscience 2016; 329: 98-111. [http://dx.doi.org/10.1016/j.neuroscience.2016.05.004] [PMID: 27167086]

[129] Maeda S, Djukic B, Taneja P, *et al.* Expression of A152T human tau causes age-dependent neuronal dysfunction and loss in transgenic mice. EMBO Rep 2016; 17(4): 530-51. [http://dx.doi.org/10.15252/embr.201541438] [PMID: 26931567]

[130] Wright AL, Zinn R, Hohensinn B, *et al.* Neuroinflammation and neuronal loss precede Aβ plaque deposition in the hAPP-J20 mouse model of Alzheimer's disease. PLoS One 2013; 8(4): e59586. [http://dx.doi.org/10.1371/journal.pone.0059586] [PMID: 23560052]

[131] Cheng IH, Scearce-Levie K, Legleiter J, *et al.* Accelerating amyloid-beta fibrillization reduces oligomer levels and functional deficits in Alzheimer disease mouse models. J Biol Chem 2007; 282(33): 23818-28. [http://dx.doi.org/10.1074/jbc.M701078200] [PMID: 17548355]

[132] Saganich MJ, Schroeder BE, Galvan V, Bredesen DE, Koo EH, Heinemann SF. Deficits in synaptic transmission and learning in amyloid precursor protein (APP) transgenic mice require C-terminal cleavage of APP. J Neurosci 2006; 26(52): 13428-36. [http://dx.doi.org/10.1523/JNEUROSCI.4180-06.2006] [PMID: 17192425]

[133] Rockenstein E, Overk CR, Ubhi K, *et al.* A novel triple repeat mutant tau transgenic model that mimics aspects of pick's disease and fronto-temporal tauopathies. PLoS One 2015; 10(3): e0121570. [http://dx.doi.org/10.1371/journal.pone.0121570] [PMID: 25803611]

[134] Rockenstein E, Mallory M, Mante M, Sisk A, Masliaha E. Early formation of mature amyloid-beta protein deposits in a mutant APP transgenic model depends on levels of Abeta(1-42). J Neurosci Res 2001; 66(4): 573-82. [http://dx.doi.org/10.1002/jnr.1247] [PMID: 11746377]

[135] Games D, Adams D, Alessandrini R, *et al.* Alzheimer-type neuropathology in transgenic mice overexpressing V717F beta-amyloid precursor protein. Nature 1995; 373(6514): 523-7. [http://dx.doi.org/10.1038/373523a0] [PMID: 7845465]

[136] Hartman RE, Izumi Y, Bales KR, Paul SM, Wozniak DF, Holtzman DM. Treatment with an amyloid-beta antibody ameliorates plaque load, learning deficits, and hippocampal long-term potentiation in a mouse model of Alzheimer's disease. J Neurosci 2005; 25(26): 6213-20. [http://dx.doi.org/10.1523/JNEUROSCI.0664-05.2005] [PMID: 15987951]

[137] Dodart JC, Meziane H, Mathis C, Bales KR, Paul SM, Ungerer A. Behavioral disturbances in transgenic mice overexpressing the V717F beta-amyloid precursor protein. Behav Neurosci 1999; 113(5): 982-90. [http://dx.doi.org/10.1037/0735-7044.113.5.982] [PMID: 10571480]

[138] Larson J, Lynch G, Games D, Seubert P. Alterations in synaptic transmission and long-term potentiation in hippocampal slices from young and aged PDAPP mice. Brain Res 1999; 840(1-2): 23-

35.
[http://dx.doi.org/10.1016/S0006-8993(99)01698-4] [PMID: 10517949]

[139] Ryan D, Koss D, Porcu E, *et al.* Spatial learning impairments in PLB1Triple knock-in Alzheimer mice are task-specific and age-dependent. Cell Mol Life Sci 2013; 70(14): 2603-19.
[http://dx.doi.org/10.1007/s00018-013-1314-4] [PMID: 23535719]

[140] Platt B, Drever B, Koss D, *et al.* Abnormal cognition, sleep, EEG and brain metabolism in a novel knock-in Alzheimer mouse, PLB1. PLoS One 2011; 6(11): e27068.
[http://dx.doi.org/10.1371/journal.pone.0027068] [PMID: 22096518]

[141] Koss DJ, Drever BD, Stoppelkamp S, Riedel G, Platt B. Age-dependent changes in hippocampal synaptic transmission and plasticity in the PLB1Triple Alzheimer mouse. Cell Mol Life Sci 2013; 70(14): 2585-601.
[http://dx.doi.org/10.1007/s00018-013-1273-9] [PMID: 23407662]

[142] Billings LM, Green KN, McGaugh JL, LaFerla FM. Learning decreases A beta*56 and tau pathology and ameliorates behavioral decline in 3xTg-AD mice. J Neurosci 2007; 27(4): 751-61.
[http://dx.doi.org/10.1523/JNEUROSCI.4800-06.2007] [PMID: 17251414]

[143] Lesné S, Koh MT, Kotilinek L, *et al.* A specific amyloid-beta protein assembly in the brain impairs memory. Nature 2006; 440(7082): 352-7.
[http://dx.doi.org/10.1038/nature04533] [PMID: 16541076]

[144] Yu H, Saura CA, Choi SY, *et al.* APP processing and synaptic plasticity in presenilin-1 conditional knockout mice. Neuron 2001; 31(5): 713-26.
[http://dx.doi.org/10.1016/S0896-6273(01)00417-2] [PMID: 11567612]

[145] Brown JT, Richardson JC, Collingridge GL, Randall AD, Davies CH. Synaptic transmission and synchronous activity is disrupted in hippocampal slices taken from aged TAS10 mice. Hippocampus 2005; 15(1): 110-7.
[http://dx.doi.org/10.1002/hipo.20036] [PMID: 15390159]

[146] Arendash GW, King DL, Gordon MN, *et al.* Progressive, age-related behavioral impairments in transgenic mice carrying both mutant amyloid precursor protein and presenilin-1 transgenes. Brain Res 2001; 891(1-2): 42-53.
[http://dx.doi.org/10.1016/S0006-8993(00)03186-3] [PMID: 11164808]

[147] Wines-Samuelson M, Schulte EC, Smith MJ, *et al.* Characterization of age-dependent and progressive cortical neuronal degeneration in presenilin conditional mutant mice. PLoS One 2010; 5(4): e10195.
[http://dx.doi.org/10.1371/journal.pone.0010195] [PMID: 20419112]

[148] Beglopoulos V, Sun X, Saura CA, Lemere CA, Kim RD, Shen J. Reduced beta-amyloid production and increased inflammatory responses in presenilin conditional knock-out mice. J Biol Chem 2004; 279(45): 46907-14.
[http://dx.doi.org/10.1074/jbc.M409544200] [PMID: 15345711]

[149] Wheeler JM, McMillan PJ, Hawk M, *et al.* High copy wildtype human 1N4R tau expression promotes early pathological tauopathy accompanied by cognitive deficits without progressive neurofibrillary degeneration. Acta Neuropathol Commun 2015; 3: 33.
[http://dx.doi.org/10.1186/s40478-015-0210-6] [PMID: 26041339]

[150] Umeda T, Yamashita T, Kimura T, *et al.* Neurodegenerative disorder FTDP-17-related tau intron 10 +16C → T mutation increases tau exon 10 splicing and causes tauopathy in transgenic mice. Am J Pathol 2013; 183(1): 211-25.
[http://dx.doi.org/10.1016/j.ajpath.2013.03.015] [PMID: 23680655]

[151] Kim Y, Choi H, Lee W, *et al.* Caspase-cleaved tau exhibits rapid memory impairment associated with tau oligomers in a transgenic mouse model. Neurobiol Dis 2016; 87: 19-28.
[http://dx.doi.org/10.1016/j.nbd.2015.12.006] [PMID: 26704708]

[152] Van der Jeugd A, Hochgräfe K, Ahmed T, *et al.* Cognitive defects are reversible in inducible mice

expressing pro-aggregant full-length human Tau. Acta Neuropathol 2012; 123(6): 787-805. [http://dx.doi.org/10.1007/s00401-012-0987-3] [PMID: 22532069]

[153] Maurin H, Chong SA, Kraev I, *et al.* Early structural and functional defects in synapses and myelinated axons in stratum lacunosum moleculare in two preclinical models for tauopathy. PLoS One 2014; 9(2): e87605. [http://dx.doi.org/10.1371/journal.pone.0087605] [PMID: 24498342]

[154] Boekhoorn K, Terwel D, Biemans B, *et al.* Improved long-term potentiation and memory in young tau-P301L transgenic mice before onset of hyperphosphorylation and tauopathy. J Neurosci 2006; 26(13): 3514-23. [http://dx.doi.org/10.1523/JNEUROSCI.5425-05.2006] [PMID: 16571759]

[155] Terwel D, Lasrado R, Snauwaert J, *et al.* Changed conformation of mutant Tau-P301L underlies the moribund tauopathy, absent in progressive, nonlethal axonopathy of Tau-4R/2N transgenic mice. J Biol Chem 2005; 280(5): 3963-73. [http://dx.doi.org/10.1074/jbc.M409876200] [PMID: 15509565]

[156] Takeuchi H, Iba M, Inoue H, *et al.* P301S mutant human tau transgenic mice manifest early symptoms of human tauopathies with dementia and altered sensorimotor gating. PLoS One 2011; 6(6): e21050. [http://dx.doi.org/10.1371/journal.pone.0021050] [PMID: 21698260]

[157] Lasagna-Reeves CA, de Haro M, Hao S, *et al.* Reduction of Nuak1 Decreases Tau and Reverses Phenotypes in a Tauopathy Mouse Model. Neuron 2016; 92(2): 407-18. [http://dx.doi.org/10.1016/j.neuron.2016.09.022] [PMID: 27720485]

[158] Yoshiyama Y, Higuchi M, Zhang B, *et al.* Synapse loss and microglial activation precede tangles in a P301S tauopathy mouse model. Neuron 2007; 53(3): 337-51. [http://dx.doi.org/10.1016/j.neuron.2007.01.010] [PMID: 17270732]

[159] Lanz TA, Carter DB, Merchant KM. Dendritic spine loss in the hippocampus of young PDAPP and Tg2576 mice and its prevention by the ApoE2 genotype. Neurobiol Dis 2003; 13(3): 246-53. [http://dx.doi.org/10.1016/S0969-9961(03)00079-2] [PMID: 12901839]

[160] Jacobsen JS, Wu CC, Redwine JM, *et al.* Early-onset behavioral and synaptic deficits in a mouse model of Alzheimer's disease. Proc Natl Acad Sci USA 2006; 103(13): 5161-6. [http://dx.doi.org/10.1073/pnas.0600948103] [PMID: 16549764]

[161] Chapman PF, White GL, Jones MW, *et al.* Impaired synaptic plasticity and learning in aged amyloid precursor protein transgenic mice. Nat Neurosci 1999; 2(3): 271-6. [http://dx.doi.org/10.1038/6374] [PMID: 10195221]

[162] Bouter Y, Dietrich K, Wittnam JL, *et al.* N-truncated amyloid β (Aβ) 4-42 forms stable aggregates and induces acute and long-lasting behavioral deficits. Acta Neuropathol 2013; 126(2): 189-205. [http://dx.doi.org/10.1007/s00401-013-1129-2] [PMID: 23685882]

[163] Chishti MA, Yang DS, Janus C, *et al.* Early-onset amyloid deposition and cognitive deficits in transgenic mice expressing a double mutant form of amyloid precursor protein 695. J Biol Chem 2001; 276(24): 21562-70. [http://dx.doi.org/10.1074/jbc.M100710200] [PMID: 11279122]

[164] Kimura R, MacTavish D, Yang J, Westaway D, Jhamandas JH. Beta amyloid-induced depression of hippocampal long-term potentiation is mediated through the amylin receptor. J Neurosci 2012; 32(48): 17401-6. [http://dx.doi.org/10.1523/JNEUROSCI.3028-12.2012] [PMID: 23197731]

[165] Schindowski K, Bretteville A, Leroy K, *et al.* Alzheimer's disease-like tau neuropathology leads to memory deficits and loss of functional synapses in a novel mutated tau transgenic mouse without any motor deficits. Am J Pathol 2006; 169(2): 599-616. [http://dx.doi.org/10.2353/ajpath.2006.060002] [PMID: 16877359]

[166] Sydow A, Van der Jeugd A, Zheng F, *et al.* Tau-induced defects in synaptic plasticity, learning, and

memory are reversible in transgenic mice after switching off the toxic Tau mutant. J Neurosci 2011; 31(7): 2511-25.
[http://dx.doi.org/10.1523/JNEUROSCI.5245-10.2011] [PMID: 21325519]

[167] Absalon S, Kochanek DM, Raghavan V, Krichevsky AM. MiR-26b, upregulated in Alzheimer's disease, activates cell cycle entry, tau-phosphorylation, and apoptosis in postmitotic neurons. J Neurosci 2013; 33(37): 14645-59.
[http://dx.doi.org/10.1523/JNEUROSCI.1327-13.2013] [PMID: 24027266]

[168] Kumar A, Singh A, Ekavali . A review on Alzheimer's disease pathophysiology and its management: an update. Pharmacol Rep 2015; 67(2): 195-203.
[http://dx.doi.org/10.1016/j.pharep.2014.09.004] [PMID: 25712639]

[169] Kametani F. Epsilon-secretase: reduction of amyloid precursor protein epsilon-site cleavage in Alzheimer's disease. Curr Alzheimer Res 2008; 5(2): 165-71.
[http://dx.doi.org/10.2174/156720508783954776] [PMID: 18393801]

[170] Klein WL. Abeta toxicity in Alzheimer's disease: globular oligomers (ADDLs) as new vaccine and drug targets. Neurochem Int 2002; 41(5): 345-52.
[http://dx.doi.org/10.1016/S0197-0186(02)00050-5] [PMID: 12176077]

[171] Moya KL, Benowitz LI, Schneider GE, Allinquant B. The amyloid precursor protein is developmentally regulated and correlated with synaptogenesis. Dev Biol 1994; 161(2): 597-603.
[http://dx.doi.org/10.1006/dbio.1994.1055] [PMID: 8314003]

[172] Mileusnic R, Lancashire CL, Johnston AN, Rose SP. APP is required during an early phase of memory formation. Eur J Neurosci 2000; 12(12): 4487-95.
[PMID: 11122359]

[173] Atwood CS, Obrenovich ME, Liu T, *et al.* Amyloid-beta: a chameleon walking in two worlds: a review of the trophic and toxic properties of amyloid-beta. Brain Res Brain Res Rev 2003; 43(1): 1-16.
[http://dx.doi.org/10.1016/S0165-0173(03)00174-7] [PMID: 14499458]

[174] Lu P, Bai XC, Ma D, *et al.* Three-dimensional structure of human γ-secretase. Nature 2014; 512(7513): 166-70.
[http://dx.doi.org/10.1038/nature13567] [PMID: 25043039]

[175] Carroll CM, Li YM. Physiological and pathological roles of the γ-secretase complex. Brain Res Bull 2016; 126(Pt 2): 199-206.
[http://dx.doi.org/10.1016/j.brainresbull.2016.04.019] [PMID: 27133790]

[176] Kane MD, Lipinski WJ, Callahan MJ, *et al.* Evidence for seeding of beta -amyloid by intracerebral infusion of Alzheimer brain extracts in beta -amyloid precursor protein-transgenic mice. J Neurosci 2000; 20(10): 3606-11.
[http://dx.doi.org/10.1523/JNEUROSCI.20-10-03606.2000] [PMID: 10804202]

[177] Ivins KJ, Thornton PL, Rohn TT, Cotman CW. Neuronal apoptosis induced by beta-amyloid is mediated by caspase-8. Neurobiol Dis 1999; 6(5): 440-9.
[http://dx.doi.org/10.1006/nbdi.1999.0268] [PMID: 10527810]

[178] Jarosz-Griffiths HH, Noble E, Rushworth JV, Hooper NM. Amyloid-β Receptors: The Good, the Bad, and the Prion Protein. J Biol Chem 2016; 291(7): 3174-83.
[http://dx.doi.org/10.1074/jbc.R115.702704] [PMID: 26719327]

[179] Lin X, Koelsch G, Wu S, Downs D, Dashti A, Tang J. Human aspartic protease memapsin 2 cleaves the beta-secretase site of beta-amyloid precursor protein. Proc Natl Acad Sci USA 2000; 97(4): 1456-60.
[http://dx.doi.org/10.1073/pnas.97.4.1456] [PMID: 10677483]

[180] Sinha S, Anderson JP, Barbour R, *et al.* Purification and cloning of amyloid precursor protein beta-secretase from human brain. Nature 1999; 402(6761): 537-40.
[http://dx.doi.org/10.1038/990114] [PMID: 10591214]

[181] Cai H, Wang Y, McCarthy D, *et al.* BACE1 is the major beta-secretase for generation of Abeta peptides by neurons. Nat Neurosci 2001; 4(3): 233-4. [http://dx.doi.org/10.1038/85064] [PMID: 11224536]

[182] Luo Y, Bolon B, Kahn S, *et al.* Mice deficient in BACE1, the Alzheimer's beta-secretase, have normal phenotype and abolished beta-amyloid generation. Nat Neurosci 2001; 4(3): 231-2. [http://dx.doi.org/10.1038/85059] [PMID: 11224535]

[183] Wang H, Megill A, Wong PC, Kirkwood A, Lee HK. Postsynaptic target specific synaptic dysfunctions in the CA3 area of BACE1 knockout mice. PLoS One 2014; 9(3): e92279. [http://dx.doi.org/10.1371/journal.pone.0092279] [PMID: 24637500]

[184] Ohno M, Sametsky EA, Younkin LH, *et al.* BACE1 deficiency rescues memory deficits and cholinergic dysfunction in a mouse model of Alzheimer's disease. Neuron 2004; 41(1): 27-33. [http://dx.doi.org/10.1016/S0896-6273(03)00810-9] [PMID: 14715132]

[185] Citron M. Strategies for disease modification in Alzheimer's disease. Nat Rev Neurosci 2004; 5(9): 677-85. [http://dx.doi.org/10.1038/nrn1495] [PMID: 15322526]

[186] Yan R. Physiological Functions of the β-Site Amyloid Precursor Protein Cleaving Enzyme 1 and 2. Front Mol Neurosci 2017; 10: 97. [http://dx.doi.org/10.3389/fnmol.2017.00097] [PMID: 28469554]

[187] Yan R, Vassar R. Targeting the β secretase BACE1 for Alzheimer's disease therapy. Lancet Neurol 2014; 13(3): 319-29. [http://dx.doi.org/10.1016/S1474-4422(13)70276-X] [PMID: 24556009]

[188] Brandt R, Lee G. Functional organization of microtubule-associated protein tau. Identification of regions which affect microtubule growth, nucleation, and bundle formation *in vitro*. J Biol Chem 1993; 268(5): 3414-9. [PMID: 8429017]

[189] Bré MH, Karsenti E. Effects of brain microtubule-associated proteins on microtubule dynamics and the nucleating activity of centrosomes. Cell Motil Cytoskeleton 1990; 15(2): 88-98. [http://dx.doi.org/10.1002/cm.970150205] [PMID: 2107033]

[190] Panda D, Goode BL, Feinstein SC, Wilson L. Kinetic stabilization of microtubule dynamics at steady state by tau and microtubule-binding domains of tau. Biochemistry 1995; 34(35): 11117-27. [http://dx.doi.org/10.1021/bi00035a017] [PMID: 7669769]

[191] Hanger DP, Anderton BH, Noble W. Tau phosphorylation: the therapeutic challenge for neurodegenerative disease. Trends Mol Med 2009; 15(3): 112-9. [http://dx.doi.org/10.1016/j.molmed.2009.01.003] [PMID: 19246243]

[192] García de Ancos J, Correas I, Avila J. Differences in microtubule binding and self-association abilities of bovine brain tau isoforms. J Biol Chem 1993; 268(11): 7976-82. [PMID: 8463318]

[193] Kosik KS. Tau protein and neurodegeneration. Mol Neurobiol 1990; 4(3-4): 171-9. [http://dx.doi.org/10.1007/BF02780339] [PMID: 2135393]

[194] Liu XA, Rizzo V, Puthanveettil SV. Pathologies of axonal transport in neurodegenerative diseases. Transl Neurosci 2012; 3(4): 355-72. [http://dx.doi.org/10.2478/s13380-012-0044-7] [PMID: 23750323]

[195] Wang JZ, Wang ZH, Tian Q. Tau hyperphosphorylation induces apoptotic escape and triggers neurodegeneration in Alzheimer's disease. Neurosci Bull 2014; 30(2): 359-66. [http://dx.doi.org/10.1007/s12264-013-1415-y] [PMID: 24627329]

[196] Liu XA, Liao K, Liu R, *et al.* Tau dephosphorylation potentiates apoptosis by mechanisms involving a failed dephosphorylation/activation of Bcl-2. J Alzheimers Dis 2010; 19(3): 953-62.

[http://dx.doi.org/10.3233/JAD-2010-1294] [PMID: 20157251]

[197] Liu XA, Song J, Jiang Q, Wang Q, Tian Q, Wang JZ. Expression of the hyperphosphorylated tau attenuates ER stress-induced apoptosis with upregulation of unfolded protein response. Apoptosis 2012; 17(10): 1039-49.
[http://dx.doi.org/10.1007/s10495-012-0744-z] [PMID: 22802092]

[198] Li HL, Wang HH, Liu SJ, *et al.* Phosphorylation of tau antagonizes apoptosis by stabilizing beta-catenin, a mechanism involved in Alzheimer's neurodegeneration. Proc Natl Acad Sci USA 2007; 104(9): 3591-6.
[http://dx.doi.org/10.1073/pnas.0609303104] [PMID: 17360687]

[199] Morris M, Knudsen GM, Maeda S, *et al.* Tau post-translational modifications in wild-type and human amyloid precursor protein transgenic mice. Nat Neurosci 2015; 18(8): 1183-9.
[http://dx.doi.org/10.1038/nn.4067] [PMID: 26192747]

[200] Cohen TJ, Guo JL, Hurtado DE, *et al.* The acetylation of tau inhibits its function and promotes pathological tau aggregation. Nat Commun 2011; 2: 252.
[http://dx.doi.org/10.1038/ncomms1255] [PMID: 21427723]

[201] Min SW, Cho SH, Zhou Y, *et al.* Acetylation of tau inhibits its degradation and contributes to tauopathy. Neuron 2010; 67(6): 953-66.
[http://dx.doi.org/10.1016/j.neuron.2010.08.044] [PMID: 20869593]

[202] Roberson ED, Scearce-Levie K, Palop JJ, *et al.* Reducing endogenous tau ameliorates amyloid beta-induced deficits in an Alzheimer's disease mouse model. Science 2007; 316(5825): 750-4.
[http://dx.doi.org/10.1126/science.1141736] [PMID: 17478722]

[203] Leroy K, Ando K, Laporte V, *et al.* Lack of tau proteins rescues neuronal cell death and decreases amyloidogenic processing of APP in APP/PS1 mice. Am J Pathol 2012; 181(6): 1928-40.
[http://dx.doi.org/10.1016/j.ajpath.2012.08.012] [PMID: 23026200]

[204] Götz J, Chen F, van Dorpe J, Nitsch RM. Formation of neurofibrillary tangles in P301l tau transgenic mice induced by Abeta 42 fibrils. Science 2001; 293(5534): 1491-5.
[http://dx.doi.org/10.1126/science.1062097] [PMID: 11520988]

[205] Giacobini E, Gold G. Alzheimer disease therapy--moving from amyloid-β to tau. Nat Rev Neurol 2013; 9(12): 677-86.
[http://dx.doi.org/10.1038/nrneurol.2013.223] [PMID: 24217510]

[206] Zhang B, Maiti A, Shively S, *et al.* Microtubule-binding drugs offset tau sequestration by stabilizing microtubules and reversing fast axonal transport deficits in a tauopathy model. Proc Natl Acad Sci USA 2005; 102(1): 227-31.
[http://dx.doi.org/10.1073/pnas.0406361102] [PMID: 15615853]

[207] Brunden KR, Zhang B, Carroll J, *et al.* Epothilone D improves microtubule density, axonal integrity, and cognition in a transgenic mouse model of tauopathy. J Neurosci 2010; 30(41): 13861-6.
[http://dx.doi.org/10.1523/JNEUROSCI.3059-10.2010] [PMID: 20943926]

[208] Lashuel HA, Hartley D, Petre BM, Walz T, Lansbury PT Jr. Neurodegenerative disease: amyloid pores from pathogenic mutations. Nature 2002; 418(6895): 291.
[http://dx.doi.org/10.1038/418291a] [PMID: 12124613]

[209] Shankar GM, Bloodgood BL, Townsend M, Walsh DM, Selkoe DJ, Sabatini BL. Natural oligomers of the Alzheimer amyloid-beta protein induce reversible synapse loss by modulating an NMDA-type glutamate receptor-dependent signaling pathway. J Neurosci 2007; 27(11): 2866-75.
[http://dx.doi.org/10.1523/JNEUROSCI.4970-06.2007] [PMID: 17360908]

[210] Nakamura T, Lipton SA. Redox regulation of mitochondrial fission, protein misfolding, synaptic damage, and neuronal cell death: potential implications for Alzheimer's and Parkinson's diseases. Apoptosis 2010; 15(11): 1354-63.
[http://dx.doi.org/10.1007/s10495-010-0476-x] [PMID: 20177970]

[211] Nixon RA, Cataldo AM. Lysosomal system pathways: genes to neurodegeneration in Alzheimer's disease. J Alzheimers Dis 2006; 9(3) (Suppl.): 277-89. [http://dx.doi.org/10.3233/JAD-2006-9S331] [PMID: 16914867]

[212] Cruz JC, Kim D, Moy LY, *et al.* p25/cyclin-dependent kinase 5 induces production and intraneuronal accumulation of amyloid beta *in vivo*. J Neurosci 2006; 26(41): 10536-41. [http://dx.doi.org/10.1523/JNEUROSCI.3133-06.2006] [PMID: 17035538]

[213] Patrick GN, Zukerberg L, Nikolic M, de la Monte S, Dikkes P, Tsai LH. Conversion of p35 to p25 deregulates Cdk5 activity and promotes neurodegeneration. Nature 1999; 402(6762): 615-22. [http://dx.doi.org/10.1038/45159] [PMID: 10604467]

[214] Cruz JC, Tsai LH. A Jekyll and Hyde kinase: roles for Cdk5 in brain development and disease. Curr Opin Neurobiol 2004; 14(3): 390-4. [http://dx.doi.org/10.1016/j.conb.2004.05.002] [PMID: 15194121]

[215] Greenberg SM, Qiu WQ, Selkoe DJ, Ben-Itzhak A, Kosik KS. Amino-terminal region of the beta-amyloid precursor protein activates mitogen-activated protein kinase. Neurosci Lett 1995; 198(1): 52-6. [http://dx.doi.org/10.1016/0304-3940(95)11944-R] [PMID: 8570096]

[216] Zhu X, Lee HG, Raina AK, Perry G, Smith MA. The role of mitogen-activated protein kinase pathways in Alzheimer's disease. Neurosignals 2002; 11(5): 270-81. [http://dx.doi.org/10.1159/000067426] [PMID: 12566928]

[217] Webster B, Hansen L, Adame A, *et al.* Astroglial activation of extracellular-regulated kinase in early stages of Alzheimer disease. J Neuropathol Exp Neurol 2006; 65(2): 142-51. [http://dx.doi.org/10.1097/01.jnen.0000199599.63204.6f] [PMID: 16462205]

[218] Zhu X, Sun Z, Lee HG, Siedlak SL, Perry G, Smith MA. Distribution, levels, and activation of MEK1 in Alzheimer's disease. J Neurochem 2003; 86(1): 136-42. [http://dx.doi.org/10.1046/j.1471-4159.2003.01820.x] [PMID: 12807433]

[219] Zhang C, Qiu HE, Krafft GA, Klein WL. A beta peptide enhances focal adhesion kinase/Fyn association in a rat CNS nerve cell line. Neurosci Lett 1996; 211(3): 187-90. [http://dx.doi.org/10.1016/0304-3940(96)12761-0] [PMID: 8817572]

[220] Guerreiro R, Wojtas A, Bras J, *et al.* TREM2 variants in Alzheimer's disease. N Engl J Med 2013; 368(2): 117-27. [http://dx.doi.org/10.1056/NEJMoa1211851] [PMID: 23150934]

[221] Jin SC, Benitez BA, Karch CM, *et al.* Coding variants in TREM2 increase risk for Alzheimer's disease. Hum Mol Genet 2014; 23(21): 5838-46. [http://dx.doi.org/10.1093/hmg/ddu277] [PMID: 24899047]

[222] Bradshaw EM, Chibnik LB, Keenan BT, *et al.* CD33 Alzheimer's disease locus: altered monocyte function and amyloid biology. Nat Neurosci 2013; 16(7): 848-50. [http://dx.doi.org/10.1038/nn.3435] [PMID: 23708142]

[223] Akiyama H, Barger S, Barnum S, *et al.* Inflammation and Alzheimer's disease. Neurobiol Aging 2000; 21(3): 383-421. [http://dx.doi.org/10.1016/S0197-4580(00)00124-X] [PMID: 10858586]

[224] Heneka MT, Carson MJ, El Khoury J, *et al.* Neuroinflammation in Alzheimer's disease. Lancet Neurol 2015; 14(4): 388-405. [http://dx.doi.org/10.1016/S1474-4422(15)70016-5] [PMID: 25792098]

[225] Kettenmann H, Hanisch UK, Noda M, Verkhratsky A. Physiology of microglia. Physiol Rev 2011; 91(2): 461-553. [http://dx.doi.org/10.1152/physrev.00011.2010] [PMID: 21527731]

[226] Bamberger ME, Harris ME, McDonald DR, Husemann J, Landreth GE. A cell surface receptor

complex for fibrillar beta-amyloid mediates microglial activation. J Neurosci 2003; 23(7): 2665-74. [http://dx.doi.org/10.1523/JNEUROSCI.23-07-02665.2003] [PMID: 12684452]

[227] Mawuenyega KG, Sigurdson W, Ovod V, *et al.* Decreased clearance of CNS beta-amyloid in Alzheimer's disease. Science 2010; 330(6012): 1774. [http://dx.doi.org/10.1126/science.1197623] [PMID: 21148344]

[228] Hickman SE, Allison EK, El Khoury J. Microglial dysfunction and defective beta-amyloid clearance pathways in aging Alzheimer's disease mice. J Neurosci 2008; 28(33): 8354-60. [http://dx.doi.org/10.1523/JNEUROSCI.0616-08.2008] [PMID: 18701698]

[229] Goldman S. Glia as neural progenitor cells. Trends Neurosci 2003; 26(11): 590-6. [http://dx.doi.org/10.1016/j.tins.2003.09.011] [PMID: 14585598]

[230] Wyss-Coray T, Loike JD, Brionne TC, *et al.* Adult mouse astrocytes degrade amyloid-beta *in vitro* and *in situ*. Nat Med 2003; 9(4): 453-7. [http://dx.doi.org/10.1038/nm838] [PMID: 12612547]

[231] Blasko I, Stampfer-Kountchev M, Robatscher P, Veerhuis R, Eikelenboom P, Grubeck-Loebenstein B. How chronic inflammation can affect the brain and support the development of Alzheimer's disease in old age: the role of microglia and astrocytes. Aging Cell 2004; 3(4): 169-76. [http://dx.doi.org/10.1111/j.1474-9728.2004.00101.x] [PMID: 15268750]

[232] Olabarria M, Noristani HN, Verkhratsky A, Rodríguez JJ. Concomitant astroglial atrophy and astrogliosis in a triple transgenic animal model of Alzheimer's disease. Glia 2010; 58(7): 831-8. [PMID: 20140958]

[233] Tseng JH, Xie L, Song S, *et al.* The Deacetylase HDAC6 Mediates Endogenous Neuritic Tau Pathology. Cell Reports 2017; 20(9): 2169-83. [http://dx.doi.org/10.1016/j.celrep.2017.07.082] [PMID: 28854366]

[234] Su JH, Anderson AJ, Cummings BJ, Cotman CW. Immunohistochemical evidence for apoptosis in Alzheimer's disease. Neuroreport 1994; 5(18): 2529-33. [http://dx.doi.org/10.1097/00001756-199412000-00031] [PMID: 7696596]

[235] Smale G, Nichols NR, Brady DR, Finch CE, Horton WE Jr. Evidence for apoptotic cell death in Alzheimer's disease. Exp Neurol 1995; 133(2): 225-30. [http://dx.doi.org/10.1006/exnr.1995.1025] [PMID: 7544290]

[236] Stadelmann C, Deckwerth TL, Srinivasan A, *et al.* Activation of caspase-3 in single neurons and autophagic granules of granulovacuolar degeneration in Alzheimer's disease. Evidence for apoptotic cell death. Am J Pathol 1999; 155(5): 1459-66. [http://dx.doi.org/10.1016/S0002-9440(10)65460-0] [PMID: 10550301]

[237] Carter J, Lippa CF. Beta-amyloid, neuronal death and Alzheimer's disease. Curr Mol Med 2001; 1(6): 733-7. [http://dx.doi.org/10.2174/1566524013363177] [PMID: 11899259]

[238] Selkoe DJ, Schenk D. Alzheimer's disease: molecular understanding predicts amyloid-based therapeutics. Annu Rev Pharmacol Toxicol 2003; 43: 545-84. [http://dx.doi.org/10.1146/annurev.pharmtox.43.100901.140248] [PMID: 12415125]

[239] Morishima M, Ihara Y. Posttranslational modifications of tau in paired helical filaments. Dementia 1994; 5(5): 282-8. [PMID: 7951685]

[240] Caughey B, Lansbury PT. Protofibrils, pores, fibrils, and neurodegeneration: separating the responsible protein aggregates from the innocent bystanders. Annu Rev Neurosci 2003; 26: 267-98. [http://dx.doi.org/10.1146/annurev.neuro.26.010302.081142] [PMID: 12704221]

[241] Gschwind M, Huber G. Apoptotic cell death induced by beta-amyloid 1-42 peptide is cell type dependent. J Neurochem 1995; 65(1): 292-300. [http://dx.doi.org/10.1046/j.1471-4159.1995.65010292.x] [PMID: 7790874]

[242] Bonda DJ, Wang X, Lee HG, Smith MA, Perry G, Zhu X. Neuronal failure in Alzheimer's disease: a view through the oxidative stress looking-glass. Neurosci Bull 2014; 30(2): 243-52. [http://dx.doi.org/10.1007/s12264-013-1424-x] [PMID: 24733654]

[243] Sims NR, Bowen DM, Neary D, Davison AN. Metabolic processes in Alzheimer's disease: adenine nucleotide content and production of 14CO2 from [U-14C]glucose *in vitro* in human neocortex. J Neurochem 1983; 41(5): 1329-34. [http://dx.doi.org/10.1111/j.1471-4159.1983.tb00829.x] [PMID: 6413656]

[244] Saito K, Elce JS, Hamos JE, Nixon RA. Widespread activation of calcium-activated neutral proteinase (calpain) in the brain in Alzheimer disease: a potential molecular basis for neuronal degeneration. Proc Natl Acad Sci USA 1993; 90(7): 2628-32. [http://dx.doi.org/10.1073/pnas.90.7.2628] [PMID: 8464868]

[245] Zhou Y, Richardson JS, Mombourquette MJ, Weil JA. Free radical formation in autopsy samples of Alzheimer and control cortex. Neurosci Lett 1995; 195(2): 89-92. [http://dx.doi.org/10.1016/0304-3940(94)11787-J] [PMID: 7478275]

[246] Donev R, Kolev M, Millet B, Thome J. Neuronal death in Alzheimer's disease and therapeutic opportunities. J Cell Mol Med 2009; 13(11-12): 4329-48. [http://dx.doi.org/10.1111/j.1582-4934.2009.00889.x] [PMID: 19725918]

[247] Busser J, Geldmacher DS, Herrup K. Ectopic cell cycle proteins predict the sites of neuronal cell death in Alzheimer's disease brain. J Neurosci 1998; 18(8): 2801-7. [http://dx.doi.org/10.1523/JNEUROSCI.18-08-02801.1998] [PMID: 9525997]

[248] Nagy Z, Esiri MM, Cato AM, Smith AD. Cell cycle markers in the hippocampus in Alzheimer's disease. Acta Neuropathol 1997; 94(1): 6-15. [http://dx.doi.org/10.1007/s004010050665] [PMID: 9224524]

[249] Perry E, Walker M, Grace J, Perry R. Acetylcholine in mind: a neurotransmitter correlate of consciousness? Trends Neurosci 1999; 22(6): 273-80. [http://dx.doi.org/10.1016/S0166-2236(98)01361-7] [PMID: 10354606]

[250] Martorana A, Koch G. Is dopamine involved in Alzheimer's disease? Front Aging Neurosci 2014; 6: 252. [http://dx.doi.org/10.3389/fnagi.2014.00252] [PMID: 25309431]

[251] Wong TP, Debeir T, Duff K, Cuello AC. Reorganization of cholinergic terminals in the cerebral cortex and hippocampus in transgenic mice carrying mutated presenilin-1 and amyloid precursor protein transgenes. J Neurosci 1999; 19(7): 2706-16. [http://dx.doi.org/10.1523/JNEUROSCI.19-07-02706.1999] [PMID: 10087083]

[252] Selkoe DJ. Alzheimer's disease is a synaptic failure. Science 2002; 298(5594): 789-91. [http://dx.doi.org/10.1126/science.1074069] [PMID: 12399581]

[253] Schliebs R, Arendt T. The significance of the cholinergic system in the brain during aging and in Alzheimer's disease. J Neural Transm (Vienna) 2006; 113(11): 1625-44. [http://dx.doi.org/10.1007/s00702-006-0579-2] [PMID: 17039298]

[254] Whitehouse PJ, Price DL, Clark AW, Coyle JT, DeLong MR. Alzheimer disease: evidence for selective loss of cholinergic neurons in the nucleus basalis. Ann Neurol 1981; 10(2): 122-6. [http://dx.doi.org/10.1002/ana.410100203] [PMID: 7283399]

[255] Apelt J, Kumar A, Schliebs R. Impairment of cholinergic neurotransmission in adult and aged transgenic Tg2576 mouse brain expressing the Swedish mutation of human beta-amyloid precursor protein. Brain Res 2002; 953(1-2): 17-30. [http://dx.doi.org/10.1016/S0006-8993(02)03262-6] [PMID: 12384234]

[256] Roy KK, Tota S, Tripathi T, Chander S, Nath C, Saxena AK. Lead optimization studies towards the discovery of novel carbamates as potent AChE inhibitors for the potential treatment of Alzheimer's disease. Bioorg Med Chem 2012; 20(21): 6313-20.

[http://dx.doi.org/10.1016/j.bmc.2012.09.005] [PMID: 23026084]

[257] Raina P, Santaguida P, Ismaila A, *et al.* Effectiveness of cholinesterase inhibitors and memantine for treating dementia: evidence review for a clinical practice guideline. Ann Intern Med 2008; 148(5): 379-97.
[http://dx.doi.org/10.7326/0003-4819-148-5-200803040-00009] [PMID: 18316756]

[258] Kavirajan H, Schneider LS. Efficacy and adverse effects of cholinesterase inhibitors and memantine in vascular dementia: a meta-analysis of randomised controlled trials. Lancet Neurol 2007; 6(9): 782-92.
[http://dx.doi.org/10.1016/S1474-4422(07)70195-3] [PMID: 17689146]

[259] Sun Y, Lai MS, Lu CJ, Chen RC. How long can patients with mild or moderate Alzheimer's dementia maintain both the cognition and the therapy of cholinesterase inhibitors: a national population-based study. Eur J Neurol 2008; 15(3): 278-83.
[http://dx.doi.org/10.1111/j.1468-1331.2007.02049.x] [PMID: 18290848]

[260] Howard R, McShane R, Lindesay J, *et al.* Donepezil and memantine for moderate-to-severe Alzheimer's disease. N Engl J Med 2012; 366(10): 893-903.
[http://dx.doi.org/10.1056/NEJMoa1106668] [PMID: 22397651]

[261] Hager K, Baseman AS, Nye JS, *et al.* Effects of galantamine in a 2-year, randomized, placebo-controlled study in Alzheimer's disease. Neuropsychiatr Dis Treat 2014; 10: 391-401.
[PMID: 24591834]

[262] Dhillon S. Rivastigmine transdermal patch: a review of its use in the management of dementia of the Alzheimer's type. Drugs 2011; 71(9): 1209-31.
[http://dx.doi.org/10.2165/11206380-000000000-00000] [PMID: 21711064]

[263] Tsang SW, Lai MK, Kirvell S, *et al.* Impaired coupling of muscarinic M1 receptors to G-proteins in the neocortex is associated with severity of dementia in Alzheimer's disease. Neurobiol Aging 2006; 27(9): 1216-23.
[http://dx.doi.org/10.1016/j.neurobiolaging.2005.07.010] [PMID: 16129514]

[264] Caccamo A, Oddo S, Billings LM, *et al.* M1 receptors play a central role in modulating AD-like pathology in transgenic mice. Neuron 2006; 49(5): 671-82.
[http://dx.doi.org/10.1016/j.neuron.2006.01.020] [PMID: 16504943]

[265] Jones CK, Brady AE, Davis AA, *et al.* Novel selective allosteric activator of the M1 muscarinic acetylcholine receptor regulates amyloid processing and produces antipsychotic-like activity in rats. J Neurosci 2008; 28(41): 10422-33.
[http://dx.doi.org/10.1523/JNEUROSCI.1850-08.2008] [PMID: 18842902]

[266] Quirion R, Wilson A, Rowe W, *et al.* Facilitation of acetylcholine release and cognitive performance by an M(2)-muscarinic receptor antagonist in aged memory-impaired. J Neurosci 1995; 15(2): 1455-62.
[http://dx.doi.org/10.1523/JNEUROSCI.15-02-01455.1995] [PMID: 7869110]

[267] Rowe WB, O'Donnell JP, Pearson D, Rose GM, Meaney MJ, Quirion R. Long-term effects of BIBN-99, a selective muscarinic M2 receptor antagonist, on improving spatial memory performance in aged cognitively impaired rats. Behav Brain Res 2003; 145(1-2): 171-8.
[http://dx.doi.org/10.1016/S0166-4328(03)00116-5] [PMID: 14529815]

[268] Quirion R, Aubert I, Lapchak PA, *et al.* Muscarinic receptor subtypes in human neurodegenerative disorders: focus on Alzheimer's disease. Trends Pharmacol Sci 1989; (Suppl.)80-4.
[PMID: 2694529]

[269] Züchner T, Perez-Polo JR, Schliebs R. Beta-secretase BACE1 is differentially controlled through muscarinic acetylcholine receptor signaling. J Neurosci Res 2004; 77(2): 250-7.
[http://dx.doi.org/10.1002/jnr.20152] [PMID: 15211591]

[270] Freund-Levi Y, Vedin I, Hjorth E, *et al.* Effects of supplementation with omega-3 fatty acids on oxidative stress and inflammation in patients with Alzheimer's disease: the OmegAD study. J

Alzheimers Dis 2014; 42(3): 823-31.
[http://dx.doi.org/10.3233/JAD-132042] [PMID: 24934544]

[271] Matias M, Silvestre S, Falcao A, Alves G. Recent Highlights on Molecular Hybrids Potentially Useful in Central Nervous System Disorders. Mini Rev Med Chem 2017; 17(6): 486-517.
[http://dx.doi.org/10.2174/1389557517666161111110121] [PMID: 27834131]

[272] Saxena AK Sr. The structural hybrids of acetylcholinesterase inhibitors in the treatment of alzheimer's disease: a review. J Alzheimers Neurodegener 2018; p. 4.

[273] Hardy J, Selkoe DJ. The amyloid hypothesis of Alzheimer's disease: progress and problems on the road to therapeutics. Science 2002; 297(5580): 353-6.
[http://dx.doi.org/10.1126/science.1072994] [PMID: 12130773]

[274] Guénette S, Strecker P, Kins S. APP protein family signaling at the synapse: insights from intracellular APP-binding proteins. Front Mol Neurosci 2017; 10: 87.
[http://dx.doi.org/10.3389/fnmol.2017.00087] [PMID: 28424586]

[275] Dominguez D, Tournoy J, Hartmann D, *et al.* Phenotypic and biochemical analyses of BACE1- and BACE2-deficient mice. J Biol Chem 2005; 280(35): 30797-806.
[http://dx.doi.org/10.1074/jbc.M505249200] [PMID: 15987683]

[276] Jonsson T, Atwal JK, Steinberg S, *et al.* A mutation in APP protects against Alzheimer's disease and age-related cognitive decline. Nature 2012; 488(7409): 96-9.
[http://dx.doi.org/10.1038/nature11283] [PMID: 22801501]

[277] Vassar R, Kovacs DM, Yan R, Wong PC. The beta-secretase enzyme BACE in health and Alzheimer's disease: regulation, cell biology, function, and therapeutic potential. J Neurosci 2009; 29(41): 12787-94.
[http://dx.doi.org/10.1523/JNEUROSCI.3657-09.2009] [PMID: 19828790]

[278] Kandalepas PC, Sadleir KR, Eimer WA, Zhao J, Nicholson DA, Vassar R. The Alzheimer's β-secretase BACE1 localizes to normal presynaptic terminals and to dystrophic presynaptic terminals surrounding amyloid plaques. Acta Neuropathol 2013; 126(3): 329-52.
[http://dx.doi.org/10.1007/s00401-013-1152-3] [PMID: 23820808]

[279] Cai J, Qi X, Kociok N, *et al.* β-Secretase (BACE1) inhibition causes retinal pathology by vascular dysregulation and accumulation of age pigment. EMBO Mol Med 2012; 4(9): 980-91.
[http://dx.doi.org/10.1002/emmm.201101084] [PMID: 22903875]

[280] May PC, Dean RA, Lowe SL, *et al.* Robust central reduction of amyloid-β in humans with an orally available, non-peptidic β-secretase inhibitor. J Neurosci 2011; 31(46): 16507-16.
[http://dx.doi.org/10.1523/JNEUROSCI.3647-11.2011] [PMID: 22090477]

[281] Ghosh AK, Osswald HL. BACE1 (β-secretase) inhibitors for the treatment of Alzheimer's disease. Chem Soc Rev 2014; 43(19): 6765-813.
[http://dx.doi.org/10.1039/C3CS60460H] [PMID: 24691405]

[282] Suzuki K, Iwata A, Iwatsubo T. The past, present, and future of disease-modifying therapies for Alzheimer's disease. Proc Jpn Acad, Ser B, Phys Biol Sci 2017; 93(10): 757-71.
[http://dx.doi.org/10.2183/pjab.93.048] [PMID: 29225305]

[283] Wolfe MS. Inhibition and modulation of gamma-secretase for Alzheimer's disease. Neurotherapeutics 2008; 5(3): 391-8.
[http://dx.doi.org/10.1016/j.nurt.2008.05.010] [PMID: 18625450]

[284] Dovey HF, John V, Anderson JP, *et al.* Functional gamma-secretase inhibitors reduce beta-amyloid peptide levels in brain. J Neurochem 2001; 76(1): 173-81.
[http://dx.doi.org/10.1046/j.1471-4159.2001.00012.x] [PMID: 11145990]

[285] Barten DM, Guss VL, Corsa JA, *et al.* Dynamics of beta-amyloid reductions in brain, cerebrospinal fluid, and plasma of beta-amyloid precursor protein transgenic mice treated with a gamma-secretase inhibitor. J Pharmacol Exp Ther 2005; 312(2): 635-43.

[http://dx.doi.org/10.1124/jpet.104.075408] [PMID: 15452193]

[286] Anderson JJ, Holtz G, Baskin PP, *et al.* Reductions in beta-amyloid concentrations *in vivo* by the gamma-secretase inhibitors BMS-289948 and BMS-299897. Biochem Pharmacol 2005; 69(4): 689-98. [http://dx.doi.org/10.1016/j.bcp.2004.11.015] [PMID: 15670587]

[287] Golde TE, Koo EH, Felsenstein KM, Osborne BA, Miele L. γ-Secretase inhibitors and modulators. Biochim Biophys Acta 2013; 1828(12): 2898-907. [http://dx.doi.org/10.1016/j.bbamem.2013.06.005] [PMID: 23791707]

[288] Best JD, Jay MT, Otu F, *et al.* Quantitative measurement of changes in amyloid-beta(40) in the rat brain and cerebrospinal fluid following treatment with the gamma-secretase inhibitor LY-411575 [N2-[(2S)-2-(3,5-difluorophenyl)-2-hydroxyethanoyl]-N1-[(7S)-5-methyl-6-oxo--,7-dihydro-5H-dibenzo[b,d]azepin-7-yl]-L-alaninamide]. J Pharmacol Exp Ther 2005; 313(2): 902-8. [http://dx.doi.org/10.1124/jpet.104.081174] [PMID: 15743924]

[289] Siemers ER, Dean RA, Friedrich S, *et al.* Safety, tolerability, and effects on plasma and cerebrospinal fluid amyloid-beta after inhibition of gamma-secretase. Clin Neuropharmacol 2007; 30(6): 317-25. [http://dx.doi.org/10.1097/WNF.0b013e31805b7660] [PMID: 18090456]

[290] Siemers ER, Quinn JF, Kaye J, *et al.* Effects of a gamma-secretase inhibitor in a randomized study of patients with Alzheimer disease. Neurology 2006; 66(4): 602-4. [http://dx.doi.org/10.1212/01.WNL.0000198762.41312.E1] [PMID: 16505324]

[291] Green RC, Schneider LS, Amato DA, *et al.* Effect of tarenflurbil on cognitive decline and activities of daily living in patients with mild Alzheimer disease: a randomized controlled trial. JAMA 2009; 302(23): 2557-64. [http://dx.doi.org/10.1001/jama.2009.1866] [PMID: 20009055]

[292] Sumner IL, Edwards RA, Asuni AA, Teeling JL. Antibody Engineering for Optimized Immunotherapy in Alzheimer's Disease. Front Neurosci 2018; 12: 254. [http://dx.doi.org/10.3389/fnins.2018.00254] [PMID: 29740272]

[293] Panza F, Frisardi V, Solfrizzi V, *et al.* Immunotherapy for Alzheimer's disease: from anti-β-amyloid to tau-based immunization strategies. Immunotherapy 2012; 4(2): 213-38. [http://dx.doi.org/10.2217/imt.11.170] [PMID: 22339463]

[294] Lee VM, Kenyon TK, Trojanowski JQ. Transgenic animal models of tauopathies. Biochim Biophys Acta 2005; 1739(2-3): 251-9. [http://dx.doi.org/10.1016/j.bbadis.2004.06.014] [PMID: 15615643]

[295] Alonso AdelC, Mederlyova A, Novak M, Grundke-Iqbal I, Iqbal K. Promotion of hyperphosphorylation by frontotemporal dementia tau mutations. J Biol Chem 2004; 279(33): 34873-81. [http://dx.doi.org/10.1074/jbc.M405131200] [PMID: 15190058]

[296] Necula M, Kuret J. Pseudophosphorylation and glycation of tau protein enhance but do not trigger fibrillization *in vitro*. J Biol Chem 2004; 279(48): 49694-703. [http://dx.doi.org/10.1074/jbc.M405527200] [PMID: 15364924]

[297] Sengupta A, Kabat J, Novak M, Wu Q, Grundke-Iqbal I, Iqbal K. Phosphorylation of tau at both Thr 231 and Ser 262 is required for maximal inhibition of its binding to microtubules. Arch Biochem Biophys 1998; 357(2): 299-309. [http://dx.doi.org/10.1006/abbi.1998.0813] [PMID: 9735171]

[298] Gong CX, Iqbal K. Hyperphosphorylation of microtubule-associated protein tau: a promising therapeutic target for Alzheimer disease. Curr Med Chem 2008; 15(23): 2321-8. [http://dx.doi.org/10.2174/092986708785909111] [PMID: 18855662]

[299] Mazanetz MP, Fischer PM. Untangling tau hyperphosphorylation in drug design for neurodegenerative diseases. Nat Rev Drug Discov 2007; 6(6): 464-79. [http://dx.doi.org/10.1038/nrd2111] [PMID: 17541419]

[300] Noble W, Planel E, Zehr C, *et al.* Inhibition of glycogen synthase kinase-3 by lithium correlates with reduced tauopathy and degeneration *in vivo*. Proc Natl Acad Sci USA 2005; 102(19): 6990-5. [http://dx.doi.org/10.1073/pnas.0500466102] [PMID: 15867159]

[301] Bali A, Jaggi AS. Anti-stress effects of a GSK-3β inhibitor, AR-A014418, in immobilization stress of variable duration in mice. J Basic Clin Physiol Pharmacol 2017; 28(4): 315-25. [http://dx.doi.org/10.1515/jbcpp-2016-0157] [PMID: 28590916]

[302] Pérez M, Hernández F, Lim F, Díaz-Nido J, Avila J. Chronic lithium treatment decreases mutant tau protein aggregation in a transgenic mouse model. J Alzheimers Dis 2003; 5(4): 301-8. [http://dx.doi.org/10.3233/JAD-2003-5405] [PMID: 14624025]

[303] Liu F, Iqbal K, Grundke-Iqbal I, Hart GW, Gong CX. O-GlcNAcylation regulates phosphorylation of tau: a mechanism involved in Alzheimer's disease. Proc Natl Acad Sci USA 2004; 101(29): 10804-9. [http://dx.doi.org/10.1073/pnas.0400348101] [PMID: 15249677]

[304] Yuzwa SA, Macauley MS, Heinonen JE, *et al.* A potent mechanism-inspired O-GlcNAcase inhibitor that blocks phosphorylation of tau *in vivo*. Nat Chem Biol 2008; 4(8): 483-90. [http://dx.doi.org/10.1038/nchembio.96] [PMID: 18587388]

[305] Wischik CM, Edwards PC, Lai RY, Roth M, Harrington CR. Selective inhibition of Alzheimer disease-like tau aggregation by phenothiazines. Proc Natl Acad Sci USA 1996; 93(20): 11213-8. [http://dx.doi.org/10.1073/pnas.93.20.11213] [PMID: 8855335]

[306] Nixon RA. Autophagy in neurodegenerative disease: friend, foe or turncoat? Trends Neurosci 2006; 29(9): 528-35. [http://dx.doi.org/10.1016/j.tins.2006.07.003] [PMID: 16859759]

[307] Keck S, Nitsch R, Grune T, Ullrich O. Proteasome inhibition by paired helical filament-tau in brains of patients with Alzheimer's disease. J Neurochem 2003; 85(1): 115-22. [http://dx.doi.org/10.1046/j.1471-4159.2003.01642.x] [PMID: 12641733]

[308] Keller JN, Hanni KB, Markesbery WR. Impaired proteasome function in Alzheimer's disease. J Neurochem 2000; 75(1): 436-9. [http://dx.doi.org/10.1046/j.1471-4159.2000.0750436.x] [PMID: 10854289]

[309] Hamano T, Gendron TF, Causevic E, *et al.* Autophagic-lysosomal perturbation enhances tau aggregation in transfectants with induced wild-type tau expression. Eur J Neurosci 2008; 27(5): 1119-30. [http://dx.doi.org/10.1111/j.1460-9568.2008.06084.x] [PMID: 18294209]

[310] Brunden KR, Trojanowski JQ, Lee VM. Advances in tau-focused drug discovery for Alzheimer's disease and related tauopathies. Nat Rev Drug Discov 2009; 8(10): 783-93. [http://dx.doi.org/10.1038/nrd2959] [PMID: 19794442]

[311] Cummings JL, Kaufer D. Neuropsychiatric aspects of Alzheimer's disease: the cholinergic hypothesis revisited. Neurology 1996; 47(4): 876-83. [http://dx.doi.org/10.1212/WNL.47.4.876] [PMID: 8857712]

[312] Whitehouse PJ, Price DL, Struble RG, Clark AW, Coyle JT, Delon MR. Alzheimer's disease and senile dementia: loss of neurons in the basal forebrain. Science 1982; 215(4537): 1237-9. [http://dx.doi.org/10.1126/science.7058341] [PMID: 7058341]

[313] Eagger S, Morant N, Levy R, Sahakian B. Tacrine in Alzheimer's disease. Time course of changes in cognitive function and practice effects. Br J Psychiatry 1992; 160: 36-40. [http://dx.doi.org/10.1192/bjp.160.1.36] [PMID: 1544011]

[314] Eagger SA, Levy R, Sahakian BJ. Tacrine in Alzheimer's disease. Lancet 1991; 337(8748): 989-92. [http://dx.doi.org/10.1016/0140-6736(91)92656-M] [PMID: 1673209]

[315] Burns A, Rossor M, Hecker J, *et al.* The effects of donepezil in Alzheimer's disease - results from a multinational trial. Dement Geriatr Cogn Disord 1999; 10(3): 237-44.

[http://dx.doi.org/10.1159/000017126] [PMID: 10325453]

[316] Rogers SL, Farlow MR, Doody RS, Mohs R, Friedhoff LT. A 24-week, double-blind, placebo-controlled trial of donepezil in patients with Alzheimer's disease. Neurology 1998; 50(1): 136-45. [http://dx.doi.org/10.1212/WNL.50.1.136] [PMID: 9443470]

[317] Maelicke A, Samochocki M, Jostock R, *et al.* Allosteric sensitization of nicotinic receptors by galantamine, a new treatment strategy for Alzheimer's disease. Biol Psychiatry 2001; 49(3): 279-88. [http://dx.doi.org/10.1016/S0006-3223(00)01109-4] [PMID: 11230879]

[318] Tariot PN, Solomon PR, Morris JC, Kershaw P, Lilienfeld S, Ding C. A 5-month, randomized, placebo-controlled trial of galantamine in AD. The Galantamine USA-10 Study Group. Neurology 2000; 54(12): 2269-76. [http://dx.doi.org/10.1212/WNL.54.12.2269] [PMID: 10881251]

[319] Wilcock GK, Lilienfeld S, Gaens E. Efficacy and safety of galantamine in patients with mild to moderate Alzheimer's disease: multicentre randomised controlled trial. Galantamine International-1 Study Group. BMJ 2000; 321(7274): 1445-9. [http://dx.doi.org/10.1136/bmj.321.7274.1445] [PMID: 11110737]

[320] Annicchiarico R, Federici A, Pettenati C, Caltagirone C. Rivastigmine in Alzheimer's disease: Cognitive function and quality of life. Ther Clin Risk Manag 2007; 3(6): 1113-23. [PMID: 18516265]

[321] Cummings J, Lefèvre G, Small G, Appel-Dingemanse S. Pharmacokinetic rationale for the rivastigmine patch. Neurology 2007; 69(4) (Suppl. 1): S10-3. [http://dx.doi.org/10.1212/01.wnl.0000281846.40390.50] [PMID: 17646618]

[322] Birks JS, Chong LY, Grimley Evans J. Rivastigmine for Alzheimer's disease. Cochrane Database Syst Rev 2015; 9: CD001191. [PMID: 26393402]

[323] Currais A, Goldberg J, Farrokhi C, *et al.* A comprehensive multiomics approach toward understanding the relationship between aging and dementia. Aging (Albany NY) 2015; 7(11): 937-55. [http://dx.doi.org/10.18632/aging.100838] [PMID: 26564964]

[324] Chen HY, Xu DP, Tan GL, *et al.* A Potent Multi-functional Neuroprotective Derivative of Tetramethylpyrazine. J Mol Neurosci 2015; 56(4): 977-87. [http://dx.doi.org/10.1007/s12031-015-0566-x] [PMID: 25982925]

[325] Prior M, Dargusch R, Ehren JL, Chiruta C, Schubert D. The neurotrophic compound J147 reverses cognitive impairment in aged Alzheimer's disease mice. Alzheimers Res Ther 2013; 5(3): 25. [http://dx.doi.org/10.1186/alzrt179] [PMID: 23673233]

[326] Hynd MR, Scott HL, Dodd PR. Glutamate-mediated excitotoxicity and neurodegeneration in Alzheimer's disease. Neurochem Int 2004; 45(5): 583-95. [http://dx.doi.org/10.1016/j.neuint.2004.03.007] [PMID: 15234100]

[327] Mattson MP, Cheng B, Davis D, Bryant K, Lieberburg I, Rydel RE. beta-Amyloid peptides destabilize calcium homeostasis and render human cortical neurons vulnerable to excitotoxicity. J Neurosci 1992; 12(2): 376-89. [http://dx.doi.org/10.1523/JNEUROSCI.12-02-00376.1992] [PMID: 1346802]

[328] Olney JW. Brain lesions, obesity, and other disturbances in mice treated with monosodium glutamate. Science 1969; 164(3880): 719-21. [http://dx.doi.org/10.1126/science.164.3880.719] [PMID: 5778021]

[329] Bezprozvanny I, Mattson MP. Neuronal calcium mishandling and the pathogenesis of Alzheimer's disease. Trends Neurosci 2008; 31(9): 454-63. [http://dx.doi.org/10.1016/j.tins.2008.06.005] [PMID: 18675468]

[330] Masliah E, Alford M, DeTeresa R, Mallory M, Hansen L. Deficient glutamate transport is associated with neurodegeneration in Alzheimer's disease. Ann Neurol 1996; 40(5): 759-66.

[http://dx.doi.org/10.1002/ana.410400512] [PMID: 8957017]

[331] Kashani A, Lepicard E, Poirel O, *et al.* Loss of VGLUT1 and VGLUT2 in the prefrontal cortex is correlated with cognitive decline in Alzheimer disease. Neurobiol Aging 2008; 29(11): 1619-30. [http://dx.doi.org/10.1016/j.neurobiolaging.2007.04.010] [PMID: 17531353]

[332] Kirvell SL, Esiri M, Francis PT. Down-regulation of vesicular glutamate transporters precedes cell loss and pathology in Alzheimer's disease. J Neurochem 2006; 98(3): 939-50. [http://dx.doi.org/10.1111/j.1471-4159.2006.03935.x] [PMID: 16893425]

[333] Chen KH, Reese EA, Kim HW, Rapoport SI, Rao JS. Disturbed neurotransmitter transporter expression in Alzheimer's disease brain. J Alzheimers Dis 2011; 26(4): 755-66. [http://dx.doi.org/10.3233/JAD-2011-110002] [PMID: 21743130]

[334] Jacob CP, Koutsilieri E, Bartl J, *et al.* Alterations in expression of glutamatergic transporters and receptors in sporadic Alzheimer's disease. J Alzheimers Dis 2007; 11(1): 97-116. [http://dx.doi.org/10.3233/JAD-2007-11113] [PMID: 17361039]

[335] Zoia C, Cogliati T, Tagliabue E, *et al.* Glutamate transporters in platelets: EAAT1 decrease in aging and in Alzheimer's disease. Neurobiol Aging 2004; 25(2): 149-57. [http://dx.doi.org/10.1016/S0197-4580(03)00085-X] [PMID: 14749132]

[336] Takahashi K, Kong Q, Lin Y, *et al.* Restored glial glutamate transporter EAAT2 function as a potential therapeutic approach for Alzheimer's disease. J Exp Med 2015; 212(3): 319-32. [http://dx.doi.org/10.1084/jem.20140413] [PMID: 25711212]

[337] Chartier-Harlin MC, Crawford F, Houlden H, *et al.* Early-onset Alzheimer's disease caused by mutations at codon 717 of the beta-amyloid precursor protein gene. Nature 1991; 353(6347): 844-6. [http://dx.doi.org/10.1038/353844a0] [PMID: 1944558]

[338] Murrell J, Farlow M, Ghetti B, Benson MD. A mutation in the amyloid precursor protein associated with hereditary Alzheimer's disease. Science 1991; 254(5028): 97-9. [http://dx.doi.org/10.1126/science.1925564] [PMID: 1925564]

[339] Pike CJ, Burdick D, Walencewicz AJ, Glabe CG, Cotman CW. Neurodegeneration induced by beta-amyloid peptides *in vitro*: the role of peptide assembly state. J Neurosci 1993; 13(4): 1676-87. [http://dx.doi.org/10.1523/JNEUROSCI.13-04-01676.1993] [PMID: 8463843]

[340] Geula C, Wu CK, Saroff D, Lorenzo A, Yuan M, Yankner BA. Aging renders the brain vulnerable to amyloid beta-protein neurotoxicity. Nat Med 1998; 4(7): 827-31. [http://dx.doi.org/10.1038/nm0798-827] [PMID: 9662375]

[341] Kuchibhotla KV, Goldman ST, Lattarulo CR, Wu HY, Hyman BT, Bacskai BJ. Abeta plaques lead to aberrant regulation of calcium homeostasis *in vivo* resulting in structural and functional disruption of neuronal networks. Neuron 2008; 59(2): 214-25. [http://dx.doi.org/10.1016/j.neuron.2008.06.008] [PMID: 18667150]

[342] Arispe N, Rojas E, Pollard HB. Alzheimer disease amyloid beta protein forms calcium channels in bilayer membranes: blockade by tromethamine and aluminum. Proc Natl Acad Sci USA 1993; 90(2): 567-71. [http://dx.doi.org/10.1073/pnas.90.2.567] [PMID: 8380642]

[343] Talantova M, Sanz-Blasco S, Zhang X, *et al.* Aβ induces astrocytic glutamate release, extrasynaptic NMDA receptor activation, and synaptic loss. Proc Natl Acad Sci USA 2013; 110(27): E2518-27. [http://dx.doi.org/10.1073/pnas.1306832110] [PMID: 23776240]

[344] Qin S, Colin C, Hinners I, Gervais A, Cheret C, Mallat M. System Xc- and apolipoprotein E expressed by microglia have opposite effects on the neurotoxicity of amyloid-beta peptide 1-40. J Neurosci 2006; 26(12): 3345-56. [http://dx.doi.org/10.1523/JNEUROSCI.5186-05.2006] [PMID: 16554485]

[345] Scimemi A, Meabon JS, Woltjer RL, Sullivan JM, Diamond JS, Cook DG. Amyloid-β1-42 slows clearance of synaptically released glutamate by mislocalizing astrocytic GLT-1. J Neurosci 2013;

33(12): 5312-8.
[http://dx.doi.org/10.1523/JNEUROSCI.5274-12.2013] [PMID: 23516295]

[346] Huang S, Tong H, Lei M, *et al.* Astrocytic glutamatergic transporters are involved in Aβ-induced synaptic dysfunction. Brain Res 2018; 1678: 129-37.
[http://dx.doi.org/10.1016/j.brainres.2017.10.011] [PMID: 29066369]

[347] Lipton SA. Failures and successes of NMDA receptor antagonists: molecular basis for the use of open-channel blockers like memantine in the treatment of acute and chronic neurologic insults. NeuroRx 2004; 1(1): 101-10.
[http://dx.doi.org/10.1602/neurorx.1.1.101] [PMID: 15717010]

[348] Lipton SA. Paradigm shift in NMDA receptor antagonist drug development: molecular mechanism of uncompetitive inhibition by memantine in the treatment of Alzheimer's disease and other neurologic disorders. J Alzheimers Dis 2004; 6(6) (Suppl.): S61-74.
[PMID: 15665416]

[349] Xia P, Chen HS, Zhang D, Lipton SA. Memantine preferentially blocks extrasynaptic over synaptic NMDA receptor currents in hippocampal autapses. J Neurosci 2010; 30(33): 11246-50.
[http://dx.doi.org/10.1523/JNEUROSCI.2488-10.2010] [PMID: 20720132]

[350] Bordji K, Becerril-Ortega J, Nicole O, Buisson A. Activation of extrasynaptic, but not synaptic, NMDA receptors modifies amyloid precursor protein expression pattern and increases amyloid-ß production. J Neurosci 2010; 30(47): 15927-42.
[http://dx.doi.org/10.1523/JNEUROSCI.3021-10.2010] [PMID: 21106831]

[351] Ray B, Banerjee PK, Greig NH, Lahiri DK. Memantine treatment decreases levels of secreted Alzheimer's amyloid precursor protein (APP) and amyloid beta (A beta) peptide in the human neuroblastoma cells. Neurosci Lett 2010; 470(1): 1-5.
[http://dx.doi.org/10.1016/j.neulet.2009.11.016] [PMID: 19948208]

[352] Beal MF, Matson WR, Storey E, *et al.* Kynurenic acid concentrations are reduced in Huntington's disease cerebral cortex. J Neurol Sci 1992; 108(1): 80-7.
[http://dx.doi.org/10.1016/0022-510X(92)90191-M] [PMID: 1385624]

[353] Ogawa T, Matson WR, Beal MF, *et al.* Kynurenine pathway abnormalities in Parkinson's disease. Neurology 1992; 42(9): 1702-6.
[http://dx.doi.org/10.1212/WNL.42.9.1702] [PMID: 1513457]

[354] Traynor BJ, Bruijn L, Conwit R, *et al.* Neuroprotective agents for clinical trials in ALS: a systematic assessment. Neurology 2006; 67(1): 20-7.
[http://dx.doi.org/10.1212/01.wnl.0000223353.34006.54] [PMID: 16832072]

[355] Gulaj E, Pawlak K, Bien B, Pawlak D. Kynurenine and its metabolites in Alzheimer's disease patients. Adv Med Sci 2010; 55(2): 204-11.
[http://dx.doi.org/10.2478/v10039-010-0023-6] [PMID: 20639188]

[356] Hartai Z, Juhász A, Rimanóczy A, *et al.* Decreased serum and red blood cell kynurenic acid levels in Alzheimer's disease. Neurochem Int 2007; 50(2): 308-13.
[http://dx.doi.org/10.1016/j.neuint.2006.08.012] [PMID: 17023091]

[357] Zwilling D, Huang SY, Sathyasaikumar KV, *et al.* Kynurenine 3-monooxygenase inhibition in blood ameliorates neurodegeneration. Cell 2011; 145(6): 863-74.
[http://dx.doi.org/10.1016/j.cell.2011.05.020] [PMID: 21640374]

[358] Kessler M, Terramani T, Lynch G, Baudry M. A glycine site associated with N-methyl-D-aspartic acid receptors: characterization and identification of a new class of antagonists. J Neurochem 1989; 52(4): 1319-28.
[http://dx.doi.org/10.1111/j.1471-4159.1989.tb01881.x] [PMID: 2538568]

[359] Majláth Z, Török N, Toldi J, Vécsei L. Memantine and Kynurenic Acid: Current Neuropharmacological Aspects. Curr Neuropharmacol 2016; 14(2): 200-9.

[http://dx.doi.org/10.2174/1570159X14666151113123221] [PMID: 26564141]

[360] Akasu T, Tsurusaki M, Shoji S. Depletion of glucose causes presynaptic inhibition of neuronal transmission in the rat dorsolateral septal nucleus. Synapse 1996; 24(2): 125-34. [http://dx.doi.org/10.1002/(SICI)1098-2396(199610)24:2<125::AID-SYN4>3.0.CO;2-H] [PMID: 8890454]

[361] Kim AY, Baik EJ. Glutamate Dehydrogenase as a Neuroprotective Target Against Neurodegeneration. Neurochem Res 2018. [http://dx.doi.org/10.1007/s11064-018-2467-1] [PMID: 29357018]

[362] Mastorodemos V, Zaganas I, Spanaki C, Bessa M, Plaitakis A. Molecular basis of human glutamate dehydrogenase regulation under changing energy demands. J Neurosci Res 2005; 79(1-2): 65-73. [http://dx.doi.org/10.1002/jnr.20353] [PMID: 15578726]

[363] Burbaeva GSh, Boksha IS, Tereshkina EB, Savushkina OK, Prokhorova TA, Vorobyeva EA. Glutamate and GABA-metabolizing enzymes in post-mortem cerebellum in Alzheimer's disease: phosphate-activated glutaminase and glutamic acid decarboxylase. Cerebellum 2014; 13(5): 607-15. [http://dx.doi.org/10.1007/s12311-014-0573-4] [PMID: 24950944]

[364] Badawi Y, Pal R, Hui D, Michaelis EK, Shi H. Ischemic tolerance in an *in vivo* model of glutamate preconditioning. J Neurosci Res 2015; 93(4): 623-32. [http://dx.doi.org/10.1002/jnr.23517] [PMID: 25421886]

[365] Vlaming H, van Leeuwen F. Crosstalk between aging and the epigenome. Epigenomics 2012; 4(1): 5-7. [http://dx.doi.org/10.2217/epi.11.113] [PMID: 22332652]

[366] Siegmund KD, Connor CM, Campan M, *et al.* DNA methylation in the human cerebral cortex is dynamically regulated throughout the life span and involves differentiated neurons. PLoS One 2007; 2(9): e895. [http://dx.doi.org/10.1371/journal.pone.0000895] [PMID: 17878930]

[367] Salminen A, Haapasalo A, Kauppinen A, Kaarniranta K, Soininen H, Hiltunen M. Impaired mitochondrial energy metabolism in Alzheimer's disease: Impact on pathogenesis *via* disturbed epigenetic regulation of chromatin landscape. Prog Neurobiol 2015; 131: 1-20. [http://dx.doi.org/10.1016/j.pneurobio.2015.05.001] [PMID: 26001589]

[368] Bustos FJ, Ampuero E, Jury N, *et al.* Epigenetic editing of the Dlg4/PSD95 gene improves cognition in aged and Alzheimer's disease mice. Brain 2017; 140(12): 3252-68. [http://dx.doi.org/10.1093/brain/awx272] [PMID: 29155979]

[369] Yamakawa H, Cheng J, Penney J, *et al.* The Transcription Factor Sp3 Cooperates with HDAC2 to Regulate Synaptic Function and Plasticity in Neurons. Cell Reports 2017; 20(6): 1319-34. [http://dx.doi.org/10.1016/j.celrep.2017.07.044] [PMID: 28793257]

[370] Sharma M, Dierkes T, Sajikumar S. Epigenetic regulation by G9a/GLP complex ameliorates amyloid-beta 1-42 induced deficits in long-term plasticity and synaptic tagging/capture in hippocampal pyramidal neurons. Aging Cell 2017; 16(5): 1062-72. [http://dx.doi.org/10.1111/acel.12634] [PMID: 28665013]

[371] Iwata A, Nagata K, Hatsuta H, *et al.* Altered CpG methylation in sporadic Alzheimer's disease is associated with APP and MAPT dysregulation. Hum Mol Genet 2014; 23(3): 648-56. [http://dx.doi.org/10.1093/hmg/ddt451] [PMID: 24101602]

[372] Mano T, Nagata K, Nonaka T, *et al.* Neuron-specific methylome analysis reveals epigenetic regulation and tau-related dysfunction of BRCA1 in Alzheimer's disease. Proc Natl Acad Sci USA 2017; 114(45): E9645-54. [http://dx.doi.org/10.1073/pnas.1707151114] [PMID: 29042514]

[373] Aisen PS, Schneider LS, Sano M, *et al.* High-dose B vitamin supplementation and cognitive decline in Alzheimer disease: a randomized controlled trial. JAMA 2008; 300(15): 1774-83.

[http://dx.doi.org/10.1001/jama.300.15.1774] [PMID: 18854539]

[374] Green KN, Steffan JS, Martinez-Coria H, *et al.* Nicotinamide restores cognition in Alzheimer's disease transgenic mice *via* a mechanism involving sirtuin inhibition and selective reduction of Thr231-phosphotau. J Neurosci 2008; 28(45): 11500-10. [http://dx.doi.org/10.1523/JNEUROSCI.3203-08.2008] [PMID: 18987186]

[375] Noh H, Seo H. Age-dependent effects of valproic acid in Alzheimer's disease (AD) mice are associated with nerve growth factor (NGF) regulation. Neuroscience 2014; 266: 255-65. [http://dx.doi.org/10.1016/j.neuroscience.2014.02.012] [PMID: 24568732]

[376] Rumbaugh G, Sillivan SE, Ozkan ED, *et al.* Pharmacological Selectivity Within Class I Histone Deacetylases Predicts Effects on Synaptic Function and Memory Rescue. Neuropsychopharmacology 2015; 40(10): 2307-16. [http://dx.doi.org/10.1038/npp.2015.93] [PMID: 25837283]

[377] Govindarajan N, Rao P, Burkhardt S, *et al.* Reducing HDAC6 ameliorates cognitive deficits in a mouse model for Alzheimer's disease. EMBO Mol Med 2013; 5(1): 52-63. [http://dx.doi.org/10.1002/emmm.201201923] [PMID: 23184605]

[378] Chuang DM, Leng Y, Marinova Z, Kim HJ, Chiu CT. Multiple roles of HDAC inhibition in neurodegenerative conditions. Trends Neurosci 2009; 32(11): 591-601. [http://dx.doi.org/10.1016/j.tins.2009.06.002] [PMID: 19775759]

[379] Kilgore M, Miller CA, Fass DM, *et al.* Inhibitors of class 1 histone deacetylases reverse contextual memory deficits in a mouse model of Alzheimer's disease. Neuropsychopharmacology 2010; 35(4): 870-80. [http://dx.doi.org/10.1038/npp.2009.197] [PMID: 20010553]

[380] Monsonego A, Nemirovsky A, Harpaz I. CD4 T cells in immunity and immunotherapy of Alzheimer's disease. Immunology 2013; 139(4): 438-46. [http://dx.doi.org/10.1111/imm.12103] [PMID: 23534386]

[381] Dodel R, Hampel H, Depboylu C, *et al.* Human antibodies against amyloid beta peptide: a potential treatment for Alzheimer's disease. Ann Neurol 2002; 52(2): 253-6. [http://dx.doi.org/10.1002/ana.10253] [PMID: 12210803]

[382] Moretto N, Bolchi A, Rivetti C, *et al.* Conformation-sensitive antibodies against alzheimer amyloid-beta by immunization with a thioredoxin-constrained B-cell epitope peptide. J Biol Chem 2007; 282(15): 11436-45. [http://dx.doi.org/10.1074/jbc.M609690200] [PMID: 17267402]

[383] Rosenblum WI. Why Alzheimer trials fail: removing soluble oligomeric beta amyloid is essential, inconsistent, and difficult. Neurobiol Aging 2014; 35(5): 969-74. [http://dx.doi.org/10.1016/j.neurobiolaging.2013.10.085] [PMID: 24210593]

[384] Hyman BT, Sorger P. Failure analysis of clinical trials to test the amyloid hypothesis. Ann Neurol 2014; 76(2): 159-61. [http://dx.doi.org/10.1002/ana.24227] [PMID: 25044380]

[385] Hye A, Riddoch-Contreras J, Baird AL, *et al.* Plasma proteins predict conversion to dementia from prodromal disease Alzheimers Dement 2014; 10(6): 799-807. e2 [http://dx.doi.org/10.1016/j.jalz.2014.05.1749]

[386] Rasmussen KL, Tybjaerg-Hansen A, Nordestgaard BG, Frikke-Schmidt R. Plasma levels of apolipoprotein E and risk of dementia in the general population. Ann Neurol 2015; 77(2): 301-11. [http://dx.doi.org/10.1002/ana.24326] [PMID: 25469919]

[387] Wolters FJ, Koudstaal PJ, Hofman A, van Duijn CM, Ikram MA. Serum apolipoprotein E is associated with long-term risk of Alzheimer's disease: The Rotterdam Study. Neurosci Lett 2016; 617: 139-42. [http://dx.doi.org/10.1016/j.neulet.2016.02.018] [PMID: 26876448]

[388] van Harten AC, Jongbloed W, Teunissen CE, Scheltens P, Veerhuis R, van der Flier WM. CSF ApoE

predicts clinical progression in nondemented APOEε4 carriers. Neurobiol Aging 2017; 57: 186-94. [http://dx.doi.org/10.1016/j.neurobiolaging.2017.04.002] [PMID: 28571653]

[389] Song F, Poljak A, Crawford J, *et al.* Plasma apolipoprotein levels are associated with cognitive status and decline in a community cohort of older individuals. PLoS One 2012; 7(6): e34078. [http://dx.doi.org/10.1371/journal.pone.0034078] [PMID: 22701550]

[390] Yasuno F, Tanimukai S, Sasaki M, *et al.* Effect of plasma lipids, hypertension and APOE genotype on cognitive decline. Neurobiol Aging 2012; 33(11): 2633-40. [http://dx.doi.org/10.1016/j.neurobiolaging.2011.12.028] [PMID: 22285757]

[391] Deguil J, Ravasi L, Lamberty Y, *et al.* Early Development of Symptomatic Drugs in AD: A Systematic Review of the Use of Biomarkers. CNS Neurol Disord Drug Targets 2016; 15(7): 823-36. [http://dx.doi.org/10.2174/1871527315666160518124759] [PMID: 27189465]

[392] Johnson KA, Fox NC, Sperling RA, Klunk WE. Brain imaging in Alzheimer disease. Cold Spring Harb Perspect Med 2012; 2(4): a006213. [http://dx.doi.org/10.1101/cshperspect.a006213] [PMID: 22474610]

[393] Li JC, Han L, Wen YX, *et al.* Increased permeability of the blood-brain barrier and Alzheimer's disease-like alterations in slit-2 transgenic mice. J Alzheimers Dis 2015; 43(2): 535-48. [http://dx.doi.org/10.3233/JAD-141215] [PMID: 25114073]

[394] Schlageter NL, Carson RE, Rapoport SI. Examination of blood-brain barrier permeability in dementia of the Alzheimer type with [68Ga]EDTA and positron emission tomography. J Cereb Blood Flow Metab 1987; 7(1): 1-8. [http://dx.doi.org/10.1038/jcbfm.1987.1] [PMID: 3100543]

[395] Starr JM, Farrall AJ, Armitage P, McGurn B, Wardlaw J. Blood-brain barrier permeability in Alzheimer's disease: a case-control MRI study. Psychiatry Res 2009; 171(3): 232-41. [http://dx.doi.org/10.1016/j.pscychresns.2008.04.003] [PMID: 19211227]

[396] Caserta MT, Caccioppo D, Lapin GD, Ragin A, Groothuis DR. Blood-brain barrier integrity in Alzheimer's disease patients and elderly control subjects. J Neuropsychiatry Clin Neurosci 1998; 10(1): 78-84. [http://dx.doi.org/10.1176/jnp.10.1.78] [PMID: 9547470]

CHAPTER 4

Alzheimer's Disease and Proteasome: The Therapeutic Development and Management

Qunxing Ding* and **Haiyan Zhu**

Department of Biological Sciences, Kent State University, East Liverpool, OH, USA

Abstract: The proteasome system is a cellular machinery that is responsible for the degradation of nearly 90% of the proteins in cells and is crucial in protein metabolism involved in physiological and pathological developments, especially in aging and aging-related disorders. Numerous reports indicate that impaired proteasome is involved in the pathological process of Alzheimer's disease (AD), which is a leading form of dementia. It is well known that the pathological hallmarks of the AD are the aggregated proteins such as plaques, tangles and Lewy bodies. The formation of these aggregates is tightly associated with the dysfunction of the proteasome system, which is responsible for the degradation of oxidized, misfolded, aged and other damaged proteins. In fact, the proteasome system plays a major role in quality and quantity control in cellular protein homeostasis, and in responses to inflammatory signals, oxidative stress, and other cellular signals. This chapter will summarize the basic information and updates on the proteasome system and related cellular complexes, such as lysosome and ribosome and their alterations during aging and AD pathogenesis. In addition, some clinical trials and practical management for the AD will be discussed to explore possible strategies for pharmaceutical and clinical development associated with the proteasome system.

Keywords: Aging, Alzheimer's disease, Clinical trial, Immune, Management, Neurodegeneration, Pharmaceutical development, Proteasome, Subunits.

INTRODUCTION

Proteasome was first identified in 1977 by Etlinger and Goldberg when they worked on rabbit reticulocytes [1]. Later studies indicate that proteasome is a highly conserved structure in all eukaryotic cells and some archaea cells [2, 3]. The 20S core complex is a 4-ring cylinder structure that contains 28 subunits, seven subunits for each ring. In eukaryotic cells, the subunits in each ring are encoded by different genes, and in archaea cells, the subunits in one ring are the same, although the inside two rings (β) and outside two rings (α) are encoded by

* **Corresponding author, Qunxing Ding:** Department of Biological Sciences, Kent State University, East Liverpool, OH, USA; Tel: 330 382 7523; E-mail: qding@kent.edu

different genes [3, 4]. In higher eukaryotic cells, the proteasome system has 11S and 19S regulatory complexes that can shuttle on one end or both ends of the cylinder of the 20S core complex [4]. In addition, some special subunits can replace the regular subunits to form immune proteasome (or immunoproteasome), working on the production of antigen peptides in an immune response. It is the major machinery for protein degradation, especially for oxidized, misfolded, aged, and other damaged proteins [3 - 5]. This machinery has multiple protease activities, including chymotrypsin-like, trypsin-like and caspase-like activities, which can digest proteins into short peptides [4, 5]. In fact, the proteasome system plays a major role in quality and quantity control in cellular protein homeostasis, and in responses to inflammatory signals, infection, oxidative stress, genetic mutation and other signals to maintain the cellular metabolism [5]. In other words, the proteasome plays critical roles in both physiological and pathological conditions, so it could be a valuable target for pharmaceutical development. In fact, it has been the target in cancer research for more than twenty years, and a group of inhibitors has been developed with anti-tumor activity and apoptotic activity. Hundreds of clinical trials related to proteasome inhibition have been conducted, and nearly 60 clinic trials are currently active. Alzheimer's disease (AD) is on the opposite side of cancer: AD deals with cell death; cancer deals with overgrowth of cells. If the strategy in cancer study is to inhibit the activity of the proteasome, obviously the strategy in AD study should be to re-activate the function of the proteasome system.

GENETICS AND STRUCTURE OF PROTEASOME

The proteasome is a dynamic system that continuously undergoes assembling, disassembling, shuttling between regulatory complexes, and delivery from one cellular location to another [8, 9]. Due to the wide range of cellular metabolic processes it involves, proteasome is highly associated with pathogenesis of many disorders including AD. The AD is currently the fourth leading cause of death worldwide. While AD mortality has increased in recent years, mortality of cardiovascular diseases, the leading cause of death, has decreased with advances in medical science and technology. The involvement of proteasome in immune function is highlighted in numerous studies. An immune proteasome is a special form of the proteasome with three β subunits replaced that plays critical roles in regulating pro-inflammatory responses, including cytokine induction, the activation of the NF-κB signal transduction pathways, fighting viral infection and oxidative stress in different conditions [6, 7]. There are elevated levels of immune subunits in human brains affected by Dementia with Lewy Body (DLB) and AD (data in preparation for publication), indicating the involvement of immune proteasome in the onset and development of neuronal degeneration, revealing the possible direction for pharmaceutical development.

Proteasomes are present in all the eukaryotic cells and exist in both the cytoplasm and nucleus. These structures may also associate with membranes like endoplasmic reticulum and cytoskeleton [8, 9]. In archaea bacteria proteasomes also exist although the genetic components are slightly different from eukaryotic cells [2, 3]. In this section, we mainly focus on the genetics of human proteasome, and some of the alternative symbols may refer to other organisms like yeast or rat [3, 5, 8].

The 20S core structure of proteasome has α and β subunits. The α subunits share higher levels of homolog, and they are critical to initiating assembly of the core complex, although they have no catalytic function. Table **1** summarizes some of the genetic features of α subunits of human proteasome (PSMA). It is clear that the human proteasome α subunits are encoded in different chromosomes including 1, 7, 11, 14, 15, 18 and 20. Chromosome 14 has two α subunit genes on it: PSMA3 and PSMA6. Some α subunits like PSMA1, PSMA3 and PSMA4 contain positively charged peptides as nuclear localization signals that can aid in transporting these subunits inside the nucleus to form proteasome complexes [10]. The α subunits form α rings that not only control the access to catalytic β rings but also connect with regulatory complexes (19S and 11S, see below). PSMA8 is a subunit specifically found in the testis that promotes degradation of histones, thereby participating actively in the exchange of histones during spermatogenesis [11]. The expression levels of α subunits PSMA1-7 are ubiquitously stable in nearly all kinds of tissues, but PSMA8 selectively expresses higher in serum, testis, ovary, lymphocytes, nasal epithelium, lung and heart, and may replace the position of PSMA7 to form the α rings in these tissues [12].

Table 1. The genetic indexes of the human proteasome α subunits.

Gene Symbol	Amino Acids	Cytogenetic Location	Genomic Coordinates	Alternative Symbols
PSMA1	263	11p15.2	11:14,504,875-4,643,633	HC2, PROS30, HEL-S-275, NU
PSMA2	234	7p14.1	7:42,916,860-42,932,205	HC3, PSC2, MU
PSMA3	255	14q23.1	14:58,244,804-58,272,008	HC8, PSC3
PSMA4	261	15q25.1	15:78,540,404-78,549,219	PSC9, HC9, HsT17706
PSMA5	241	1p13.3	1:109,399,030-109,426,485	PSC Z, PSC5
PSMA6	246	14q13.2	14:35,278,557-35,317,478	PSC i., PROS27, p27K
PSMA7	248	20q13.33	20:62,136,726-62,143,457	XAPC7, PS α-4, C6, RC6-1, XAPC7
PSMA8	256	18q11.2	18:26,133,836-26,193,355	PSMA7L

*The table information is collected from https://www.ncbi.nlm.nih.gov/omim and https://www.genecards.org/, Numerous references are not cited here but can be found in the websites.

Human proteasomal β subunits diverge more than α subunits in the sequence of amino acids. In regard to the genomic distribution, the β subunits form a few groups: PSMB1, PSMB8, and PSMB9 are located on the chromosome 6, and PSMB8 and PSMB9 are even tightly linked with ~10 kb apart. PSMB3 and PSMB6 locate on chromosome 17, and PSMB5 and PSMB11 on chromosome 14 with only ~ 7kb apart (Table **2**). The genetic linkage of β subunits indicates the different regulation pattern of gene transcription, and the expression of β subunits is more synergic and synchronic than α subunits. Six of the β subunits (PSMB5, PSMB6, PSMB7; PSMB8, PSMB9, PSMB10) have proteolytic activities that can be divided into two groups: PSMB5, PSMB6, and PSMB7 are constitutive subunits; and PSMB8, PSMB9, and PSMB10 are inducible subunits, which only express when γ-interferon and other inducers are present. PSMB8, PSMB9, and PSMB10 may replace PSMB5, PSMB6, and PSMB7 to form 20S core complex, which is the immune proteasome that has been mentioned previously. The immune proteasome is involved in the production of antigen display by the major histocompatibility complex class I (MHC) proteins on the surface of antigen-presenting cells [6]. PSMB11, which is also a catalytic subunit that was reported to express exclusively in cortical thymic epithelial cells, may replace the position of PSMB5 or PSMB8 [13].

Table 2. The genetic indexes of the human proteasome β subunits.

Gene Symbol	Amino Acids	Cytogenetic Location	Genomic Coordinates	Alternative Symbols
PSMB1	241	6q27	6:170,535,115-170,553,328	PSC5, HC5
PSMB2	201	1p34.3	1:35,599,540-35,641,843	PS β-4, HC7-I
PSMB3	205	17q12	17:38,752,712-38,764,230	PS β-3, HC10-II
PSMB4	264	1q21.3	1:151,399,564-151,401,935	PS β-7, HN3, HsN3, PROS26
PSMB5	263	14q11.2	14:23,016,542-23,035,219	PS X, PS β-5, LMPX, MB1
PSMB6	239	17p13	17:4,796,144-4,798,503	LMPY, PS β-1, DELTA
PSMB7	277	9q33.3	9:124,353,464-124,415,472	PS β-2, PS Z
PSMB8	276	6p21.32	6:32,840,716-32,844,934	RING 10, PS β-5i, ALDD, D6S216, D6S216E, JMP, LMP7
PSMB9	219	6p21.32	6:32,854,160-32,859,850	RING12, LMP2, PS β-1i
PSMB10	273	16q22.1	16:67,934,503-67,936,876	PS MECL1, PS β-2i
PSMB11	300	14q11.2	14:23,042,166-23,044,059	PS β-5t, EC 3.4.25.1

*The table information is collected from https://www.ncbi.nlm.nih.gov/omim and https://www.genecards.org/, Numerous references are not cited here but can be found in the websites.

Two 19S regulatory complexes and the 20S core complex form the 26S proteasome. The 26S proteasome is the most common form of the proteasome in human cells and can quickly degrade ubiquitinated proteins. The 19S regulatory complex is also called PA700, comprised of two sub-complexes: base and lid. The 19S base sub-complex includes six 19S subunits (Table **3**, PSMC1-6) with ATPase activity to form a heterohexameric ring that directly associated with 20S core complex, to support the quick unfolding of peptides for degradation with the energy supply from ATP. The 19S lid sub-complex is composed of subunits without ATPase activity listed in Table **4**. In the subunits with ATPase activity, only PSMC1 and PSMC6 are on the same chromosome (chromosome 6) and the others are located on different chromosomes individually, even though PSMC3 and PSMC4 are 57% identical. With ATPase activity, PSMC subunits are normally more than 400 aa, only PSMC6 has 389 aa. These subunits are generally larger than PSMA and PSMB subunits that are generally less than 300 amino acids (aa). The expression levels of all PSMC are ubiquitously stable in all tissues, and their activities are critical to the degradation of ubiquitinated proteins, which is ATP-dependent. Interestingly, these proteasomal subunits can be ubiquitinated *in-situ* as well [14]. Some of these ATPase may have proteasome-independent functions. For example, PSMC1 may directly interact with ataxin-7, a protein that is involved in the pathogenesis of a neurodegenerative disorder: Spinocerebellar ataxia type 7 [15], while PSMC2 may directly interact with TATA box-binding protein (TBP; 600075), the general transcription factors IIB (GFT2B; 189963), IIH (GTF2H1; 189972), and IIF (GTF2F1; 189968) to regulate gene expression [16]. Moreover, PSMC5 strongly interacted with retinoid X receptor-alpha (RXRA; 180245) and with Thrb in the presence of thyroid hormone [17].

Table 3. The genetic indexes of the human proteasome 19S regulatory subunits with ATPase activity.

Gene Symbol	Amino Acids	Cytogenetic Location	Genomic Coordinates	Alternative Symbols
PSMC1	440	14q32.11	14:90,256,549-90,272,624	S4, P56
PSMC2	433	7q22.1	7:103,344,404-103,369,394	MSS1, S7, Nbla10058
PSMC3	439	11p11.2	11:47,418,768-47,426,472	p50, TBP1, TSP Li42
PSMC4	418	19q13.2	19:39,971,004-39,981,763	TBP7, S6, RPT3,MIP224
PSMC5	406	17q23.3	17:63,827,409-63,832,026	TRIP1, SUG1,S8, P45
PSMC6	389	14q22.1	14:52,707,162-52,727,997	p42, P44,CADP44, SUG2

*The table information is collected from https://www.ncbi.nlm.nih.gov/omim and https://www.genecards.org/, Numerous references are not cited here but can be found in the websites.

The 19S non-ATPase subunits form the lid sub-complex in the 19S regulatory complex that controls the unfolding and deubiquitination of ubiquitinated proteins. The PSMD5, PSMD9 and PSMD10 have chaperone activity and work together with PSMC1, PSMC2, PSMC4 and PSMC5 to control the entrance of proteasome. Chromosome 17 has seven subunit genes, PSMD3, PSMD11, PSMD12, PSMB2, PSMB6, PSMC5, and PSME3, although only PSMD3 and PSME3 are tightly linked. Chromosome 19 has two linked subunit genes, PSMD4 and PSMD8, in addition to PSMC4. Chromosome 2 has three proteasomal subunit genes, PSMD1, PSMD14, and PSME4. Chromosome 3 has two proteasomal subunit genes, PSMD2 and PSMD6, all the others are on different chromosomes. Regarding the size of the protein, PSMD11 and PSMD12 have more than 400 aa, and PSMD3 and PSMD5 have more than 500 aa, PSMD1 and PSMD2 have more than 900 aa. With 953 aa the PSMD1 is the second largest proteasomal subunit. Some PSMD subunits also have proteasome-independent functions: PSMD10 interacts with MDM2 to regulate the stability of p53 and plays important roles in RAS-induced tumorigenesis [18].

Table 4. The genetic indexes of the human proteasome 19S regulatory subunits without ATPase activity.

Gene Symbol	Amino Acids	Cytogenetic Location	Genomic Coordinates	Alternative Symbols
PSMD1	953	2q37.1	2:231925993-231925993	P112, Rpn2, S1
PSMD2	908	3q27.1	3:184,299,097-184,309,053	P97, Rpn1, S2, TRAP2
PSMD3	534	17q21.1	17:39,980,768 - 39,997,960	P58, Rpn3, S3, TSTA2
PSMD4	377	19q13.2	19:39,971,004-39,981,763	AF-1, ASF, MCB1, Rpn10, S5A
PSMD5	504	9q33.2	9:120,814,779 -120,843,021	S5B, KIAA0072
PSMD6	389	3p14.1	3:64,010,549 - 64,024,010	p42A,Rpn7,S10, PFAAP4
PSMD7	324	16q23.1	16:74,296,775 -74,306,288	S12, P40, Rpn8, MOV34L
PSMD8	350	19q13.2	19:38,374,536 - 38,383,824	P31,S14, HIP6, Nin1p
PSMD9	223	12q24.31	12:121,888,731-121,918,297	P27, Rpn4
PSMD10	226	Xq22.3	X:108,084,205-108,091,644	P28, Gankyrin, DJ889N15.2
PSMD11	422	17q11.2	17:32,444,261-32,483,319	S9,Rpn6, P44.5
PSMD12	456	17q24.2	17:67,337,916-67,366,627	P55, Rpn5
PSMD13	376	11p15.5	11:236,546-252,984	S11, Rpn9, P40.5, HSPC027
PSMD14	310	2q24.2	2:161,308,038 -161,411,717	PAD1,Rpn11,POH1

*The table information is collected from https://www.ncbi.nlm.nih.gov/omim and https://www.genecards.org/. Numerous references are not cited here but can be found in the websites.

The 26S proteasome is ubiquitin-dependent and ATP-dependent. Besides the 19S regulatory complex, there is another complex called 11S or PA28, which can bind with 20S core complex to perform proteolysis that is ubiquitin-independent and ATP-independent. The 11S complex is a hetero-heptametrical comprising PSME1 and PSME2, which are highly linked on chromosome 14, share 50% homolog

(Table **5**). Chromosome 14 has eight proteasomal subunit genes, PSMA3, PSMA6, PSMB5, PSMB11, PSMC1, PSMC6, PSME1 and PSME2. PSME3 is not only involved in the activation of the proteasome, but also plays roles in immune response especially in bacterial infection: it was induced by NF-κB and feedforward to activate NF-κB, and interacted with p53 and mdm2 [19, 20]. PSME4 is also called PA200, the largest proteasomal subunit with 1843 aa, it can work by itself to activate proteasome. In fact, PSME1/PSME2, PSME3, and PSME4 activate proteasome in different patterns: PSME1/PSME2 stimulated all three enzymatic activities of the proteasome, but PSME3 specifically enhanced the trypsin-like activity but inhibited the chymotrypsin-like activity; while the PSME4 mainly stimulated the caspase-like activity. In addition, PSME4 may locate in the nucleus and involve in DNA repair [21].

Table 5. The genetic indexes of the human proteasome 11S regulatory subunits.

Gene Symbol	Amino Acids	Cytogenetic Location	Genomic Coordinates	Alternative Symbols
PSME1	249	14q12	14:24,136,158-24,138,967	PA28A, REG α, IGUP I-5111
PSME2	239	14q12	14:24,143,362-24,147,570	PA28B, REG β
PSME3	254	17q21.31	17:42,824,385-42,843,760	PA28G, Ki, REG γ3
PSME4	1843	2p16.2	2:53,864,067 -53,970,840	PA200, KIAA0077

*The table information is collected from https://www.ncbi.nlm.nih.gov/omim and https://www.genecards.org/, Numerous references are not cited here but can be found in the websites.

The proteasome sometimes is also called ubiquitin proteasome system (UPS) due to the fact that the majority of proteins that are degraded by proteasome are conjugated with a small protein ubiquitin. The human ubiquitin gene is coded by four genes as listed in Table **6**. UBA52 is a fusion protein comprising ubiquitin and ribosomal large subunit L40, and RPS27A is a fusion protein comprising ubiquitin and ribosomal small subunit S27a. After co-translational processing, the free ubiquitin will be released from L40 and S27 to play enormous roles in cellular metabolism, especially proteasome pathway. It is still not clear what the biological significance is of the fusion of ubiquitin to the ribosomal proteins, but it was reported to contribute to gametogenesis and reproductive success [22]. The genes UBB and UBC are also ubiquitin encoding genes with poly-ubiquitin sequences: the UBB has three ubiquitin peptides connected the head to tail, and the UBC has nine ubiquitin peptides tandemly fused together. UBB and UBC genes are translated into poly-ubiquitin precursors, which will be processed into single ubiquitin proteins. Ubiquitin is a protein with 76 aa, containing seven lysines: Lys 6, Lys 11, Lys27, Lys29, Lys33, Lys48, Lys63. Proteins can be conjugated with mono-ubiquitin or poly-ubiquitin for different purposes, which rely on the location of amino acid Lys residue in ubiquitin: if a protein conjugated ubiquitin at Lys48, then it may be delivered to the 26S proteasome for degradation; if at Lys29, it may be degraded by lysosome; if at Lys11, it may be degraded by an endoplasmic reticulum associated process and involved in cell cycle regulation; if at Lys6, it may be involved in DNA remodeling and repair; if at Lys63, this protein may involve in endocytosis, activation of NF-κB and DNA repair [23].

Table 6. The genetic indexes of the human ubiquitin genes.

Gene Symbol	Amino Acids	Cytogenetic Location	Genomic Coordinates	Alternative Symbols
UBA52	128	19p13.11	19:18,563,766-18,577,550	CEP52, RPL40
RPS27A	156	2p16.1	2:55,231,903-55,235,853	UBA80, HEL112,S27A
UBB	229	17p11.2	17:16,380,793-16,382,745	HEL-S-50
UBC	685	12q24.31	12:124,911,604-124,917,368	HMG20

*The table information is collected from https://www.ncbi.nlm.nih.gov/omim and https://www.genecards.org/. Numerous references are not cited here but can be found in the websites.

The conjugation of ubiquitin to a protein requires three groups of enzymes: ubiquitin-activating enzymes (E1), ubiquitin-conjugating enzymes (E2), and ubiquitin ligases (E3). E1 needs ATP to be conjugated with ubiquitin, and E2 will replace E1 conjugating with ubiquitin and deliver it to E3. E3 will transfer ubiquitin to the target proteins. The human genome has more than seven E1 genes, more than 40 E2 genes, and more than 600 E3 genes [24]. The number of E3 genes reveals the complexity of ubiquitination, which largely depends on the E3 activities. The forms of ubiquitination, including single mono-ubiquitin, multiple mono-ubiquitin, linear chain ubiquitin, and branched chain ubiquitin, have different functions in different metabolic processes. The ubiquitination is a special pathway that involves in a vast range of cellular metabolism, including cell cycle control, cell degeneration and death, biogenesis of ribosome and other organelles, immune response, DNA transcript and repair. Proteasome degradation is only one portion of the function of ubiquitination, and the complete review of ubiquitination has been published elsewhere [22 - 24], only some related issues will be discussed in the following sections.

It is obvious that two chromosomes have the most proteasomal subunits genes: chromosome 14 and 17. Chromosomes 1, 2, 6, 11, 19 each has three proteasomal subunit genes, chromosome 3, 7, 9, 16 each has two proteasomal subunit genes and chromosome 12, 15, 18, 20 and X each has only one subunit gene (Table **7**). All the other chromosomes do not contain proteasome subunit genes.

Table 7. The Chromosome distribution of proteasomal subunit genes.

Chromosome	Subunits
X	PSMD10
1	PSMA5, PSMB2, PSMB4
2	PSMD1, PSMD14, PSME4
3	PSMD2, PSMD6
6	PSMB1, PSMB8, PSMB9*
7	PSMA2, PSMC2
9	PSMB7, PSMD5
11	PSMA1, PSMC3, PSMD13
12	PSMD9
14	PSMA3, PSMA6, PSMB5, PSMB11*, PSMC1, PSMC6, PSME1, PSME2*
15	PSMA4
16	PSMB10, PSMD7
17	PSMB3, PSMB6, PSMC5, PSMD3, PSMD11, PSMD12, PSME3
18	PSMA8
19	PSMC4, PSMD4, PSMD8
20	PSMA7

*PSMB8 and PSMB9 are linked; PSMB5 and PSMB11 are linked; PSME1 and PSME2 are linked.
The table information is collected from https://www.ncbi.nlm.nih.gov/omim and https://www.genecards.org. Numerous references are not cited here but can be found on the websites.

ASSOCIATION BETWEEN PROTEASOME AND LYSOSOME

Lysosome is another cellular machinery that can degrade proteins, although it also involves in many other functions like secretion, membrane repair, defence, energy metabolism and signal transduction [25]. As the degradation machinery, it catalyzes not only proteins, but also carbohydrates, lipids and even organelles. The lysosomal enzymes that normally degrade proteins include cathepsins, which mostly work in acidic condition. The proteasome and lysosome usually work together to keep the balance of cellular proteins, and remove/recycle the proteins that are misfolded, oxidized, aggregated or damaged in another way. Their cooperation is critical to the quality and quantity control of cellular proteins to keep cellular homeostasis. Evidence indicated that the function of proteasome was correlated with the function of the lysosome. For example, UBR4, a ubiquitin ligase, promoted both N-degron-dependent proteasomal degradation and lysosomal cargo degradation [26]. In Parkinson's disease (PD), the dysfunction of proteasome and lysosome was synergistic [27], the wild type α-synuclein was degraded by both proteasome and lysosome independently [28]. In addition, the proteasome and lysosome interacted with one another to degrade advanced glycation end products (AGE) [29]. It is also reported that chronic low-level proteasome inhibition leads to an excessive activation of the lysosomal system [30]. In AD and DLB, the reduced proteasomal activity is highly associated with increased lysosomal activity, specifically, the activity of cathepsin B [31]. Proteasome inhibitors induced autophagy effects [30], and the dysfunction of both lysosome and proteasome could occur simultaneously: the lysosome system was disturbed in heart and skeleton muscle; and the proteasome system had reduced function in brain, kidney, liver and lung in HD transgenic mice [32]. Under chronic low level proteasome inhibition, the autophagy was induced in cultured cells resulted in apoptosis through class III PI3K pathway possibly [32, 33]. Autophagy was significantly elevated along with aging [34] and such lysosomal elevation usually was coupled with decreased proteasomal function. In certain case inhibition of deubiquitination also blocked autophagy [35]. The connection or crosstalk between proteasome and lysosome is based on different signal transduction pathways, for example the fusion protein of glutathionine S-transferase N-terminal to betaine-homocysteine S-methyltransferase reporter may play a role [36] and glycogen synthase kinase 3β may also deliver the signals [37]. Interestingly, such signaling pathways varied along with age [38]. The interplay between proteasome and lysosome systems might be based on the upstream metabolic signaling pathways or the downstream substrate signals. In summary, the cellular location of proteasome and lysosome may not be associated physically; their functions are cooperative and synergistic.

ASSOCIATION BETWEEN PROTEASOME AND RIBOSOME

Ribosome is the machinery of protein synthesis, comprising a large sub-complex (60S) and a small sub-complex (40S) that can be dissociated in and after the translation process. The ribosomal subunits contain ribosomal RNA and proteins to form the complex structure. The 60S sub-complex is composed of a 5S RNA (120 nucleotides), a 28S RNA (4700 nucleotides), a 5.8S RNA (160 nucleotides) subunits and 46 proteins, and the 40S sub-complex has a 18S RNA subunit (1540 nucleotides) bound to 21 proteins [39]. In human cells, the ribosomes can bound to membrane (endoplasmic reticulum) to form clusters and work together in translation, or individually free in the cytosol that can also work in protein translation. Both free and membrane bound ribosome can synthesize peptides that may be post-translationally modified in different ways or delivered to different locations. As discussed previously, the ubiquitin is genetically linked and co-translated with 60S ribosomal protein L40 and 40S ribosomal protein S27, indicating a genetic correlation between ribosome and proteasome system. In addition, the functions of proteasome and ribosome are tightly associated as well.

After translation the newly synthesized peptides need to fold properly for right conformation and function, more than 50% of nascent protein molecules from ribosome may bear an amino-terminal degradation signal, which can be degraded co-translationally by proteasome before proper folding and maturation [40]. One of the machinery that help newly synthesized peptides to fold properly is nascent polypeptide-associated complex (NAC), which associates with ribosomes and nascent peptide chains in an apparent 1:1 stoichiometry [41]. The tight association between proteasome and ribosome was also evidenced by a ribosome-linked E3 ubiquitin ligase Not4p [42], and ribosome-linked E2 conjugation enzyme Ubc4p [43]. Conversely, one of the components of NAC, Egd2p, was associated with proteasome [44]. If the ribosome can be called the factory of protein production, the proteasome should be the quality control of products. Furthermore, in neurodegenerative conditions, the inhibition of proteasome is correlated with decreased rRNA expression, increased rRNA oxidation and functional decline of ribosome [45, 46]. In a cultured cell line, proteasome inhibition impaired neuronal protein synthesis, and such impairment is dose-dependent, and reversible in the first six hours of treatment. Interestingly, such impairment is cell-dependent, purified ribosome functioned well in the presence of proteasome inhibitors [47]. Such interaction was also confirmed in plant leaf adaxial determination. Mutation in the proteasomal subunit gene and ribosomal protein gene share similarity in leaf development with an outgrowth formed on the distal part of the leaf abaxial side [48]. Therefore, some cellular signalling pathways were involved in the crosstalk between proteasome and ribosome. For example, the ribosomal biogenesis factor WBSCR22 is regulated and tightly controlled by proteasome [49], translation initiation factor 3 (eIF3e) had direct interaction with both ribosomal subunits and proteasome subunits [50]. Proteasome controls many factors in ribosome biogenesis that may set up the connection between protein synthesis and degradation [51]. These data indicated important functional interplay between proteasome and ribosome. In other words, the protein synthesis and degradation may have fundamental association that contribute to aging and age-related pathogenesis. The association is dynamic, and the regulation of one system might affect the other system significantly, which provides potentials and convenience for drug development.

IMPAIRMENT OF PROTEASOME IN AGING AND AD

AD is the leading dementia especially in elder population, and it counts for nearly 70% of all dementia cases. Currently, the cause of AD is still not fully understood, although a group of genetic factors have been identified: the risk genes like ApoE, the deterministic genes like APP, PS1 and PS2. Even though the genetic factors only contribute to about 1% of AD cases. The most significant factor in statistics that associate with AD is aging, which leads to the debate on whether AD is a specific disease or part of regular aging: AD incidence changes dramatically with age----about 10% of people of 65-74 years old, about 20% of people in the range of 75-84 years old and about 40% of the people above 85. The point is, if the human life span increases enough, would the majority, if not all, of the people get AD?

Among all the pathogenesis study, it is reported that the proteasome system played a critical role. For example, the proteasomal activities and the expression of its subunits declined along with aging in epidermis cells [52], such functional decline was also found in heart tissue associated with decreased 20S proteasome content [53]. More data have been reported that impaired proteasome function was associated with the process of aging, and the function of proteasome system played the role in modulating aging rate [54]. On the other hand, the declined proteasome function contributes to the development of aging-associated disorders. For example, genetic depletion of proteasome induced accumulation of mitochondrial inclusions and neurodegeneration [55], and proteasome inhibition is sufficient to induce mitochondrial dysfunction, increase generation of reactive oxygen species (ROS), elevate RNA and DNA oxidation, and to promote protein oxidation [56]. Furthermore, elevated proteasome assembling factor UMP1 exhibited enhanced viability during stationary-phase aging [57], and increased content and activities of proteasome could extend the lifespan of *C. elegans* [58] and mice [59].

The β-amyloid (Aβ) is one of the causative factors for AD that have been densely investigated. Growing evidence indicates that dysfunction of proteasome system induced Aβ accumulation and the accumulated Aβ reversely inhibits the activities of proteasome system [60]. Evidence indicated that impaired proteasome function occurred at very young age of an AD mouse model (APPswe/PS1dE9) before plaque formation and cognitive problems, revealing the causative role of the proteasome system in the development of AD [61]. In a mice model of MPTP-induced Parkinson's disease (PD), the expression of proteasomal genes Uchl3, Ubr7, Ube3c, Usp39, Ube2k, Ube2d3, Ube2g1 were reduced at pre-symptomatic stage and Uchl3, Ube3c, Usp39, Ube2k, Ube2m were reduced at an early symptomatic stage [62]. Proteasomal dysfunction was also reported in neuroblastoma, kidney cells, and in the cortex and striatum of Huntington's disease (HD) transgenic mice [32]. Furthermore, an elevated expression level of proteasome subunit gene PMSE3 was found in multiple pathological conditions such as cancer, rheumatoid arthritis, Sjogren's syndrome, and connective-tissue diseases [63].

In summary, the function of proteasome is tightly associated with aging and aging-related disorders; the early occurrence of proteasome dysfunction in these conditions indicates the causal role of proteasome system. Nevertheless, the cause(s) of proteasomal dysfunction is widely investigated and oxidative stress is one of the factors identified. Most likely, proteasomal alteration may be part of the aging process. In other words, proteasomal function decline occurs regularly along with aging. Evidence indicates that oxidative stress plays a critical role in aging and aging related disorders. Consequently, the proteasome system is involved in the generation of oxidative stress. Due to cellular respiration, there is constant oxidative damage in cellular proteins, and the majority of oxidized proteins are cleaned up by the proteasome system. The inhibition of proteasome function induced oxidative stress and elevated levels of oxidized and ubiquitinated proteins [64]. Conversely, the inhibition of proteasome activity could also be induced by oxidized substrate proteins and oxidative damage in proteasome subunits [65]. The oxidative stress and proteasome inhibition could be synergistic [66]. In pathological conditions, inhibition of proteasome sometimes showed protective effects: the cardiac superoxide dismutase 1 and 2 were increased, the autophagic response was triggered and inflammation was delayed [67]. Therefore, the correlation between oxidative stress and proteasome dysfunction might be another chicken-egg paradox. The actual interaction between proteasome inhibition and oxidative stress may vary along with different cellular conditions in the aging process.

Protein aggregation occurs commonly in aging and aging related disorders. The senile plaques and tangles in AD, Lewy bodies and Lewy threads in PD and DLB, and the mutant huntingtin aggregates in HD are well documented examples of protein aggregation. Inhibition of proteasome and lysosome systems could induce α-synuclein aggregation directly [68], and protein aggregation could induce proteasome dysfunction as well [69]. Nevertheless, proteasomal subunits could also form aggregates [70]. Although the proteasome impairment and protein aggregation mostly occur in pathological conditions [70, 71], protein aggregation could form in healthy cells without inhibition of proteasome and may have detox function [72]. In summary, dysfunction of proteasome is sufficient to induce protein aggregation and even cell death; conversely, protein aggregation could induce proteasome inhibition in selected conditions. Generally, proteasome is responsible to remove protein aggregation, but their interaction is not a simple two-element game; other factors including oxidative stress and ubiquitination/deubiquitination might also take part in the interaction.

UBIQUITINATION, SUMOYLATION AND NEDDYLATION IN AD

In proteasome system, the proteins are degraded through ubiquitin independent and ubiquitin-dependent pathways and the latter is the major process. Generally, ubiquitination is the process in which a protein is modified for degradation or other metabolic processes like cell cycle control and cell death as described above [24]. The ubiquitin marking process is conducted by a series of enzymes (E1, E2, E3, deubiquitinases (DUB)). The alteration of ubiquitin and the related enzymes dramatically affects the proteasome function. For example, ubiquitin, E1, E2 and E3 had increased expression levels after treatment with oxidative low-density lipoprotein (ox-LDL) [73], and overexpression of ubiquitin could reduce the protein aggregates and extend the lifespan of HD transgenic mice [74]. On the contrary, mutation in ubiquitin activating enzyme E1 could significantly reduce the lifespan of Drosophila [75]. Mutation of ubiquitin is directly associated with Aβ accumulation and deposition in AD [60]. The mutation in ubiquitin and associated enzymes is involved in the development of multiple diseases including Angelman syndrome [76], Paget's disease-like disorder [77], and Charcot-Mari--Tooth disease [78]. These data indicated the critical position of ubiquitination in proteasome system as well as in other cellular metabolism pathways.

Ubiquitination associates with AD directly. It is reported that higher level of ubiquitin may be used as a diagnostic marker of AD, which is comparable to other identified markers like Aβ42 and tau, or apolipoprotein Eε4 [79]. Ubiquitin carboxyl-terminal hydrolase L1 (UCHL1) is a DUB enzyme, which interacts with APP, regulates Aβ production, and increases free ubiquitin level to accelerate the lysosomal degradation of APP. Overexpression of UCHL1 reduced Aβ production, inhibited neuronal plaque formation, and improved memory deficits in AD [80].

In addition, human AD brains had elevated level of histone protein H3/H4 and their acetylation, which was correlated with elevated ubiquitin level [81]. An E3 ubiquitin ligase, HRD1 was reported to have lower level in AD brains due to its insolubility, which was induced by oxidative stress, contributed to increased Aβ production, endoplasmic reticulum stress and apoptosis [82]. It is clear that a genetic analysis indicated that protein ubiquitination was one of the prime targets for AD therapeutic development [83].

Related to ubiquitination, sumoylation is another process of post-translational protein modification that is involved in the regulation of gene expression, protein stability, stress response and cell cycle control. SUMO represents Small Ubiquitin-like Modifier, which is a group of small proteins that can covalently associate with other proteins to alter their structure and function. Similar to ubiquitination, sumoylation also needs a group of enzymes to finish the modification. In contrast to ubiquitination, sumoylation is not involved in protein degradation but involved in the pathogenesis of AD. A SUMO enzyme SENP3 had significant decreased expression in sporadic AD patients [84], acute proteasome inhibition leads to decreased sumoylation and increased ubiquitination of protein tau, which is another causal protein as Aβ in AD [85]. Interestingly, overexpression of SUMO2 greatly reduced Aβ production, but inhibition of sumoylation did not affect either APP or Aβ levels [86, 87]. So sumoylation may indirectly affect APP processing. For example, the GTPase dynamin related protein (DRP1) is required for mitochondrial fission, sumoylation of DRP1 protected the protein from degradation and localizes DRP1 in cytosol. It is reported that the DRP1 levels were significantly reduced, leading to abnormal mitochondrial morphology and distribution in AD brains [88]. In return, the onset of AD could dramatically alter sumoylation in varied directions [89, 90].

Another process that associates with ubiquitination is neddylation, which utilizes a small protein NEDD8 to covalently modify other proteins. NEDD8 shares 60% homology with ubiquitin and usual conjugates to limited substrate proteins, including culins, which are a family of hydrophobic proteins providing a scaffold for ubiquitin ligases E3. APP is also a substrate of NEDD8 in the intracellular domain, and the neddylation of APP inhibited its signaling by reducing the interaction between APP and FE65 [91]. Neddylation has been involved in AD pathogenesis. NEDD8 is located in cytoplasm in AD hippocampal neurons and located in nucleus in age-matched control subjects [92]. The neurofibrillary tangles and senile plaques from patients with AD contains NEDD8 [93], which could be erroneously incorporated into ubiquitin chains by the ubiquitination enzymes, especially under stress conditions and when the NEDD8/ubiquitin ratio is increased [94].

An ubiquitinated protein can be deubiquitinated as well, which is a process called deubiquitination. The enzymes that catalyze deubiquitination is known as DUB, and there are nearly 100 DUB in human genome, including the ubiquitin C-terminal hydrolases (UCH), ubiquitin specific proteases (USP), Machado-Joseph disease proteases (MJD), Otubain (OTU) Proteases (cysteine proteases), and JAB1/MPN/Mov34 Metallo-enzyme (JAMM) proteases (zinc-dependent metallo-proteases). These enzymes can completely remove ubiquitin from the substrate protein and recycle the free ubiquitin, or modify the polyubiquitin chain for different metabolic pathways [112]. The constitutive 19S proteasomal subunit, PSMD14, has DUB activity. Other DUB (such as USP14, and UCHL5) may also associate with the proteasome. They play roles in the process of protein degradation, and the removed ubiquitin could be used again in ubiquitination [113]. Recent reports indicated that ubiquitin may bind to Rpn11 (a yeast counterpart of PSMD14) to induce a conformational switch of Rpn11's Insert-1 loop from an inactive closed state to an active β hairpin, and to ensure the poly-ubiquitin chains are removed before the degradation of committed substrates [114]. One of the abundant DUB in human brain is UCHL1, reached almost 2%

of total protein [115]. UCHL1 protein level was reduced in the hippocampus of a mouse model of AD [116] and human AD brains [117]. Overexpression of UCHL1 could restore synaptic plasticity and cognitive defects [116], revealing its importance in the development of AD onset. DUB is also involved in other neurodegenerative disorders. For example, a mutation in UCHL1 caused family PD in human [118], and another DUB (USP9X) gene had altered expression in a mouse model of PD [119]. Triple mutation in a DUB (ataxin-3) directly lead to a neurodegenerative disorder Spinocerebellar Ataxia Type 3 (SCA3), also known as Machado-Joseph Disease [120].

IMMUNOPROTEASOME IN AGING AND AD

As described above, there are three inducible proteasome subunits (PSMB8, 9 and 10) that can replace three constitutive subunits (PSMB 5, 6 and 7) to form a special type of proteasome, so-called immunoproteasome. The immunoproteasome has similar catalytic activities as a regular proteasome, with functions specifically in immune responses. Generally, the immunoproteasome is critical in MHC class I antigen presentation, responsible for oxidative stress [95], and regulated by redox state [96]. Mutation in immunoproteasome subunits largely reduced the capacity to deal with oxidative stress [95] and knocking out PSMB8, 9 and 10 dramatically reduced the MHC class I antigen presentation in transgenic mice [97]. Impairment of immunoproteasome could also induce illness such as enterovirus myocarditis [6, 98]. On the other hand, oxidative stress, injury and aging could increase the expression of immunoproteasome [7, 99]. In addition, the accumulation of AGE (advanced glycation end products) could induce immunoproteasome through RAGE (receptor for AGE) signaling, and the long-living species had elevated immunoproteasome levels that indicated the possible role of immunoproteasome in longevity of mice [100]. In the rat hippocampus region, the content of immunoproteasome was increased along with aging [101] and this observation was confirmed in human [34]. It is believed that the elevated immunoproteasome was associated with chronic inflammation during pathological development [101]. It is well documented that immune dysfunction is coupled with aging, so the inducible proteasome subunits (PSMB 8, 9 and 10) are easy targets for genetic engineering and therapeutic development to improve immune function, aging and aging associated disorders.

THERAPEUTIC STUDY RELATED TO PROTEASOME

As discussed above, the proteasome system is involved in physiological and pathological processes, especially aging and aging related disorders. Therefore, the proteasome system becomes an active therapeutic target for disease, aging and related conditions. With biological and chemical agents, the proteasome system can be activated to extend lifespan or attenuate diseases [102]. As a hormone, ghrelin enhanced the activities of proteasome [103], and a receptor agonist (baclofen) could also elevate the proteasome activities to promote cell viability and improve HD symptoms in transgenic mice [104]. Overexpression of one proteasome subunit could enhance the expression of other proteasome subunits to promote the survival rate of culture cells under oxidative stress [105]. In another report, upregulation of proteasome catalytic subunits could not only restore the proteasomal activities but also extend the lifespan of skin cells [106]. Upregulation of a chaperone (POMP) that involves in proteasome complex assembling could improve proteasome function and resistance to oxidative stress [107]. Expressing a peptide (proteasome-activating peptide 1, PAP1) in cultured cells could improve the proteasome activity, and reduce oxidative damage and protein aggregation [108]. Furthermore, some chemical proteasome inhibitors like MLN9708 could increase antioxidant enzyme transcripts to elevate the cellular antioxidant levels including glutathione, gamma-globin, and Hb F [109]. Algae extract from *Phaeodactylum tricornutum* could preserve proteasome activities and reduce the oxidative damage from ultra violet irradiation [110]. A novel proteasome inhibitor VR23 was evidenced to reduce proteasome activities, and kill cancer cells selectively [111]. Bortezomib (PS-341) and carfilzomib (PR-171) are two inhibitors that can inhibit the activity of the 20S proteasomal complex, used as a treatment option for multiple myeloma and mantle cell lymphoma [112, 121]. These studies indicate the proteasome system is an effective target for therapeutic development with multiple approaches. For example, it is reported that inhibition of a DUB enzyme, USP14, could enhance the clearance of disease-related proteins, including tau (related to AD), TDP-43 (AD and Amyotrophic Lateral Sclerosis), and ataxin-3 (SCA3), so a special USP14 inhibitor was screened and identified, 1-[1-(4-fluorophenyl)-2,5-dimethylpropyl-3-yl]- 2-pyrrolidin-1-ylethanone (abbreviated as IU1), which can specifically reduce the catalytic activity of USP14 [122]. It has been found that hyperphosphorylated tau oligomers accumulated in synaptic neurons, which induced the dysfunction of proteasome [123]. Protein kinase A (PKA) was found to activate the assembling and activities of proteasome by the phosphorylation of proteasome subunit PSMD11 through cAMP signaling pathways [124]. Furthermore, as a phosphodiesterase inhibitor, rolipram could increase cAMP and PKA levels and subsequently enhance the proteasome activity to improve cognition [125]. New reports revealed new conformation changes of the proteasomal subunits and novel interaction proteins, which may also be the targets for therapeutic development [126].

SOME CLINICAL TRAILS FOR AD

Currently, there is no cure for AD, and the approved medicines are mainly focused on the symptomatic, short-term benefits, which could not affect the pathogenic mechanisms of the disease. The medicines include cholinesterase inhibitors (donepezil, rivastigmine, galantamine), and the NMDA receptor antagonist, memantine. These drugs may provide neuronal protection but cannot counteract the development of AD [127, 128]. Therefore, developing disease-specific drugs is critical for the treatment of AD. Presently nearly 2000 clinical trials related with AD have been conducted worldwide and among them, there are more than 200 active clinical trials to explore the different therapeutic strategies that may deal with protein misfolding, Aβ clearance, neurotransmitter signaling, and other metabolic pathways. The following are some examples of AD clinical trials.

Clinical Trials for Verubecestat (MK-8931)

MK-8931 has been reported to selectively inhibit the activity of β-secretase, so the production of Aβ could be reduced. It has been tested in AD mice model and human patients [129]. There are five clinical trials for MK-8931: phase I (NCT01496170), covered 32 patients from 2011 to 2012, used a dose of 12 or 40 mg orally, once per day for 7 days; phase II and III (NCT01739348) had more than 2000 patients enrolled from 2012 to 2017; the continued clinical trial (NCT01953601) has more than 1000 patients enrolled and will be finished in 2019. Participants had been randomized to receive placebo, or 12 mg to 40 mg verubecestat, once daily. This trial is conducted by the test of the Clinical Dementia Rating scale-Sum of Boxes (CDR-SB) score at 104 weeks, and a long term double-blind extension to assess efficacy and safety of verubecestat administered for up to an additional 260 weeks. The other two clinical trials (NCT01537757, NCT02910739) had fewer patients (12, 16) enrolled and were conducted in short times (3 months, 6 months).

Clinical Trials for Pinitol (NIC5-15)

Pinitol is a natural product in soy and several other plants, having β-secretase inhibition and mild insulin sensitizing effects [130]. The first clinical trial (NCT00470418) involving pinitol covered 15 patients who received escalating doses of 1500, 3000 and 5000 mg daily over the course of the study (2007-2010). The second clinical trial (NCT01928420) covered 40 patients (2010-2013). The results showed encouraging data but lacked statistical significance due to the number of subjects.

Clinical Trials for EVP-0962

EVP-0962 was reported as the γ-secretase inhibitor that involved in the production of Aβ and modulation of cathepsin B. The clinical trial

(NCT01661673) has two parts, the first part was to evaluate its safety and tolerability in healthy subjects and the second part was to evaluate similar indexes in patients with mild cognitive impairment (MCI) or early AD. The doses were 10, 50 100 and 200 mg administered once-daily for 14 days. It was conducted from 2012 to 2013, and the enrollment was 52.

Clinical Trials for EGCG (Epigallocatechin-Gallate)

EGCG is a natural product found in tea, apples, pecans and onions *etc* [131]. It is believed to have an antioxidant effect and can promote the activity of α-secretase. There have been two clinical trials for EGCG: One was for AD (NCT00951834) and was conducted from 2009 to 2015, with 21 people enrolled. The maximum dose was two cups of black tea/diet and no more than 500 ml/diet of grapefruit juice. Another was for Down Syndrome (NCT01699711) and was conducted from 2012 to 2015, enrolling 87 patients who were given oral doses containing 9 mg/kg (range 6.9-12.7) of EGCG for 12 months.

Clinical Trials for Tramiprosate (3APS)

3APS is a synthetic compound with GABAergic activity that may have anti-aggregation effects [132, 133]. It is analogous to taurine, but with an extra carbon in its chain. It can resemble the effects of GABA. The clinical trial (NCT00088673) started in 2004 with about 950 AD patients to "evaluate the efficacy and safety of 3APS as an add-on therapy to most standard medication for Alzheimer's disease." It was followed by a clinical trial (NCT00217763) conducted in Europe to further evaluate its efficacy. About 940 mild/moderate AD patients were enrolled from 2005 to 2007. Under the same sponsor (Bellus Health Inc.) another clinical trial (NCT00314912) started in 2006 to study the long-term safety and efficacy of 3APS with 650 AD patients enrolled.

Clinical Trials for Bexarotene

Bexarotene is a third-generation retinoid that has been used in lung cancer and breast cancer [134, 135] and may help in ApoE activation and Aβ clearance. One clinical trial (NCT01782742) had 20 patients enrolled in 2013-2014 to evaluate its efficacy and safety in mild/moderate AD patients. Another one (CT02061878) had 12 people enrolled in 2014. The subjects were administered three (3, 75 mg/capsule) capsules twice daily (450 mg/day) for five days.

Clinical Trials for Estrogen

Estrogen is a hormone in all vertebrates and some insects [136] that has vast functions in development and metabolism. There are 11 clinic trials for AD on record. Nine of them are completed and two remain active: NCT01982578 started in 2013 and will be completed in 2018. It has about 50 people enrolled to investigate the effect of 60 mg BID of genistein administration during 180 days in AD patients. The NCT03101085 started in 2017 and will be completed in 2019. It is designed to study the compound S-equol, which acts like estrogen in human body, to see if it can improve the mitochondrial activity and cognition. About 40 people are enrolled in this study.

Clinical Trials for Azeliragon

Azeliragon is a selective inhibitor for RAGE (receptor for advanced glycation end products), which is a membrane-anchored protein involved in the pro-inflammatory response of many pathologic developments, including AD [137]. There are three clinical trials on record focusing on Azeliragon, also termed PF 04494700 or TTP488. One trial (NCT00566397) started in 2007 and is expected to complete in 2010, with about 402 AD patients involved to evaluate its safety and efficacy of cognitive function. Another one (NCT02080364) started in 2015 and will complete in 2019, with about 800 enrollments. Patients will receive either azeliragon or placebo lasting approximately 18 months. The other one (NCT02916056) started in 2016 and will complete in 2020, with 640 patients involved.

Clinical Trials for Valproic Acid

Valproic acid is a medicine used to treat epilepsy and bipolar disorder, and to prevent migraine headaches [138]. It is also reported that valproic acid may enhance the activity of neprilysin (NEP), a peptidase that can degrade Aβ [139]. A clinical trial (NCT01729598) was conducted from 2012 to 2014 with 12 normal people enrolled. Two doses of valproate were used (250 mg PO bid, followed by 500 mg PO bid) to evaluate the safety and effects of valproic acid. Another clinical trial (NCT00071721) had 303 AD patients enrolled, and was conducted during 2003-2009, tried to "demonstrate whether valproate therapy delays the emergence of agitation and/or psychosis in outpatients with probable Alzheimer's disease (AD) who have not experienced agitation and psychosis in their illness." The third clinical trial (NCT00088387) had 35 AD patients enrolled, was conducted in 2004-2005, "to examine the acute effects of lithium alone and/or in combination with divalproex on surrogate measures of neuroprotective activity in patients with Alzheimer's disease." The last clinic trial (NCT00375557) was withdrawn before it really started.

Clinical Trials for Bapineuzumab

Bapineuzumab is an antibody that could recognize Aβ. There are 14 clinical trials for it but all of them were completed or stopped before/in 2013, and none of them obtained significant data to remove Aβ in AD patients [140]. In addition, patients receiving higher doses were found developing abnormal brain imaging, such as increased brain fluid [141].

Clinical Trials for Lithium

Lithium salts were reported to inhibit the activity of the enzyme glycogen synthase kinase-3beta (GSK3), which was found overactive in AD patients [142], so lithium is proposed for the treatment of AD. GSK3 is involved in the hyperphosphorylation of tau protein and the production of beta-amyloid peptide, the chronic lithium administration is associated with a decrement in the expected prevalence of dementia. So far there are six clinical trials on record, the earliest one (NCT00870311) had only 28 people enrolled, started in 1996 and completed in 2004. Two clinical trials were conducted in a short period: NCT00088387 had 35 patients involved, started in 2004 and completed in 2005; another one (NCT02204969) had 100 people enrolled, started in January and completed in December of 2015. There are three clinical trials still active: NCT01055392 had 80 people enrolled and started in 2007 but no further results reported; NCT02129348 also has 80 people involved, started in 2014 and will complete in 2019; the last one (NCT03185208) has 80 people enrolled, will start in 2017 and complete in 2022.

Clinical Trial for Methylene Blue

Methylene blue is a dye used for urinary tract infection, cyanide poisoning and methemoglobinemia [143]. A recent study indicated that methylene blue has important neuroprotective effects to reduce tau oligomerization [144]. The clinic trial (NCT02380573) started in 2015 and will complete in 2019. There are 240 patients enrolled and more patients are being recruited.

Clinical Trial for Rilapladib

Rilapladib is an inhibitor for Lipoprotein-Associated Phospholipase A2, which is reported to involve in many pathological conditions including hyperlipidaemia, stroke, Type 1 and Type 2 diabetes mellitus, and AD [145]. A clinic trial (NCT01428453) started in 2011, with 124 people enrolled, completed in 2013. A followed clinic trial (NCT02130661) was withdrawn before it started.

Besides the clinic trials listed above, there are many more clinic trials that focused on different aspects of AD pathogenesis, including anti-inflammatory, anti-oxidative stress, glia cell modulation, mitochondria dysfunction, and multiple-targets agents. Most of the completed clinic trials have limited or no significance, and some ongoing clinic trials have encouraging data but still need further evidence. As we have discussed above, the proteasome is highly involved in the development and onset of AD, but currently there are no clinical trials focused on proteasome, lysosome or ubiquitin pathways. One reason is that the proteasome system is not controlled by one gene or one factor, and traditional clinic trials used to focus on a single compound, which may not have significant effects. The second reason is that AD patients have decreased proteasomal activity, and it is hard to find a simple strategy to enhance it; on the contrary, it is easy to find an inhibitor. The third reason is that most of the clinical trials recruited patients after the onset of AD, which may be too late to show significance, so the early diagnosis and biomarker development for AD is one of the key factors for pharmaceutical development. The last reason is that the complexity of human body, personal index, lifestyle, diet and many other factors may interact with the drug administration.

AD MANAGEMENT: DIET

Food is the source of the energy and nutrients for the human body, but it also can be the source of disease. Issues like "what kind of food," "how much of it," "how to eat it," and "when to eat it" may affect one's health dramatically. A diet with enriched vegetables could reduce the risk of AD [146], nutrients like folic acid, vitamin B12, choline, zinc, selenium, dietary polyphenols are believed to interact with epigenetic mechanisms and alter gene expression profile so the vulnerability of neurons in human brain may be affected and the incidence of AD would change [147]. The Mediterranean diet, which has a higher level of vegetables and lower level of meat, could significantly reduce the incidence of MCI and AD by 33% and reduce the chance to progress MCI to AD [148]. In addition, a lower-copper diet could be an effective prevention for AD [149]. Moreover, alcohol consumption, meat and rice content in the diet correlated highly with AD incidence [150]. Omega-3 fatty acids were reported to slow down the progress of AD [151]. There are 10 clinical trials to test the effects of omega-3 fatty acids in AD. The earliest one started in 2000 and three active clinical trials are still in progress (NCT02541929, NCT01953705, NCT02719327). In animal models, high-fat diets had rapid and long-lasting effects on the memory [152], which supports the observation in human subjects. Furthermore, some researchers believe that intestinal microbial flora is associated with the initiation of AD pathogenesis, so keeping a healthy intestinal ecosystem is very important in the prevention of AD [153], and a high dose of vitamin D is also beneficial [154]. In summary, a general diet guideline to reduce the risk of AD is as follows:

1. Reduce the intake of saturated fats and trans-fats, and increase the intake of omega-3 fats. Basically, limit the intake of red meat, dairy products, fried food,

coconut oil and palm oil; use fish instead.

2. Increase the intake of fresh vegetables, especially leafy vegetables, and plant-derived products (grains, beans, lentils fruits, *etc.*) rather than animal-derived products (meats, dairy, *etc.*).
3. Increase the intake of vitamin A, vitamin E, vitamin D and B12. Good sources are plant seeds, nuts, green leafy vegetables, and whole grains.
4. Minimize the intake and exposure to iron, copper and aluminium. Pay attention to the mineral components in supplements and multiple vitamins, baking powder, *etc.*
5. Increase the intake of water, not soda. Pay attention to the hardness of the water in your home.
6. Reduce the total calorie intake by 15-30%. Calorie restriction (CR) is the most common and supported strategy to reduce the incidence and delay the onset of AD. Interestingly, CR is also effective for preventing cancers.
7. Reduce the calorie amount of dinner and increased the calorie amount of breakfast, even the daily calorie amount will not change. Such relocation of food will reduce the digestive interruption in sleeping, improve the quality of sleeping and neuronal functions.

AD MANAGEMENT: SLEEPING

Sleeping is an important part of human life, and is critical to the normal function of human brain. The sleep-wake cycle has significant influence on the onset and progress of AD, and sleep disorders or deprivation contributed to Aβ deposition. On the contrary, adequate sleep reduces plaque formation in human brain [155]. About 45% of AD patients suffer from sleep disruption, which reveals the association between sleep and AD. Hypocretin is the regulator of arousal and wakefulness, increased Aβ deposition was observed in hypocretin knock-out mice although overexpression of hypocretin did not affect the Aβ deposition [156]. In a mouse model of AD, the slow-wave activity was severely altered and induced Aβ-dependent impairment in the neocortex, thalamus and hippocampus [157]. The reduced neuron number in the hypothalamic ventrolateral preoptic nucleus in AD may contribute to the fragmented sleeping of AD patients [158]. In animal experiments, sleep deprivation had a significant decline in their learning and memory, significant increase of insoluble tau fraction, lower levels of postsynaptic density protein-95 and increased glial fibrillary acidic protein levels [159]. The sleep deprivation associated with a progressive increase in the resting level of Ca^{2+}, which interfered with the rhythm rheostat that associated with the accumulation of Aβ oligomers, further deregulated Ca^{2+} signaling and inflammatory response [160]. Interestingly, a carefully orchestrated light/dark pattern has been conducted in AD patients and control people, was evidenced to be a powerful non-pharmacological tool to improve sleep efficiency and consolidation [161]. Melatonin is an endogenous human hormone that regulates the sleep-wake cycle. It is reported that melatonin is decreased in AD patients and the add-on of 2mg melatonin to AD patients had positive effects on cognitive functioning and sleep maintenance in AD patients compared with placebo [162], and two clinical trials related with melatonin (NCT00940589, NCT00000171) had been conducted. Improving the quality and quantity of sleep would reduce the risk of amyloid pathology as well as improve cognitive function. Compared to the expense of other therapy (if any), this should ultimately be a priority in AD management.

AD MANAGEMENT: LIFESTYLE

Lifestyle is another factor that may contribute to the onset and development of AD. A systematic analysis indicated that smoking is highly associated with the risk of AD, caffeine consumption has mild association, and physical activity shows protective effects [163]. A seven-year follow-up study indicated strong association between AD risk and current smoking/daily drinking in 3170 elderly men [164], and the baseline body mineral density, bone loss rate, current smoking, and daily drinking were associated with increased risk of AD [165]. Although some statistic data indicated alcohol consuming and smoking did not increase the AD risk, the odds ratio was 1.1 for alcohol and 0.7 for smoking [166]. In fact, the amount of alcohol consumption and smoking really made a difference: moderate alcohol consumption was associated with lower risk of AD [167], and heavy smoking in midlife doubled the risk of dementia and AD [168]. Furthermore, the risk for smoking is associated with the ApoE status. The patients without the allele ApoEϵ4 had an odds ratio 4.6 while the patients with that allele had an odds ratio only 0.6 [169]. In addition, religious people had much lower risk of dementia and AD [170]. Such data indicate the complexity of human body, and a linear, simple analysis may not be able to discover the underlined mechanisms.

AD MANAGEMENT: GENDER

The incidence of AD differs in different genders: at age 65, the odds of getting AD is about 1/6 in females and 1/11 in males. In the United Kingdom, about 15% women died due to AD and other dementia in 2015 [171]. Some studies reported that mitochondria dysfunction and decreased estrogen level in elder females may play a role in the gender difference, but the detailed mechanism is still unclear [172]. Ten clinical trials for estrogen have been completed, but none of them showed significant difference and one more clinical trial is still active (as discussed above), while few of them reported gender difference. It is reported that features of pathological progress were different in psychotic AD patients in the frontal cortex: in females, phosphorylated tau was much higher and in male the presence of α-synuclein pathology was more obvious [173]. Females had accelerated age-related myelin breakdown compared to males [174], and acute psychosocial stressor caused memory impairment in women only [175]. In addition, a polymorphism of the BDNF gene (Met66) that may reduce BDNF transport was associated with increased AD risk in women but not in men [176]. Meanwhile, males had much more neuropsychiatric symptoms than females [177], more severe periventricular white matter hyperintensities, and poorer global cognitive function [178]. The genetic variants of the reelin (RELN) gene (rs528528 T/T and rs607755 A/A) were associated with the susceptibility to AD only in males [179], and cataract associated with AD only in male elders [180]. After the onset of AD, the rate of cognitive decline is different: the females progressed much faster than males [181]. Therefore, the genetic, physiological, psychological and environmental factors may all contribute to the vulnerability of female to AD, and further clinical trials should design new experimental strategies to recognize the gender difference for conclusive results.

AD MANAGEMENT: ASSOCIATION WITH OTHER DISEASES

AD patients usually share a lot of common issues with other pathological conditions. For example, AD and type 2 diabetes both have impaired glucose uptake, defective insulin release and signaling, amyloidosis, abnormal lipid peroxidation, brain atrophy, increased AGE formation and tau phosphorylation, impaired lipid metabolism and mitochondrial dysfunction [182]. In fact, diabetes is a risk factor for AD [183], and insulin therapy in diabetes could reduce the risk of AD [184]. Immune-mediated diseases like psoriasis, and Crohn disease had genetic overlap with AD [185]. Heart failure may contribute to the dysfunction of the neurovascular unit and cause an energy crisis in neurons and increase AD risk [186]. AD patients had impaired endothelial function that correlated with the severe level of AD, revealed the vascular issues in AD pathogenesis [187], and the cognitive regression is correlated with cardiovascular risk factors [188]. In addition, high systolic blood pressure and serum cholesterol concentration was associated with increased AD risk [189]. On the contrary, AD has inverse relationship with cancer. The P53 signaling, expression of neurotrophins and growth factors, growth and proliferation pathways, cAMP, EGFR, Bcl-2, apoptosis pathways, IGF-1, HSV, TDP-43, APOE variants, Carbonic anhydrases, HSPs, and SAPK are down regulated in AD but upregulated in cancer [190].

Besides the classified pathological conditions, the risk of AD is also associated with general infection. In a meta-analysis, the incidence of AD increased by ten-fold with spirochetal infection, increased by five-fold with *C. pneumoniae* infection [191], early-life or life-long exposure to infectious agents may increase the risk to develop AD at a later age [192]. Specifically, chronic *T. gondii* infection induced neuro-inflammation through cytokine networks and resulted in pathological progression of AD [193]. Higher AD prevalence and more pronounced cognitive impairment were correlated with the infection of *H. pylori* [194]. HSV-1 infection upregulated the expression of neprilysin and glycogen synthase kinase 3β, which are involved in the Aβ deposition and tau hyperphosphorylation [195]. The number of senescent T cells, and the formation of neurofibrillary tangles was highly associated with the presence of CMV in AD patients [196]. Furthermore, fungal infection was detected in AD brain samples [197], and the fungal cells were internalized inside the neuron cells [198], revealing the possible involvement of fungal infection in AD pathogenesis.

FUTURE DIRECTIONS

The Alzheimer's Association published a report to summarize the current condition of research and clinic progress in AD [199]. It is estimated that 5.4 million Americans have AD. In United States about every 66 seconds a person displays AD onset, and by 2050, possibly every 33 second one person would develop AD. In 2013, there were 84,767 AD death records in United States, and in 2016, an estimated 700,000 Americans may die with AD. In 2016, the leading causes of death were heart disease, cancer (malignant neoplasms), chronic lower respiratory disease, accidents (unintentional injuries), stroke (cerebrovascular diseases), and AD. Between 2000 and 2013, the mortality rate resulting from stroke, and heart disease decreased by 23%, and 14%, respectively; meanwhile, the mortality rate for AD increased by 71%. Total payments in 2016 for health care, long-term care and hospice services for people with dementia were estimated to be $236 billion, Medicaid payments for each dementia patient were 19 times as great as all beneficiaries without dementia. So the challenge from AD and other forms of dementia is getting severe. The dramatic increase in the number of research articles and clinical trials for AD indicates our urgent concern to AD that may need new, creative strategies to move forward the study and pharmaceutic development of AD. As we have discussed above, the hallmark of AD is the aggregated proteins (plaques, tangles, and Lewy bodies, *etc.*) so the proteasome and lysosome systems should play an important role in the therapeutic study. Of course, it is still not clear if the oligo Aβ and hyperphosphorylated tau are the actual initiating cause of AD, even though removal or decrease of the aggregation will definitely move us one step closer to the cure of AD. Due to the complex homeostatic feature of human body, which is a balanced system, any single input would induce the change of multiple pathways; that may be one of the reasons that a lot of clinical trials did not get positive results. We propose some considerations to aid in the experimental and clinical design in AD study:

1. Numerous clinical trials indicated that after the onset of AD, it is very difficult

to stop or slow down the cascade of pathological progress. Therefore, early diagnosis is critical for the prevention and treatment of AD, and developing useful biomarkers is the priority of AD study.

2. Focus on some proteasomal subunits that have been downregulated in AD, such as PSMB8. PSMB8 is an inducible subunit and is closely related with immune function, overexpress PSMB8 would be a feasible choice since the proteasome is inhibited in AD and overexpression of the proteasomal subunits may put the protein metabolism back to balance. In addition, some 19S regulatory subunits like PSMD10, ubiquitin enzymes like E1, and autophagy inducers may also be good targets to regain the normal function of proteasome and lysosome.
3. Some proteasome activating agents like POMP, and PAP1 could be valuable targets to develop therapies.
4. Design new strategies for clinical trials: find the key step in signaling pathways, avoid linear simple input, grouping participants in a way with consideration of gender, personal characters, lifestyles, and diet supply, *etc.*
5. One unique issue in human is the individual diversity due to different lifestyles and personal characteristics that may put each patient in a specific condition. So a treatment may need to consider the individual physiological and pathological profile for every patient to design a therapeutic strategy. One possible idea is to conduct genetic screening on each patient, identify a special causal gene, and then using genetic engineering techniques to manipulate its expression (miRNA *etc.*) based on the screening results. A similar strategy may also apply to causal peptides to induce individual patient-specific antibody.
6. Neurodegeneration basically is cell death and cancer is cell outgrowth. A lot of target genes have been identified from cancer research like cell cycle control factors, which may be used in the AD brain to promote neuron regeneration.
7. Neurodegeneration is generally protein metabolic dysfunction, and we have discussed that protein synthesis and degradation are tightly associated. Factors that can improve the quality of protein synthesis like protein chaperones, NAC components, ubiquitin and ubiquitin-like molecules can be genetically modified and used to promote the ribosomal function.
8. Develop nutrition and lifestyle training/education procedure, reduce the AD risk of elder population. Based on the research data we have discussed, diet and lifestyle dramatically affect one's health, so modifying the diet and lifestyle based on each person's individual condition would significantly reduce the AD risk and delay the onset time.

CONSENT FOR PUBLICATION

Not applicable.

CONFLICT OF INTEREST

The authors declare no conflict of interest, financial or otherwise.

ACKNOWLEDGEMENTS

Professor Matthew Stewart from English department have edited and proofread the manuscript, and provided valuable discussion and help.

REFERENCES

[1] Etlinger JD, Goldberg AL. A soluble ATP-dependent proteolytic system responsible for the degradation of abnormal proteins in reticulocytes. Proc Natl Acad Sci USA 1977; 74: 54-8. [http://dx.doi.org/10.1073/pnas.74.1.54]

[2] Hershko A, Ciechanover A. The ubiquitin system. Annu Rev Biochem 1998; 67: 425-79. [http://dx.doi.org/10.1146/annurev.biochem.67.1.425]

[3] Anjum RS, Bray SM, *et al.* Involvement of a eukaryotic-like ubiquitin-related modifier in the proteasome pathway of the archaeon Sulfolobus acidocaldarius. Nat Commun 2015; 6: 8163. [http://dx.doi.org/10.1038/ncomms9163]

[4] Goldberg AL, Akopian TN, Kisselev AF, Lee DH, Rohrwild M. New insights into the mechanisms and importance of the proteasome in intracellular protein degradation. Biol Chem 1997; 378: 131-40.

[5] Ding Q, Dimayuga E, Keller JN. Oxidative damage, protein synthesis, and protein degradation in Alzheimer's disease. Curr Alzheimer Res 2007; 4: 73-9. [http://dx.doi.org/10.2174/156720507779939788]

[6] Warnatsch A, Bergann T, Krüger E. Oxidation matters: the ubiquitin proteasome system connects innate immune mechanisms with MHC class I antigen presentation. Mol Immunol 2013; 55: 106-9. [http://dx.doi.org/10.1016/j.molimm.2012.10.007]

[7] Basler M, Kirk CJ, Groettrup M. The immunoproteasome in antigen processing and other immunological functions. Curr Opin Immunol 2013; 25: 74-80. [http://dx.doi.org/10.1016/j.coi.2012.11.004]

[8] Rivett AJ, Palmer A, Knecht E. Electron microscopic localization of the multicatalytic proteinase complex in rat liver and in cultured cells. J Histochem Cytochem 1992; 40(8): 1165-72. [http://dx.doi.org/10.1177/40.8.1619280]

[9] Scherrer K, Bey F. The prosomes (multicatalytic proteinases; proteasomes) and their relationship to the untranslated messenger ribonucleoproteins, the cytoskeleton, and cell differentiation. Prog Nucleic Acid Res Mol Biol 1994; 49: 1-64. [http://dx.doi.org/10.1016/S0079-6603(08)60047-1]

[10] Tanaka K, Yoshimura T, Tamura T, Fujiwara T, Kumatori A, Ichihara A. Possible mechanism of nuclear translocation of proteasomes. FEBS Lett 1990; 271(1-2): 41-6. [http://dx.doi.org/10.1016/0014-5793(90)80367-R]

[11] de Mateo S, Castillo J, Estanyol JM, Ballescà JL, Oliva R. Proteomic characterization of the human sperm nucleus. Proteomics 2011; 11(13): 2714-26. [http://dx.doi.org/10.1002/pmic.201000799]

[12] Qian MX, Pang Y, Liu CH, *et al.* Acetylation-mediated proteasomal degradation of core histones during DNA repair and spermatogenesis. Cell 2013; 153(5): 1012-24. [http://dx.doi.org/10.1016/j.cell.2013.04.032] [PMID: 23706739]

[13] Ohigashi I, Ohte Y, Setoh K, *et al.* A human PSMB11 variant affects thymoproteasome processing and CD8+ T cell production. JCI Insight 2017; 2(10): 93664.

[http://dx.doi.org/10.1172/jci.insight.93664]

[14] Jacobson AD, MacFadden A, Wu Z, Peng J, Liu CW. Autoregulation of the 26S proteasome by in situ ubiquitination. Mol. Biocell 2014; 25(12): 1824-35.

[15] Matilla A, Gorbea C, Einum DD, *et al.* Association of ataxin-7 with the proteasome subunit S4 of the 19S regulatory complex. Hum Mol Genet 2001; 10: 2821-31. [http://dx.doi.org/10.1093/hmg/10.24.2821]

[16] Yanagi S, Shimbara N, Tamura T. Tissue and cell distribution of a mammalian proteasomal ATPase, MSS1, and its complex formation with the basal transcription factors. Biochem Biophys Res Commun 2000; 279: 568-73. [http://dx.doi.org/10.1006/bbrc.2000.3969]

[17] Lee JW, Choi HS, Gyuris J, Brent R, Moore DD. Two classes of proteins dependent on either the presence or absence of thyroid hormone for interaction with the thyroid hormone receptor. Molec Endocr 1995; 9: 243-54.

[18] Qiu W, Wu J, Walsh EM, *et al.* Retinoblastoma protein modulates gankyrin-MDM2 in regulation of p53 stability and chemosensitivity in cancer cells. Oncogene 2008; 27(29): 4034-43. [http://dx.doi.org/10.1038/onc.2008.43]

[19] Sun J, Luan Y, Xiang D, *et al.* The 11S proteasome subunit PSME3 is a positive feedforward regulator of NF-κB and important for host defense against bacterial pathogens. Cell Reports 2016; 14(4): 737-49. [http://dx.doi.org/10.1016/j.celrep.2015.12.069]

[20] Zhang Z, Zhang R. Proteasome activator PA28 gamma regulates p53 by enhancing its MDM2-mediated degradation. EMBO J 2008; 27(6): 852-64. [http://dx.doi.org/10.1038/emboj.2008.25]

[21] Ustrell V, Hoffman L, Pratt G, Rechsteiner M. PA200, a nuclear proteasome activator involved in DNA repair. EMBO J 2002; 21(13): 3516-25. [http://dx.doi.org/10.1093/emboj/cdf333]

[22] Wang Q, Chen L, Wang Y, Li W, He L, Jiang H. Expression characteristics of two ubiquitin/ribosomal fusion protein genes in the developing testis, accessory gonad and ovary of Chinese mitten crab, Eriocheir sinensis. Mol Biol Rep 2012; 39(6): 6683-92. [http://dx.doi.org/10.1007/s11033-012-1474-6]

[23] Park CW, Ryu KY. Cellular ubiquitin pool dynamics and homeostasis. BMB Rep 2014; 47(9): 475-82. [http://dx.doi.org/10.5483/BMBRep.2014.47.9.128]

[24] Li W, Bengtson MH, Ulbrich A, *et al.* Genome-wide and functional annotation of human E3 ubiquitin ligases identifies MULAN, a mitochondrial E3 that regulates the organelle's dynamics and signaling. PLoS One 2008; 3(1): e1487. [http://dx.doi.org/10.1371/journal.pone.0001487]

[25] Settembre C, Fraldi A, Medina DL, Ballabio A. Signals from the lysosome: a control centre for cellular clearance and energy metabolism. Nat Rev Mol Cell Biol 2013; 14(5): 283-96. [http://dx.doi.org/10.1038/nrm3565]

[26] Kim ST, Tasaki T, Zakrzewska A, *et al.* The N-end rule proteolytic system in autophagy. Autophagy 2013; 9(7): 1100-3. [http://dx.doi.org/10.4161/auto.24643]

[27] Yong-Kee CJ, Warre R, Monnier PP, Lozano AM, Nash JE. Evidence for synergism between cell death mechanisms in a cellular model of neurodegeneration in Parkinson's disease. Neurotox Res 2012; 22(4): 355-64. [http://dx.doi.org/10.1007/s12640-012-9325-8]

[28] Vogiatzi T, Xilouri M, Vekrellis K, Stefanis L. Wild type alpha-synuclein is degraded by chaperone-mediated autophagy and macroautophagy in neuronal cells. J Biol Chem 2008; 283(35): 23542-56.

[http://dx.doi.org/10.1074/jbc.M801992200]

[29] Uchiki T, Weikel KA, Jiao W, *et al.* Glycation-altered proteolysis as a pathobiologic mechanism that links dietary glycemic index, aging, and age-related disease (in nondiabetics). Aging Cell 2012; 11(1): 1-13.
[http://dx.doi.org/10.1111/j.1474-9726.2011.00752.x]

[30] Ding Q, Dimayuga E, Martin S, *et al.* Characterization of chronic low-level proteasome inhibition on neural homeostasis. J Neurochem 2003; 86(2): 489-97.
[http://dx.doi.org/10.1046/j.1471-4159.2003.01885.x]

[31] Ding Q, Zhu H. 2017.Proteolytic alteration in the brain of dementia with Lewy Bodies (in preparation).

[32] Her LS, Lin JY, Fu MH, *et al.* The differential profiling of ubiquitin-proteasome and autophagy systems in different tissues before the onset of huntington's disease models. Brain Pathol 2015; 25: 481-90.
[http://dx.doi.org/10.1111/bpa.12191]

[33] Liu D, Gao M, Yang Y, Qi YU, Wu K, Zhao S. Inhibition of autophagy promotes cell apoptosis induced by the proteasome inhibitor MG-132 in human esophageal squamous cell carcinoma EC9706 cells. Oncol Lett 2015; 9: 2278-82.
[http://dx.doi.org/10.3892/ol.2015.3047]

[34] Keller JN, Dimayuga E, Chen Q, Thorpe J, Gee J, *et al.* Autophagy, proteasomes, lipofuscin, and oxidative stress in the aging brain. Int J Biochem Cell Biol 2004; 36: 2376-91.
[http://dx.doi.org/10.1016/j.biocel.2004.05.003]

[35] Drießen S, Berleth N, Friesen O, Löffler AS, Böhler P, *et al.* Deubiquitinase inhibition by WP1130 leads to ULK1 aggregation and blockade of autophagy. Autophagy 2015; 11: 1458-70.
[http://dx.doi.org/10.1080/15548627.2015.1067359]

[36] Rui YN, Xu Z, Chen Z, Zhang S. The GST-BHMT assay reveals a distinct mechanism underlying proteasome inhibition-induced macroautophagy in mammalian cells. Autophagy 2015; 11: 812-32.
[http://dx.doi.org/10.1080/15548627.2015.1034402]

[37] Marchand B, Arsenault D, Raymond-Fleury A, Boisvert FM, Boucher MJ. Glycogen synthase kinase-3 (GSK3) inhibition induces prosurvival autophagic signals in human pancreatic cancer cells. J Biol Chem 2015; 290(9): 5592-605.
[http://dx.doi.org/10.1074/jbc.M114.616714]

[38] Gavilan E, Pintado C, Gavilan MP, Daza P, Sanchez-Aguayo I, *et al.* Age-related dysfunctions of the autophagy lysosomal pathway in hippocampal pyramidal neurons under proteasome stress. Neurobiol Aging 2015; 36: 1953-63.
[http://dx.doi.org/10.1016/j.neurobiolaging.2015.02.025]

[39] Ben-Shem A, Garreau de Loubresse N, Melnikov S, Jenner L, Yusupova G, Yusupov M. The structure of the eukaryotic ribosome at 3.0 Å resolution. Science 2011; 334(6062): 1524-9.
[http://dx.doi.org/10.1126/science.1212642]

[40] Turner GC, Varshavsky A. Detecting and measuring cotranslational protein degradation in vivo. Science 2000; 289(5487): 2117-20.
[http://dx.doi.org/10.1126/science.289.5487.2117]

[41] Fünfschilling U, Rospert S. Nascent polypeptide-associated complex stimulates protein import into yeast mitochondria. Mol Biol Cell 1999; 10(10): 3289-99.
[http://dx.doi.org/10.1091/mbc.10.10.3289]

[42] Laribee RN, Shibata Y, Mersman DP, *et al.* CCR4/NOT complex associates with the proteasome and regulates histone methylation. Proc Natl Acad Sci USA 2007; 104(14): 5836-41.
[http://dx.doi.org/10.1073/pnas.0607996104]

[43] Chuang SM, Madura K. Saccharomyces cerevisiae Ub-conjugating enzyme Ubc4 binds the

proteasome in the presence of translationally damaged proteins. Genetics 2005; 171(4): 1477-84. [http://dx.doi.org/10.1534/genetics.105.046888]

[44] Panasenko OO, David FP, Collart MA. Ribosome association and stability of the nascent polypeptide-associated complex is dependent upon its own ubiquitination. Genetics 2009; 181(2): 447-60. [http://dx.doi.org/10.1534/genetics.108.095422]

[45] Ding Q, Markesbery WR, Cecarini V, Keller JN. Decreased RNA, and increased RNA oxidation, in ribosomes from early Alzheimer's disease. Neurochem Res 2006; 31: 705-10. [http://dx.doi.org/10.1007/s11064-006-9071-5]

[46] Ding Q, Markesbery WR, Chen Q, Li F, Keller JN. Ribosome dysfunction is an early event in Alzheimer's disease. J Neurosci 2005; 25: 9171-5. [http://dx.doi.org/10.1523/JNEUROSCI.3040-05.2005]

[47] Ding Q, Dimayuga E, Markesbery WR, Keller JN. Proteasome inhibition induces reversible impairments in protein synthesis. FASEB J 2006; 20(8): 1055-63. [http://dx.doi.org/10.1096/fj.05-5495com]

[48] Ling Q, Yao Y, Huang H. A model for the 26S proteasome and ribosome actions in leaf polarity formation. Plant Signal Behav 2008; 3: 804-5. [http://dx.doi.org/10.4161/psb.3.10.5877]

[49] Õunap K, Leetsi L, Matsoo M, Kurg R. The stability of ribosome biogenesis factor WBSCR22 is regulated by interaction with TRMT112 *via* ubiquitin-proteasome pathway. PLoS One 2015; 10: e0133841. [http://dx.doi.org/10.1371/journal.pone.0133841]

[50] Paz-Aviram T, Yahalom A, Chamovitz DA. Arabidopsis eIF3e interacts with subunits of the ribosome, Cop9 signalosome and proteasome. Plant Signal Behav 2008; 3: 409-11. [http://dx.doi.org/10.4161/psb.3.6.5434]

[51] Stavreva DA, Kawasaki M, Dundr M, Koberna K, Muller WG, *et al.* Potential roles for ubiquitin and the proteasome during ribosome biogenesis. Mol Cell Biol 2006; 26: 5131-45. [http://dx.doi.org/10.1128/MCB.02227-05]

[52] Bulteau AL, Petropoulos I, Friguet B. Age-related alterations of proteasome structure and function in aging epidermis. Exp Gerontol 2000; 35: 767-77. [http://dx.doi.org/10.1016/S0531-5565(00)00136-4]

[53] Bulteau AL, Szweda LI, Friguet B. Age-dependent declines in proteasome activity in the heart. Arch Biochem Biophys 2002; 397: 298-304. [http://dx.doi.org/10.1006/abbi.2001.2663]

[54] Chondrogianni N, Gonos ES. Proteasome function determines cellular homeostasis and the rate of aging. Adv Exp Med Biol 2010; 694: 38-46. [http://dx.doi.org/10.1007/978-1-4419-7002-2_4]

[55] Paine SM, Anderson G, Bedford K, Lawler K, Mayer RJ, *et al.* Pale body-like inclusion formation and neurodegeneration following depletion of 26S proteasomes in mouse brain neurones are independent of alpha-synuclein. PLoS One 2013; 8: e54711. [http://dx.doi.org/10.1371/journal.pone.0054711]

[56] Ding Q, Dimayuga E, Keller JN. Proteasome regulation of oxidative stress in aging and age-related diseases of the CNS. Antioxid Redox Signal 2006; 8: 163-72. [http://dx.doi.org/10.1089/ars.2006.8.163]

[57] Chen Q, Thorpe J, Dohmen JR, Li F, Keller JN. Ump1 extends yeast lifespan and enhances viability during oxidative stress: central role for the proteasome. Free Radic Biol Med 2006; 40: 120-6. [http://dx.doi.org/10.1016/j.freeradbiomed.2005.08.048]

[58] Chondrogianni N, Georgila K, Kourtis N, Tavernarakis N, Gonos ES. 20S proteasome activation promotes life span extension and resistance to proteotoxicity in Caenorhabditis elegans. FASEB J

2015; 29: 611-22.
[http://dx.doi.org/10.1096/fj.14-252189]

[59] Pickering AM, Lehr M, Miller RA. Lifespan of mice and primates correlates with immunoproteasome expression. J Clin Invest 2015; 125: 2059-68.
[http://dx.doi.org/10.1172/JCI80514]

[60] Hong L, Huang HC, Jiang ZF. Relationship between amyloid-beta and the ubiquitin-proteasome system in Alzheimer's disease. Neurol Res 2014; 36: 276-82.
[http://dx.doi.org/10.1179/1743132813Y.0000000288]

[61] Liu Y, Hettinger CL, Zhang D, Rezvani K, Wang X, *et al.* The proteasome function reporter GFPu accumulates in young brains of the APPswe/PS1dE9 Alzheimer's disease mouse model. Cell Mol Neurobiol 2014; 34: 315-22.
[http://dx.doi.org/10.1007/s10571-013-0022-9]

[62] Filatova EV, Shadrina MI, Alieva AK, Kolacheva AA, Slominsky PA, *et al.* Expression analysis of genes of ubiquitin-proteasome protein degradation system in MPTP-induced mice models of early stages of Parkinson's disease. Dokl Biochem Biophys 2014; 456: 116-8.
[http://dx.doi.org/10.1134/S1607672914030107]

[63] Gruner M, Moncsek A, Rodiger S, Kuhnhardt D, Feist E, *et al.* Increased proteasome activator 28 gamma (PA28gamma) levels are unspecific but correlate with disease activity in rheumatoid arthritis. BMC Musculoskelet Disord 2014; 15: 414-74.
[http://dx.doi.org/10.1186/1471-2474-15-414]

[64] Derouiche F, Bole-Feysot C, Naimi D, Coeffier M. Hyperhomocysteinemia induced oxidative stress differentially alters proteasome composition and activities in heart and aorta. Biochem Biophys Res Commun 2014; 452: 740-5.
[http://dx.doi.org/10.1016/j.bbrc.2014.08.141]

[65] Bulteau AL, Dancis A, Gareil M, Montagne JJ, Camadro JM, *et al.* Oxidative stress and protease dysfunction in the yeast model of Friedreich ataxia. Free Radic Biol Med 2007; 42: 1561-70.
[http://dx.doi.org/10.1016/j.freeradbiomed.2007.02.014]

[66] Vallelian F, Deuel JW, Opitz L, Schaer CA, Puglia M, *et al.* Proteasome inhibition and oxidative reactions disrupt cellular homeostasis during heme stress. Cell Death Differ 2015; 22: 597-611.
[http://dx.doi.org/10.1038/cdd.2014.154]

[67] Adams B, Mapanga RF, Essop MF. Partial inhibition of the ubiquitinproteasome system ameliorates cardiac dysfunction following ischemiareperfusion in the presence of high glucose. Cardiovasc Diabetol 2015; 14: 94.
[http://dx.doi.org/10.1186/s12933-015-0258-4]

[68] Wang R, Zhao J, Zhang J, Liu W, Zhao M, *et al.* Effect of lysosomal and ubiquitin-proteasome system dysfunction on the abnormal aggregation of alpha-synuclein in PC12 cells. Exp Ther Med 2015; 9: 2088-94.
[http://dx.doi.org/10.3892/etm.2015.2432]

[69] Liu J, Tang M, Mestril R, Wang X. Aberrant protein aggregation is essential for a mutant desmin to impair the proteolytic function of the ubiquitinproteasome system in cardiomyocytes. J Mol Cell Cardiol 2006; 40: 451-4.
[http://dx.doi.org/10.1016/j.yjmcc.2005.12.011]

[70] Ge P, Luo Y, Liu CL, Hu B. Protein aggregation and proteasome dysfunction after brain ischemia. Stroke 2007; 38: 3230-6.
[http://dx.doi.org/10.1161/STROKEAHA.107.487108]

[71] Hai J, Lin Q, Su SH, Zhang L, Wan JF, *et al.* Chronic cerebral hypoperfusion in rats causes proteasome dysfunction and aggregation of ubiquitinated proteins. Brain Res 2011; 1374: 73-81.
[http://dx.doi.org/10.1016/j.brainres.2010.12.030]

[72] Maisonneuve E, Fraysse L, Moinier D, Dukan S. Existence of abnormal protein aggregates in healthy Escherichia coli cells. J Bacteriol 2008; 190: 887-93. [http://dx.doi.org/10.1128/JB.01603-07]

[73] Zhou C, Wang P, Zhang Y, Liu C. Changes of ubiquitin-proteasome system in human umbilical vein endothelial cells induced by oxidative low density lipoprotein. Zhonghua Yi Xue Za Zhi 2014; 94: 3269-72.

[74] Safren N, El Ayadi A, Chang L, Terrillion CE, Gould TD, *et al.* Ubiquilin-1 overexpression increases the lifespan and delays accumulation of Huntingtin aggregates in the R6/2 mouse model of Huntington's disease. PLoS One 2014; 9: e87513. [http://dx.doi.org/10.1371/journal.pone.0087513]

[75] Liu HY, Pfleger CM. Mutation in E1, the ubiquitin activating enzyme, reduces Drosophila lifespan and results in motor impairment. PLoS One 2013; 8: e32835. [http://dx.doi.org/10.1371/journal.pone.0032835]

[76] Bai JL, Qu YJ, Zou LP, Yang XY, Liu LJ, *et al.* A novel missense mutation of the ubiquitin protein ligase E3A gene in a patient with Angelman syndrome. Chin Med J (Engl) 2011; 124: 84-8.

[77] Daroszewska A, van't Hof RJ, Rojas JA, Layfield R, Landao-Basonga E, *et al.* A point mutation in the ubiquitin-associated domain of SQSMT1 is sufficient to cause a Paget's disease-like disorder in mice. Hum Mol Genet 2011; 20: 2734-44. [http://dx.doi.org/10.1093/hmg/ddr172]

[78] Guernsey DL, Jiang H, Bedard K, Evans SC, Ferguson M, *et al.* Mutation in the gene encoding ubiquitin ligase LRSAM1 in patients with Charcot-MarieTooth disease. PLoS Genet 2010; 6: e1001081. [http://dx.doi.org/10.1371/journal.pgen.1001081]

[79] Kandimalla RJ, Anand R, Veeramanikandan R, *et al.* CSF ubiquitin as a specific biomarker in Alzheimer's disease. Curr Alzheimer Res 2014; 11(4): 340-8. [http://dx.doi.org/10.2174/1567205011666140331161027]

[80] Zhang M, Cai F, Zhang S, Zhang S, Song W. Overexpression of ubiquitin carboxyl-terminal hydrolase L1 (UCHL1) delays Alzheimer's progression in vivo. Sci Rep 2014; 4: 7298. [http://dx.doi.org/10.1038/srep07298]

[81] Narayan PJ, Lill C, Faull R, Curtis MA, Dragunow M. Increased acetyl and total histone levels in post-mortem Alzheimer's disease brain. Neurobiol Dis 2015; 74: 281-94. [http://dx.doi.org/10.1016/j.nbd.2014.11.023]

[82] Saito R, Kaneko M, Kitamura Y, *et al.* Effects of oxidative stress on the solubility of HRD1, a ubiquitin ligase implicated in Alzheimer's disease. PLoS One 2014; 9(5): e94576. [http://dx.doi.org/10.1371/journal.pone.0094576]

[83] International Genomics of Alzheimer's Disease Consortium (IGAP). Convergent genetic and expression data implicate immunity in Alzheimer's disease. Alzheimers Dement 2015; 11(6): 658-71. [http://dx.doi.org/10.1016/j.jalz.2014.05.1757]

[84] Weeraratna AT, Kalehua A, Deleon I, *et al.* Alterations in immunological and neurological gene expression patterns in Alzheimer's disease tissues. Exp Cell Res 2007; 313(3): 450-61. [http://dx.doi.org/10.1016/j.yexcr.2006.10.028]

[85] Dorval V, Fraser PE. Small ubiquitin-like modifier (SUMO) modification of natively unfolded proteins tau and alpha-synuclein. J Biol Chem 2006; 281(15): 9919-24. [http://dx.doi.org/10.1074/jbc.M510127200]

[86] Li Y, Wang H, Wang S, Quon D, Liu YW, Cordell B. Positive and negative regulation of APP amyloidogenesis by sumoylation. Proc Natl Acad Sci USA 2003; 100(1): 259-64. [http://dx.doi.org/10.1073/pnas.0235361100]

[87] Dorval V, Mazzella MJ, Mathews PM, Hay RT, Fraser PE. Modulation of Abeta generation by small ubiquitin-like modifiers does not require conjugation to target proteins. Biochem J 2007; 404(2): 309-16.
[http://dx.doi.org/10.1042/BJ20061451]

[88] Wang X, Su B, Lee HG, *et al.* Impaired balance of mitochondrial fission and fusion in Alzheimer's disease. J Neurosci 2009; 29(28): 9090-103.
[http://dx.doi.org/10.1523/JNEUROSCI.1357-09.2009]

[89] Haass C, Selkoe DJ. Soluble protein oligomers in neurodegeneration: lessons from the Alzheimer's amyloid beta-peptide. Nat Rev Mol Cell Biol 2007; 8(2): 101-12.
[http://dx.doi.org/10.1038/nrm2101]

[90] Mucke L, Selkoe DJ. Neurotoxicity of amyloid β-protein: synaptic and network dysfunction. Cold Spring Harb Perspect Med 2012; 2(7): a006338.
[http://dx.doi.org/10.1101/cshperspect.a006338]

[91] Lee MR, Lee D, Shin SK, Kim YH, Choi CY. Inhibition of APP intracellular domain (AICD) transcriptional activity via covalent conjugation with Nedd8. Biochem Biophys Res Commun 2008; 366(4): 976-81.
[http://dx.doi.org/10.1016/j.bbrc.2007.12.066]

[92] Chen Y, Liu W, McPhie DL, Hassinger L, Neve RL. APP-BP1 mediates APP-induced apoptosis and DNA synthesis and is increased in Alzheimer's disease brain. J Cell Biol 2003; 163(1): 27-33.
[http://dx.doi.org/10.1083/jcb.200304003]

[93] Mori F, Nishie M, Piao YS, *et al.* Accumulation of NEDD8 in neuronal and glial inclusions of neurodegenerative disorders. Neuropathol Appl Neurobiol 2005; 31(1): 53-61.
[http://dx.doi.org/10.1111/j.1365-2990.2004.00603.x]

[94] Hjerpe R, Thomas Y, Kurz T. NEDD8 overexpression results in neddylation of ubiquitin substrates by the ubiquitin pathway. J Mol Biol 2012; 421(1): 27-9.
[http://dx.doi.org/10.1016/j.jmb.2012.05.013]

[95] Pickering AM, Koop AL, Teoh CY, Ermak G, Grune T, *et al.* The immunoproteasome, the 20S proteasome and the PA28alphabeta proteasome regulator are oxidative-stress-adaptive proteolytic complexes. Biochem J 2010; 432: 585-94.
[http://dx.doi.org/10.1042/BJ20100878]

[96] Zhang Y, Liu S, Zuo Q, Wu L, *et al.* Oxidative challenge enhances REGgamma-proteasom--dependent protein degradation. Free Radic Biol Med 2015; 82: 42-9.
[http://dx.doi.org/10.1016/j.freeradbiomed.2015.01.024]

[97] Kincaid EZ, Che JW, York I, Escobar H, Reyes-Vargas E, *et al.* Mice completely lacking immunoproteasomes show major changes in antigen presentation. Nat Immunol 2011; 13: 129-35.
[http://dx.doi.org/10.1038/ni.2203]

[98] Opitz E, Koch A, Klingel K, Schmidt F, Prokop S, *et al.* Impairment of immunoproteasome function by beta5i/LMP7 subunit deficiency results in severe enterovirus myocarditis. PLoS Pathog 2011; 7: e1002233.
[http://dx.doi.org/10.1371/journal.ppat.1002233]

[99] Ferrington DA, Hussong SA, Roehrich H, Kapphahn RJ, Kavanaugh SM, *et al.* Immunoproteasome responds to injury in the retina and brain. J Neurochem 2008; 106: 158-69.
[http://dx.doi.org/10.1111/j.1471-4159.2008.05345.x]

[100] Grimm S, Ott C, Hörlacher M, Weber D, Höhn A, *et al.* Advancedglycation-end-product-induced formation of immunoproteasomes: involvement of RAGE and Jak2/STAT1. Biochem J 2012; 448: 127-39.
[http://dx.doi.org/10.1042/BJ20120298]

[101] Gavilan MP, Castano A, Torres M, Portavella M, Caballero C, *et al.* Age-related increase in the

immunoproteasome content in rat hippocampus: molecular and functional aspects. J Neurochem 2009; 108(1): 260-72.
[http://dx.doi.org/10.1111/j.1471-4159.2008.05762.x]

[102] Chondrogianni N, Voutetakis K, Kapetanou M, Delitsikou V, Papaevgeniou N, *et al.* Proteasome activation: An innovative promising approach for delaying aging and retarding age-related diseases. Ageing Res Rev 2015; 23: 37-55.
[http://dx.doi.org/10.1016/j.arr.2014.12.003]

[103] Cecarini V, Bonfili L, Cuccioloni M, Keller JN, *et al.* Effects of ghrelin on the proteolytic pathways of alzheimer's disease neuronal cells. Mol Neurobiol 2015.

[104] Kim W, Seo H. Baclofen, a GABAB receptor agonist, enhances ubiquitinproteasome system functioning and neuronal survival in Huntington's disease model mice. Biochem Biophys Res Commun 2014; 443: 706-11.
[http://dx.doi.org/10.1016/j.bbrc.2013.12.034]

[105] Chondrogianni N, Tzavelas C, Pemberton AJ, Nezis IP, Rivett AJ. Overexpression of proteasome beta5 assembled subunit increases the amount of proteasome and confers ameliorated response to oxidative stress and higher survival rates. J Biol Chem 2005; 280: 11840-50.
[http://dx.doi.org/10.1074/jbc.M413007200]

[106] Hwang JS, Hwang JS, Chang I, Kim S. Age-associated decrease in proteasome content and activities in human dermal fibroblasts: restoration of normal level of proteasome subunits reduces aging markers in fibroblasts from elderly persons. J Gerontol A Biol Sci Med Sci 2007; 62: 490-9.
[http://dx.doi.org/10.1093/gerona/62.5.490]

[107] Chondrogianni N, Gonos ES. Overexpression of hUMP1/POMP proteasome accessory protein enhances proteasome-mediated antioxidant defence. Exp Gerontol 2007; 42: 899-903.
[http://dx.doi.org/10.1016/j.exger.2007.01.012]

[108] Dal Vechio FH, Cerqueira F, Augusto O, Lopes R, Demasi M. Peptidesth at activate the 20S proteasome by gate opening increased oxidized protein removal and reduced protein aggregation. Free Radic Biol Med 2014; 67: 304-13.
[http://dx.doi.org/10.1016/j.freeradbiomed.2013.11.017]

[109] Pullarkat V, Meng Z, Tahara SM, Johnson CS, Kalra VK. Proteasome inhibition induces both antioxidant and hb f responses in sickle cell disease via the nrf2 pathway. Hemoglobin 2014; 38: 188-95.
[http://dx.doi.org/10.3109/03630269.2014.898651]

[110] Bulteau AL, Moreau M, Saunois A, Nizard C, Friguet B. Algae extractmediated stimulation and protection of proteasome activity within human keratinocytes exposed to UVA and UVB irradiation. Antioxid Redox Signal 2006; 8: 136-43.
[http://dx.doi.org/10.1089/ars.2006.8.136]

[111] Pundir S, Vu HY, Solomon VR, McClure R, Lee H. VR23: a quinolinesulfonyl hybrid proteasome inhibitor that selectively kills cancer via cyclin E-mediated centrosome amplification. Cancer Res 2015; 75: 4164-75.
[http://dx.doi.org/10.1158/0008-5472.CAN-14-3370]

[112] Clague MJ, Barsukov I, Coulson JM, Liu H, Rigden DJ, Urbé S. Deubiquitylases from genes to organism. Physiol Rev 2013; 93(3): 1289-315.
[http://dx.doi.org/10.1152/physrev.00002.2013]

[113] Ristic G, Wei-Ling Tsou WL, Todi SV. An optimal ubiquitin-proteasome pathway in the nervous system: the role of deubiquitinating enzymes. Front Mol Neurosci 2014; 7: 72.
[http://dx.doi.org/10.3389/fnmol.2014.00072]

[114] Wilkinson KD, Deshpande S, Larsen CN. Comparisons of neuronal (PGP 9.5) and non-neuronal ubiquitin C-terminal hydrolases. Biochem Soc Trans 1992; 20(3): 631-7.
[http://dx.doi.org/10.1042/bst0200631]

[115] Gong B, Cao Z, Zheng P, *et al.* Ubiquitin hydrolase Uch-L1 rescues beta-amyloid-induced decreases in synaptic function and contextual memory. Cell 2006; 126(4): 775-88. [http://dx.doi.org/10.1016/j.cell.2006.06.046]

[116] Setsuie R, Wada K. The functions of UCH-L1 and its relation to neurodegenerative diseases. Neurochem Int 2007; 51(2-4): 105-11. [http://dx.doi.org/10.1016/j.neuint.2007.05.007]

[117] Leroy E, Anastasopoulos D, Konitsiotis S, Lavedan C, Polymeropoulos MH. Deletions in the Parkin gene and genetic heterogeneity in a Greek family with early onset Parkinson's disease. Hum Genet 1998; 103(4): 424-7. [http://dx.doi.org/10.1007/s004390050845]

[118] Zhang X, Zhou JY, Chin MH, *et al.* Region-specific protein abundance changes in the brain of MPTP-induced Parkinson's disease mouse model. J Proteome Res 2010; 9(3): 1496-509. [http://dx.doi.org/10.1021/pr901024z]

[119] Costa Mdo C, Paulson HL. Toward understanding Machado-Joseph disease. Prog Neurobiol 2012; 97(2): 239-57. [http://dx.doi.org/10.1016/j.pneurobio.2011.11.006]

[120] Mujtaba T, Dou QP. Advances in the understanding of mechanisms and therapeutic use of bortezomib. Discov Med 2011; 12(67): 471-80.

[121] Lee BH, Lee MJ, Park S, *et al.* Enhancement of proteasome activity by a small-molecule inhibitor of USP14. Nature 2010; 467(7312): 179-84. [http://dx.doi.org/10.1038/nature09299]

[122] Min JW, Lü L, Freeling JL, Martin DS, Wang H. USP14 inhibitor attenuates cerebral ischemia/reperfusion-induced neuronal injury in mice. J Neurochem 2017; 140(5): 826-33. [http://dx.doi.org/10.1111/jnc.13941]

[123] Tai HC, Serrano-Pozo A, Hashimoto T, Frosch MP, Spires-Jones TL, Hyman BT. The synaptic accumulation of hyperphosphorylated tau oligomers in Alzheimer disease is associated with dysfunction of the ubiquitin-proteasome system. Am J Pathol 2012; 181(4): 1426-35. [Erratum in: Am J Pathol. 2012 Nov;181]. [5]. [:1889-90. PMID: 22867711]. [http://dx.doi.org/10.1016/j.ajpath.2012.06.033]

[124] Lokireddy S, Kukushkin NV, Goldberg AL. cAMP-induced phosphorylation of 26S proteasomes on Rpn6/PSMD11 enhances their activity and the degradation of misfolded proteins. Proc Natl Acad Sci USA 2015; 112(52): E7176-85. [http://dx.doi.org/10.1073/pnas.1522332112]

[125] Myeku N, Clelland CL, Emrani S, *et al.* Tau-driven 26S proteasome impairment and cognitive dysfunction can be prevented early in disease by activating cAMP-PKA signaling. Nat Med 2016; 22(1): 46-53. [http://dx.doi.org/10.1038/nm.4011]

[126] VanderLinden RT, Hemmis CW, Yao T, Robinson H, Hill CP. Structure and energetics of pairwise interactions between proteasome subunits RPN2, RPN13, and ubiquitin clarify a substrate recruitment mechanism. J Biol Chem 2017; 292(23): 9493-504. [http://dx.doi.org/10.1074/jbc.M117.785287]

[127] Klafki HW, Staufenbiel M, Kornhuber J, Wiltfang J. Therapeutic approaches to Alzheimer's disease. Brain 2006; 129(Pt 11): 2840-55. [http://dx.doi.org/10.1093/brain/awl280]

[128] Nordberg A. Mechanisms behind the neuroprotective actions of cholinesterase inhibitors in Alzheimer disease. Alzheimer Dis Assoc Disord 2006; 20: S12-8. [http://dx.doi.org/10.1097/01.wad.0000213804.59187.2d]

[129] Kennedy ME, Stamford AW, Chen X, *et al.* The BACE1 inhibitor verubecestat (MK-8931) reduces

CNS β-amyloid in animal models and in Alzheimer's disease patients. Sci Transl Med 2016; 8(363): 363ra150.
[http://dx.doi.org/10.1126/scitranslmed.aad9704]

[130] Anderson AB, MacDonald DL, Fischer HOL. The structure of pinitol. J Am Chem Soc 1952; 74(6): 1479.
[http://dx.doi.org/10.1021/ja01126a036]

[131] EFSA NDA Panel Panel (EFSA Panel on Dietetic Products, Nutrition and Allergies). Scientific Opinion on the substantiation of health claims related to Camellia sinensis (L.) Kuntze (tea), including catechins in green tea, and improvement of endothelium-dependent vasodilation (ID 1106, 1310), maintenance of normal blood pressure. EFSA Journal European Food Safety Authority 2011; 9(4): 2055.

[132] Lednicer D. The Organic Chemistry of Drug Synthesis. 7th ed. Hoboken: John Wiley & Sons 2008; p. 15.

[133] Caltagirone C, Ferrannini L, Marchionni N, Nappi G, Scapagnini G, Trabucchi M. The potential protective effect of tramiprosate (homotaurine) against Alzheimer's disease: a review. Aging Clin Exp Res 2012; 24(6): 580-7.

[134] Dragnev KH, Petty WJ, Shah SJ, *et al.* A proof-of-principle clinical trial of bexarotene in patients with non-small cell lung cancer. Clin Cancer Res 2007; 13(6): 1794-800.
[http://dx.doi.org/10.1158/1078-0432.CCR-06-1836]

[135] Esteva FJ, Glaspy J, Baidas S, *et al.* Multicenter Phase II Study of Oral Bexarotene for Patients With Metastatic Breast Cancer. J Clin Oncol 2003; 21(6): 999-1006.
[http://dx.doi.org/10.1200/JCO.2003.05.068]

[136] Mechoulam R, Brueggemeier RW, Denlinger DL. Estrogens in insects. Cell Mol Life Sci 2005; 40(9): 942-4.
[http://dx.doi.org/10.1007/BF01946450]

[137] Zhu H, Ding Q. Lower expression level of two RAGE alternative splicing isoforms in Alzheimer's disease. Neurosci Lett 2015; 597: 66-70.
[http://dx.doi.org/10.1016/j.neulet.2015.04.032]

[138] Owens MJ, Nemeroff CB. Pharmacology of valproate. Psychopharmacol Bull 2003; 37 (Suppl. 2): 17-24.

[139] Webster CI, Burrell M, Olsson LL, *et al.* Engineering neprilysin activity and specificity to create a novel therapeutic for Alzheimer's disease. PLoS One 2014; 9(8): e104001.
[http://dx.doi.org/10.1371/journal.pone.0104001]

[140] Salloway S, Sperling R, Fox NC, *et al.* Two phase 3 trials of bapineuzumab in mild-to-moderate Alzheimer's disease. N Engl J Med 2014; 370(4): 322-33.
[http://dx.doi.org/10.1056/NEJMoa1304839]

[141] DiFrancesco JC, Longoni M, Piazza F. Anti-Aβ Autoantibodies in Amyloid Related Imaging Abnormalities (ARIA): Candidate Biomarker for Immunotherapy in Alzheimer's Disease and Cerebral Amyloid Angiopathy. Frontiers in Neurology. 2015; 6: p. 207.

[142] Jing P, Zhang JY, Ouyang Q, Wu J, Zhang XJ. Lithium treatment induces proteasomal degradation of over-expressed acetylcholinesterase (AChE-S) and inhibit GSK3β. Chem Biol Interact 2013; 203(1): 309-13.
[http://dx.doi.org/10.1016/j.cbi.2012.08.010]

[143] Joint Formulary Committee. British National Formulary: BNF 69. British Medical Association 2015.

[144] Stack C, Jainuddin S, Elipenahli C, *et al.* Methylene blue upregulates Nrf2/ARE genes and prevents tau-related neurotoxicity. Hum Mol Genet 2014; 23(14): 3716-32.
[http://dx.doi.org/10.1093/hmg/ddu080]

[145] Tawakol A, Singh P, Rudd JH, *et al.* Effect of treatment for 12 weeks with rilapladib, a lipoprotein-associated phospholipase A2 inhibitor, on arterial inflammation as assessed with 18F-fluorodeoxyglucose-positron emission tomography imaging. J Am Coll Cardiol 2014; 63(1): 86-8. [http://dx.doi.org/10.1016/j.jacc.2013.07.050]

[146] Morris MC, Tangney CC, Wang Y, Sacks FM, Bennett DA, Aggarwal NT. MIND diet associated with reduced incidence of Alzheimer's disease. Alzheimers Dement 2015; 11(9): 1007-14. [http://dx.doi.org/10.1016/j.jalz.2014.11.009]

[147] Sezgin Z, Dincer Y. Alzheimer's disease and epigenetic diet. Neurochem Int 2014; 78: 105-16. [http://dx.doi.org/10.1016/j.neuint.2014.09.012]

[148] Singh B, Parsaik AK, Mielke MM, *et al.* Association of mediterranean diet with mild cognitive impairment and Alzheimer's disease: a systematic review and meta-analysis. J Alzheimers Dis 2014; 39(2): 271-82. [http://dx.doi.org/10.3233/JAD-130830]

[149] Squitti R, Siotto M, Polimanti R. Low-copper diet as a preventive strategy for Alzheimer's disease. Neurobiol Aging 2014; (Suppl. 2)S40-50. [http://dx.doi.org/10.1016/j.neurobiolaging.2014.02.031]

[150] Grant WB. Trends in diet and Alzheimer's disease during the nutrition transition in Japan and developing countries. J Alzheimers Dis 2014; 38(3): 611-20. [http://dx.doi.org/10.3233/JAD-130719]

[151] Thomas J, Thomas CJ, Radcliffe J, Itsiopoulos C. Omega-3 Fatty Acids in Early Prevention of Inflammatory Neurodegenerative Disease: A Focus on Alzheimer's Disease. BioMed Res Int 2015; 2015: 172801. [http://dx.doi.org/10.1155/2015/172801]

[152] Knight EM, Martins IV, Gümüsgöz S, Allan SM, Lawrence CB. High-fat diet-induced memory impairment in triple-transgenic Alzheimer's disease (3xTgAD) mice is independent of changes in amyloid and tau pathology. Neurobiol Aging 2014; 35(8): 1821-32. [http://dx.doi.org/10.1016/j.neurobiolaging.2014.02.010]

[153] Hu X, Wang T, Jin F. Alzheimer's disease and gut microbiota. Sci China Life Sci 2016; 59(10): 1006-23. [http://dx.doi.org/10.1007/s11427-016-5083-9]

[154] Petterson JA. Does high dose vitamin D supplementation enhance cognition? A randomized trial in healthy adults. Exp Gerontol 2017; 90: 90-7. [http://dx.doi.org/10.1016/j.exger.2017.01.019]

[155] The sleep-wake cycle and Alzheimer's disease: what do we know? Neurodegener Dis Manag 2014; 4(5): 351-62. [http://dx.doi.org/10.2217/nmt.14.33]

[156] Roh JH, Jiang H, Finn MB, *et al.* Potential role of orexin and sleep modulation in the pathogenesis of Alzheimer's disease. J Exp Med 2014; 211(13): 2487-96. [http://dx.doi.org/10.1084/jem.20141788]

[157] Busche MA, Kekuš M, Adelsberger H, *et al.* Rescue of long-range circuit dysfunction in Alzheimer's disease models. Nat Neurosci 2015; 18(11): 1623-30. [http://dx.doi.org/10.1038/nn.4137]

[158] Lim AS, Ellison BA, Wang JL, *et al.* Sleep is related to neuron numbers in the ventrolateral preoptic/intermediate nucleus in older adults with and without Alzheimer's disease. Brain 2014; 137(Pt 10): 2847-61. [http://dx.doi.org/10.1093/brain/awu222]

[159] Di Meco A, Joshi YB, Praticò D. Sleep deprivation impairs memory, tau metabolism, and synaptic integrity of a mouse model of Alzheimer's disease with plaques and tangles. Neurobiol Aging 2014;

35(8): 1813-20.
[http://dx.doi.org/10.1016/j.neurobiolaging.2014.02.011]

[160] Berridge MJ. Calcium regulation of neural rhythms, memory and Alzheimer's disease. J Physiol 2014; 592(2): 281-93.
[http://dx.doi.org/10.1113/jphysiol.2013.257527]

[161] Hanford N, Figueiro M. Light therapy and Alzheimer's disease and related dementia: past, present, and future. J Alzheimers Dis 2013; 33(4): 913-22.
[http://dx.doi.org/10.3233/JAD-2012-121645]

[162] Wade AG, Farmer M, Harari G, *et al.* Add-on prolonged-release melatonin for cognitive function and sleep in mild to moderate Alzheimer's disease: a 6-month, randomized, placebo-controlled, multicenter trial. Clin Interv Aging 2014; 18(9): 947-61.

[163] Beydoun MA, Beydoun HA, Gamaldo AA, Teel A, Zonderman AB, Wang Y. Epidemiologic studies of modifiable factors associated with cognition and dementia: systematic review and meta-analysis. BMC Public Health 2014; 14: 643.
[http://dx.doi.org/10.1186/1471-2458-14-643]

[164] Zhou S, Zhou R, Zhong T, Li R, Tan J, Zhou H. Association of smoking and alcohol drinking with dementia risk among elderly men in China. Curr Alzheimer Res 2014; 11(9): 899-907.

[165] Zhou R, Deng J, Zhang M, Zhou HD, Wang YJ. Association between bone mineral density and the risk of Alzheimer's disease. J Alzheimers Dis 2011; 24(1): 101-8.
[http://dx.doi.org/10.3233/JAD-2010-101467]

[166] Hebert LE, Scherr PA, Beckett LA, *et al.* Relation of smoking and alcohol consumption to incident Alzheimer's disease. Am J Epidemiol 1992; 135(4): 347-55.
[http://dx.doi.org/10.1093/oxfordjournals.aje.a116296]

[167] Campdelacreu J. Parkinson disease and Alzheimer disease: environmental risk factors. Neurologia 2014; 29(9): 541-9.
[http://dx.doi.org/10.1016/j.nrl.2012.04.001]

[168] Rusanen M, Kivipelto M, Quesenberry CP Jr, Zhou J, Whitmer RA. Heavy smoking in midlife and long-term risk of Alzheimer disease and vascular dementia. Arch Intern Med 2011; 171(4): 333-9.
[http://dx.doi.org/10.1001/archinternmed.2010.393]

[169] Ott A, Slooter AJ, Hofman A, *et al.* Smoking and risk of dementia and Alzheimer's disease in a population-based cohort study: the Rotterdam Study. Lancet 1998; 351(9119): 1840-3.
[http://dx.doi.org/10.1016/S0140-6736(97)07541-7]

[170] Norton MC, Dew J, Smith H, *et al.* Lifestyle behavior pattern is associated with different levels of risk for incident dementia and Alzheimer's disease: the Cache County study. J Am Geriatr Soc 2012; 60(3): 405-12.
[http://dx.doi.org/10.1111/j.1532-5415.2011.03860.x]

[171] England and Wales; Mortality Statistics: Deaths Registered in England and Wales (Series DR). Scotland: National Records of Scotland Vital Events Reference Tables. Northern Ireland; Northern Ireland Statistic and Research Agency Registrar General Annual Report, 2015

[172] Viña J, Lloret A. Why women have more Alzheimer's disease than men: gender and mitochondrial toxicity of amyloid-beta peptide. J Alzheimers Dis 2010; (Suppl. 2)S527-33.
[http://dx.doi.org/10.3233/JAD-2010-100501]

[173] Koppel J, Acker C, Davies P, *et al.* Psychotic Alzheimer's disease is associated with gender-specific tau phosphorylation abnormalities. Neurobiol Aging 2014; 35(9): 2021-8.
[http://dx.doi.org/10.1016/j.neurobiolaging.2014.03.003]

[174] Lane RM, He Y. Butyrylcholinesterase genotype and gender influence Alzheimer's disease phenotype. Alzheimers Dement 2013; 9(2): e1-e73.
[http://dx.doi.org/10.1016/j.jalz.2010.12.005]

[175] Almela M, Hidalgo V, Villada C, *et al.* Salivary alpha-amylase response to acute psychosocial stress: the impact of age. Biol Psychol 2011; 87: 421-9. [http://dx.doi.org/10.1016/j.biopsycho.2011.05.008]

[176] Fukumoto N, Fujii T, Combarros O, *et al.* Sexually dimorphic effect of the Val66Met polymorphism of BDNF on susceptibility to Alzheimer's disease: new data and meta-analysis. Am J Med Genet B Neuropsychiatr Genet 2010; 153B: 235-42.

[177] Eriksdotter M, Vedin I, Falahati F, *et al.* Plasma Fatty Acid Profiles in Relation to Cognition and Gender in Alzheimer's Disease Patients During Oral Omega-3 Fatty Acid Supplementation: The OmegAD Study. J Alzheimers Dis 2015; 48(3): 805-12. [http://dx.doi.org/10.3233/JAD-150102]

[178] Kim S, Kim MJ, Kim S, *et al.* Gender differences in risk factors for transition from mild cognitive impairment to Alzheimer's disease: A CREDOS study. Compr Psychiatry 2015; 62: 114-22. [http://dx.doi.org/10.1016/j.comppsych.2015.07.002]

[179] Fehér Á, Juhász A, Pákáski M, Kálmán J, Janka Z. Genetic analysis of the RELN gene: Gender specific association with Alzheimer's disease. Psychiatry Res 2015; 230(2): 716-8. [http://dx.doi.org/10.1016/j.psychres.2015.09.021]

[180] Lai SW, Lin CL, Liao KF. Cataract may be a non-memory feature of Alzheimer's disease in older people. Eur J Epidemiol 2014; 29(6): 405-9. [http://dx.doi.org/10.1007/s10654-014-9903-6]

[181] Lin KA, Choudhury KR, Rathakrishnan BG, Marks DM, Petrella JR, Doraiswamy PM. Marked gender differences in progression of mild cognitive impairment over 8 years. Alzheimers Dement (N Y) 2015; 1(2): 103-10. [http://dx.doi.org/10.1016/j.trci.2015.07.001]

[182] Adeghate E, Donáth T, Adem A. Alzheimer disease and diabetes mellitus: do they have anything in common? Curr Alzheimer Res 2013; 10(6): 609-17. [http://dx.doi.org/10.2174/15672050113109990009]

[183] Huang CC, Chung CM, Leu HB, *et al.* Diabetes mellitus and the risk of Alzheimer's disease: a nationwide population-based study. PLoS One 2014; 9(1): e87095. [http://dx.doi.org/10.1371/journal.pone.0087095]

[184] Does insulin therapy for type 1 diabetes mellitus protect against Alzheimer's disease? Pharmacotherapy 2014; 34(12): 1317-23. [http://dx.doi.org/10.1002/phar.1494]

[185] Yokoyama JS, Wang Y, Schork AJ, *et al.* Association Between Genetic Traits for Immune-Mediated Diseases and Alzheimer Disease. JAMA Neurol 2016; 73(6): 691-7. [http://dx.doi.org/10.1001/jamaneurol.2016.0150]

[186] Cermakova P, Eriksdotter M, Lund LH, Winblad B, Religa P, Religa D. Heart failure and Alzheimer's disease. J Intern Med 2015; 277(4): 406-25. [http://dx.doi.org/10.1111/joim.12287]

[187] Dede DS, Yavuz B, Yavuz BB, *et al.* Assessment of endothelial function in Alzheimer's disease: is Alzheimer's disease a vascular disease? J Am Geriatr Soc 2007; 55(10): 1613-7. [http://dx.doi.org/10.1111/j.1532-5415.2007.01378.x]

[188] Cardiovascular risk factors as potential markers for mild cognitive impairment and Alzheimer's disease. Psychiatr Danub 2011; 23(4): 340-6.

[189] Midlife vascular risk factors and Alzheimer's disease in later life: longitudinal, population based study. BMJ 2001; 322(7300): 1447-51. [http://dx.doi.org/10.1136/bmj.322.7300.1447]

[190] Shafi O. Inverse relationship between Alzheimer's disease and cancer, and other factors contributing

to Alzheimer's disease: a systematic review. BMC Neurol 2016; 16(1): 236. [http://dx.doi.org/10.1186/s12883-016-0765-2]

[191] Maheshwari P, Eslick GD. Bacterial infection and Alzheimer's disease: a meta-analysis. J Alzheimers Dis 2015; 43(3): 957-66. [http://dx.doi.org/10.3233/JAD-140621]

[192] Lim SL, Rodriguez-Ortiz CJ, Kitazawa M. Infection, systemic inflammation, and Alzheimer's disease. Microbes Infect 2015; 17(8): 549-56. [http://dx.doi.org/10.1016/j.micinf.2015.04.004]

[193] Mahmoudvand H, Sheibani V, Shojaee S, *et al.* Toxoplasma gondii Infection Potentiates Cognitive Impairments of Alzheimer's Disease in the BALB/c Mice. J Parasitol 2016; 102(6): 629-35. [http://dx.doi.org/10.1645/16-28]

[194] Roubaud Baudron C, Varon C, Mégraud F, Salles N. Alzheimer's disease and Helicobacter pylori infection: a possible link? Geriatr Psychol Neuropsychiatr Vieil 2016; 14(1): 86-94.

[195] Civitelli L, Marcocci ME, Celestino I, *et al.* Herpes simplex virus type 1 infection in neurons leads to production and nuclear localization of APP intracellular domain (AICD): implications for Alzheimer's disease pathogenesis. J Neurovirol 2015; 21(5): 480-90. [http://dx.doi.org/10.1007/s13365-015-0344-0]

[196] Lurain NS, Hanson BA, Martinson J, *et al.* Virological and immunological characteristics of human cytomegalovirus infection associated with Alzheimer disease. J Infect Dis 2013; 208(4): 564-72. [http://dx.doi.org/10.1093/infdis/jit210]

[197] Alonso R, Pisa D, Marina AI, Morato E, Rábano A, Carrasco L. Fungal infection in patients with Alzheimer's disease. J Alzheimers Dis 2014; 41(1): 301-11. [http://dx.doi.org/10.3233/JAD-132681]

[198] Pisa D, Alonso R, Juarranz A, Rábano A, Carrasco L. Direct visualization of fungal infection in brains from patients with Alzheimer's disease. J Alzheimers Dis 2015; 43(2): 613-24. [http://dx.doi.org/10.3233/JAD-141386]

[199] 2016 Alzheimer's disease facts and figures. Alzheimers Dement 2016; 12(4): 459-509. [http://dx.doi.org/10.1016/j.jalz.2016.03.001]

CHAPTER 5

Alzheimer´s Disease: Fundamental Concepts, Novel Findings and Therapeutics Outcomes Coming from the Ca^{2+}/cAMP Signalling Interaction

Leandro Bueno Bergantin[*]

Department of Pharmacology, Universidade Federal de São Paulo (UNIFESP) Rua Pedro de Toledo, 669 - Vila Clementino - São Paulo-SP, Brazil

Abstract: The evidences that a dysregulation of the intracellular Ca^{2+} homeostasis increases the incidence of the neurodegenerative diseases, such as Alzheimer´s disease (AD), have been increasing. Thus, several findings have been reinforcing the concept that a reduction of a cytosolic Ca^{2+} excess, achieved due to the L-type Ca^{2+} channel blockers (CCBs), could be an interesting pharmacological goal to alleviate the AD symptoms. In addition, aging along with a healthy brain can be endorsed by daily exercise, a self-control in caloric ingestion and participating in intellectually challenging events. Indeed, these lifestyle issues may alleviate the Ca^{2+} excess from neurons achieved through a Ca^{2+} homeostasis dysregulation. Furthermore, several studies have been indicating that increasing cAMP levels may produce neuroprotective effects, thus alleviating the AD symptoms. From these concepts in mind, we discovered that the manipulation by medicines of the Ca^{2+}/cAMP signalling through the mutual therapy involving CCBs, and cAMP-accumulating compounds, could be a novel plausible target to treat the AD. Then, this chapter discusses the fundamental concepts and current therapies to treat AD, including therapeutics outcomes coming from the pharmacological interference on the interaction between Ca^{2+} and cAMP signalling.

Keywords: Alzheimer's Disease, Ca^{2+}/cAMP Signalling Interaction, Ca^{2+} Dysregulations Neurodegenerative Diseases, Rolipram.

INTRODUCTION

Considered as one of the most common issues related to the older people, Alzheimer's disease (AD) is characterized by synaptic dysfunctions and by a dynamic deterioration related to aging of the human cognitive abilities, including memory and other intellectual issues. In 2015, it was registered about 30 million of cases of AD in worldwide, and its prevalence can reach about 81 million

[*] **Corresponding author, Leandro Bueno Bergantin:** Department of Pharmacology Universidade Federal de São Paulo (UNIFESP) Rua Pedro de Toledo, 669 - Vila Clementino - São Paulo-SP, Brazil, Zip Code: 04039-032; Tel: 551155764973; Email: leanbio39@yahoo.com.br

Atta-ur-Rahman (Ed.)

persons by 2040 due to an increasing in the lifetime of the global population. Unfortunately, no treatments can prevent or disrupt the progression of AD. However, some pharmacological treatments may temporally improve the AD symptoms [1, 2].

Since its discovery in 1906 by the German psychiatrist and pathologist Alois Alzheimer, the causes of AD are yet poorly understood. The pathological hallmarks of AD are characterized by neuritic plaques and neurofibrillary tangles, then the deposit of the β-amyloid peptide (Aβ) in the tissues from brains is highly related to the disease [1 - 3]. This Aβ accumulation provokes a dysfunction of neurons and death of the cells, then dramatically compromising the function of the medial temporal lobe and associative neocortical structures in AD patients. The amyloid hypothesis assumes that the Aβ overproduction results from the disruption of homeostatic processes that modulate the proteolytic cleavage of the amyloid precursor protein (APP). Environmental, genetic and age-related factors endorse a metabolic change, then supporting an amyloidogenic processing of APP instead of the physiological secretory pathway [1 - 3]. In addition, successive cleavages of APP by beta (β)-secretase (BACE-1) and gamma (γ)-secretase produce Aβ peptides, which have been recently considered as portions of the presenilin complex [1]. Aβ peptide presents a neurotoxic potential which results from its biochemical issues that endorse an aggregation into insoluble oligomers and protofibrils [1, 2]. Thus, these further result into fibrillary Aβ species that deposit into senile and neuritic plaques. Among several Aβ isoforms that are considered as refined differences, depending on the number of C-terminal amino acids, Aβ endorses a pivotal part in the pathogenesis of AD [1 - 6]. The Aβ deposit in the brain and cytoskeletal modifications result from the hyperphosphorylation of a microtubule-associated Tau protein in neurons [1, 2]. These processes, including a decrease of an Aβ clearance from the brain, result into the extracellular accumulation of Aβ, and the ensuing an activation of neurotoxic cascades that finally result into cytoskeletal changes, producing a synaptic dysfunction and a progressive global decline of cognitive abilities due to a dysfunction of neurons, and death [1 - 6]. In addition, metal complexes (for example: iridium(III) and rhodium(III)) are considered as inhibitors of the amyloid deposit process, including a potential use as luminescent probes for Aβ peptide [7 - 9].

In accordance with current propositions, it may be defined three clinical stages of AD: (i) pre-symptomatic (or pre-clinical) AD, in which the high deposit of Aβ in the brain results into a critical level, and it may be prolonged for several years or decades; (ii) pre-dementia stage of AD (well-suited with the classification of progressive, amnestic mild cognitive impairment), in which the early-stage pathology is existing, extending from a mild neuronal dystrophy to an early-stage

Braak pathology, and may be prolonged for several years according to an individual resilience, and a brain reserve; (iii) clinically well-defined as dementia stage of AD, in which a cognitive and functional loss is severe enough to surmount the dementia threshold; at this stage there is a significant deposit of neuritic plaques and neurofibrillary tangles in the affected brain areas, bearing a relationship with the magnitude of a global impairment [2 - 6].

Novel technologies based on the structural and functional neuroimaging, and on the biochemical analysis of a cerebrospinal fluid, may represent correlations of a brain amyloidosis in individuals with a mild, pre-dementia symptoms. These methods are generally mentioned to as AD-related biomarkers, and the combination of clinical and biological information yields a good diagnostic accuracy to identify individuals at a high risk for AD. In other words, the classification of the pathogenic Aβ by means of biochemical analysis of biological fluids, or by a molecular neuroimaging, are offered as diagnostic tools to help identify the AD cases at the earliest stages of the disease process. The early diagnosis may contribute decisively to the success of pharmacological interventions to slow-down or interrupt the progression of the AD symptoms [2 - 10].

Therapies pointing the modification of the amyloid-related cascades may be viewed as promising approaches to attenuate or even to stop the dementia. Therefore, the increasing knowledge on the AD pathogenesis derived from the basic science models will hopefully be converted into a clinical practice in the forthcoming years. Advances in the understanding of this early phase of neurodegenerative diseases will lead to the identification of biomarkers of neurodegeneration and its progression. These biomarkers will help to identify the ideal population to be included, and the most appropriate outcomes to be assessed in clinical trials of medicines. The initial diagnostic of AD offers a chance for therapies, for example: those aimed to interpose or preventing the progression of this disease, and its many complications side effects, could be of more advantage. At the present moment, therapies to modify the AD pathology by an intervention in the amyloid accumulation have been ineffective or inconclusive [2]. Thus, revealing the mechanisms of neurodegeneration from the initial stages could lead to the development of new interventions, whose therapeutic potential will need to be evaluated in adequately designed clinical trials [1 - 10].

Actually, the therapeutic strategy of AD consists in the attenuation of the synaptic dysfunctions, and cognitive deficit, by the use of drugs that modify the synaptic transmission involved in the cognitive function. This function is finely regulated by several neurotransmitters and neuromodulators, especially the acetylcholine (ACh). Then, cholinergic dysfunctions have been implicated in the cognitive deficit related to the AD [11]. These dysfunctions caused by a neurodegeneration, and death of cholinergic neurons in the AD brain, can be attenuated by the treatment with pharmacological agents that facilitate the cholinergic neurotransmission, such as the acetylcholinesterase (AChE) inhibitors and the allosteric agonists of nicotinic cholinergic receptors (nAChR) [11]. AChE inhibitors, or anti-AChE drugs such as tacrine, donepezil, rivastigmine and its derivates, inactivate an enzymatic degradation of ACh by AChE, producing an increment of a synaptic concentration of ACh released by the cholinergic nerves that results in an increase of the cholinergic neurotransmission [11]. Allosteric agonists of nAChR with a moderate anti-AChE activity, such as galantamine, increase the cholinergic neurotransmission due to an increment of response of nAChR to the ACh released in the cholinergic synapses [12]. However, this pharmacological strategy to facilitate the cholinergic neurotransmission may temporally improve the AD symptoms. The therapeutic efficacy of these cholinergic agonists to prevent or to attenuate the cognitive deficit in AD patients is limited [8]. In addition, the severity of multiple adverse effects compromises prolonged use of these drugs in the AD therapy [2, 11, 12].

Attempts to prevent an Aβ-induced neurotoxicity have led to the development of neuroprotective pharmacological strategies aimed at blocking the receptors implicated in this neuronal response, such as the N-methyl-D-aspartate (NMDA) receptors. The Aβ overproduction increases the vulnerability of neurons to a NMDA-mediated excitotoxicity, contributing to a cognitive deficit due to a neuronal death in AD [11]. Thus, a blockade of the NMDA receptors with memantine, and its derivates, has also been used to attenuate a neuronal excitotoxicity [11]. However, this pharmacological strategy has been ineffective to interrupt or to prevent the progression of AD. In addition, the complexity of adverse effects of these antagonists of NMDA receptors makes difficult their prolonged use in the AD patients [2 - 10].

Numerous lines of scientific investigation have supported that an age-related deregulation of a neuronal Ca^{2+} homeostasis is intimately involved in the pathogenesis of neurodegenerative diseases, including AD [13]. Thus, the precise understanding of the molecular mechanisms involved in the pathophysiological role of the neuronal Ca^{2+} homeostasis in the neurodegenerative diseases became crucial for the development of novel pharmacological strategies for the AD therapy [2 - 10].

PATHOPHYSIOLOGICAL ROLE OF THE NEURONAL CA^{2+} HOMEOSTASIS IN AD

The neuron uses the Ca^{2+} ions as intracellular messengers in multiple cellular responses, including in: the neurotransmitter release, the neuronal growth, the gene expression, the apoptosis and others [14, 15]. Several cellular mechanisms involving different proteins and intracellular messengers, and cellular organelles, actively participate in the neuronal Ca^{2+} homeostasis [14, 16]. Plasma membrane Ca^{2+} channels, such as voltage-activated Ca^{2+} channels (VACC) and the transient receptor potential (TRP) channels, regulate the Ca^{2+} flux from the extracellular space into the cytosol [14, 16]. Ca^{2+} channels regulated by IP_3 (IP_3R) and ryanodine (RyR) receptors located in the endoplasmic reticulum (ER) membrane regulate the Ca^{2+} flux from the ER into the cytosol [14, 16]. Thus, a Ca^{2+} release from the ER can be stimulated by an IP_3R activated by the IP_3, produced following an activation of metabotropic receptors coupled to the phospholipase C, and by a RyR activated by Ca^{2+} in response to a Ca^{2+} influx through the VACC [14, 16].

In addition to the ER, other cellular organelles such as mitochondria also participate of the neuronal Ca^{2+} homeostasis [14, 15]. Mitochondrial Ca^{2+} uniporter (MCU) regulates a Ca^{2+} flux into the matrix mitochondrial, and a mitochondrial Na^+/Ca^{2+}-ATPase (mNCX) [14, 15]. These mechanisms of Ca^{2+} transport play an important role in the neuronal physiology by stimulating a mitochondrial metabolism and increasing a mitochondrial energy production [14, 15]. However, a Ca^{2+} accumulation into the mitochondrial matrix activates a permeability transition pore (PTP) and stimulates the apoptosis [14, 15]. Owing to its importance for the neuronal function, the intracellular Ca^{2+} signalling is tightly compartmentalized, and finely regulated within signalling microdomains which involve, for example, a functional coupling between the VACC, the ER Ca^{2+} channels regulated by an IP3R and RyR, MCU and mNCX [14, 15].

In the past two decades, an increasing number of evidences have indicated that AD, and other neurodegenerative diseases, is the result of an age-related deregulation of the neuronal Ca^{2+} homeostasis [13, 16]. This deregulation that causes a neuronal dysfunction, and death, due to a cytosolic Ca^{2+} overload is mainly resulting from an enhanced Ca^{2+} influx through the VACC, an impaired ability of mitochondria to buffer or cycle Ca^{2+}, a perturbed Ca^{2+} regulation in the ER Ca^{2+}stores regulated by IP3R and RyR[16]. The expression of an array of neuronal Ca^{2+}-handling systems has been studied by a gene array and proteomic analyses. Studies using brains obtained from AD patients, and animal AD models, have revealed significant alterations in genes and proteins directly involved in the neuronal Ca^{2+} homeostasis [16]. Many of the molecular mechanisms involved in this deregulation described in normal aging can be reproduced by subjecting neurons to an oxidative and metabolic stress in culture or *in vivo*, suggesting important contributions of these fundamental aging processes to the deregulation of neuronal Ca^{2+} homeostasis in AD [13, 16]. In addition, Aβ interaction with the components of the plasma membrane increases the cytosolic Ca^{2+} overload, aggravating the vulnerability of the neurons to an excitotoxicity [2, 16]. It was shown that the oligomeric forms of Aβ42 cause a Ca^{2+}-mediated toxicity in cultured cells [16]. In addition, degenerative changes occur in neurites associated with Aβ deposits in some APP mutant mice, suggesting the involvement of an *in vivo* Ca^{2+}-mediated Aβ neurotoxicity in AD [16].

Amyloidogenic processing of APP also perturbs the neuronal Ca^{2+} homeostasis in AD by decreasing the production of a secreted form of APP (sAPPα) that activates K^+ channels, and by generating an APP intracellular domain that affects an ER Ca^{2+} release by regulating the expression of genes involved in the neuronal Ca^{2+} homeostasis [13, 16]. Aβ may also increase a Ca^{2+} influx by introducing into the plasma membrane and establishing ion-conducting pores. Neurotoxic forms of Aβ are oligomers that share structural and functional homology with pore-forming bacterial toxins, and the cytotoxic lymphocyte protein perforin. The capacity of Aβ to associate with membranes and establishing channels is improved by an exposure of phosphatidylserine on the cell surface [2, 16]. Because a cell surface exposure of phosphatidylserine is usually suggestive of apoptotic or energy-deprived cells, it is possible that age-related mitochondrial dysfunctions may rise surface phosphatidylserine levels in affected neurons, and promote Aβ-mediated pore formation, persistently enhancing a Ca^{2+} influx that causes a neuronal death due to a cytosolic Ca^{2+} overload. Indeed, neurons with a decreased cytosolic ATP concentration and an enhanced surface phosphatidylserine are particularly vulnerable to an Aβ toxicity. The surface exposure of phosphatidylserine may also result from an activation of a Ca^{2+}-sensitive phospholipid scrambalase 1 (PLSCR1), which facilitates a rapid trans-bilayer reorganization of plasma membrane phospholipids [16].

Aβ can directly interrupt the neuronal Ca^{2+} homeostasis in synaptic terminals by producing a membrane-associated oxidative stress [13, 16]. Consistent with a major role for Aβ in the synaptic damage in AD, there are data showing a loss of dendritic spines in dendrites associated with Aβ deposits in some APP mutant mice. Aβ also perturbs the neuronal Ca^{2+} homeostasis by inducing a membrane lipid peroxidation. During a peptide oligomer formation, Aβ generates a hydrogen peroxide, a process enhanced by iron (Fe^{2+}) and copper (Cu^+). Hydrogen peroxide is then converted into a hydroxyl radical, which initiates a lipid peroxidation resulting in the generation of toxic lipid aldehydes such as 4-hydroxynonenal, which impairs the function of ion-motive ATPases, and glutamate and glucose transporters, resulting into a cytosolic Ca^{2+} overload, a synaptic dysfunction, a neuronal degeneration and a cognitive impairment [16]. Because extreme and continuous increases of cytosolic Ca^{2+} enhance a free radical production (by altering a mitochondrial oxidative phosphorylation and stimulating oxygenases), it is likely that a perturbed neuronal Ca^{2+} homeostasis subsidizes the increased neuronal oxidative stress in AD, resulting in a self-amplifying cascade of free radical- and Ca^{2+}-mediated degenerative processes.

Aβ also causes a down-regulation of the expression of calcineurin, a Ca^{2+}-activated phosphatase known to play fundamental roles in the synaptic plasticity. Aβ oligomers caused a rapid decrease in the membrane expression of NMDA and EphB2 receptors, followed by an abnormal dendritic spine morphology and degeneration of spines [13, 16]. It is well established that Aβ increases the vulnerability of neurons to an excitotoxicity mediated by the NMDA receptor. The latter properties of Aβ are prevented by treatment with a NMDA receptor antagonist, signifying a major role for the Ca^{2+} influx in the dendritic dystrophy. Due to multiple actions of Aβ on the neuronal Ca^{2+} homeostasis, Aβ-targeting drug development could prevent a synaptic dysfunction, and restore the cognitive function in AD. However, the drug development to modify the AD pathology by an intervention in the amyloid accumulation has been ineffective or inconclusive. Due to an importance of the pathophysiological role of the neuronal Ca^{2+} homeostasis in the neurodegenerative diseases, the proteins involved in the cellular Ca^{2+} homeostasis became strategic targets of a new pharmacotherapy for AD. The following Fig. (**1**) summarizes the previous discussion.

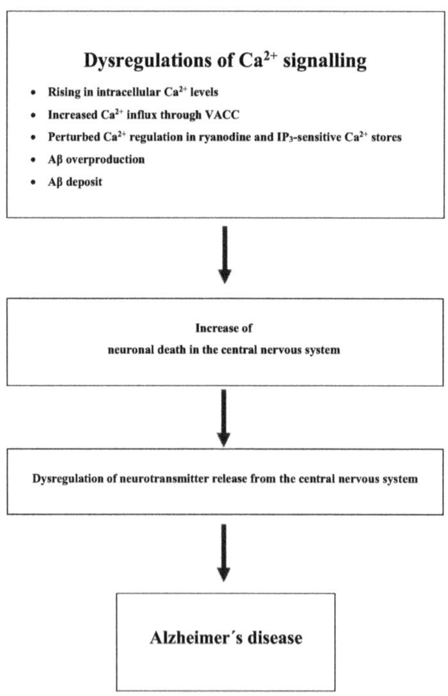

Fig. (1). The dysregulations of Ca^{2+} signalling and the pathogenesis of Alzheimer's disease.

NEURONAL CA^{2+} SIGNALLING AS A POTENTIAL TARGET FOR THE PHARMACOTHERAPY OF AD

Synaptic terminals are particularly vulnerable to a Ca^{2+}-mediated degeneration because they experience repeated bouts of a Ca^{2+} influx and have unusually high energy requirements to support their ion-homeostatic and signalling systems. Due to their physiological importance in the synaptic plasticity and memory, and their involvement in the neurodegenerative process, the L-type VACC (also named as $Ca_v1.2$) have become a strategic target for the AD pharmacotherapy. In fact, alterations of expression and function of several proteins involved in the regulation of neuronal Ca^{2+} homeostasis, especially L-type VACC have been described in AD and in other neurodegenerative diseases [17]. In addition, a brain Aβ accumulation in AD dramatically increases the L-type VACC in somatodendrites and axons in the hippocampus and cortex, contributing to a neurodegeneration of these brain regions. Thus, a pharmacological blockade of the L-type VACC to prevent a neuronal dysfunction, and death, caused by a cytosolic Ca^{2+} overload could be a promising therapeutic strategy for AD [2, 3].

Pharmacologically, the L-type VACC are blockade by drugs classified as L-type Ca^{2+} channel blockers (CCB). Classically used in the pharmacotherapy of arterial hypertension to produce a vasodilation and a reduction of arterial pressure, the L-type CCB inhibit the Ca^{2+} influx through the L-type VACC by reducing the cytosolic Ca^{2+} concentration ($[Ca^{2+}]_c$) [2, 3]. Numerous epidemiological studies performed since the 1990s support that the use of L-type CCB during antihypertensive therapy prevents, or slows, the rate of progression of dementia in the hypertensive patients [17 - 28]. These studies also suggest that a chronic hypertension could be associated with an increased risk for a cognitive decline, and dementia. Thus, the use of L-type CCB in the antihypertensive therapy not only lowers the high arterial pressure, but also has positive effects on preventing dementia [17 - 28]. Although this association between hypertension and dementia remains poorly understood, the antihypertensive therapy with the L-type CCB might have a preventive effect on dementia. The molecular mechanisms involved in the preventive effects of the L-type CCB on the incidence of dementia, or cognitive decline, are unclear.

Several lines of investigation support that the L-type CCB prevent an Aβ-induced neuronal decline and attenuate a neurodegeneration, producing a neuroprotection in AD [2, 17]. In addition to preventing a cytosolic Ca^{2+} overload, leading to a neuronal dysfunction and death in the neurodegenerative diseases, a selective blockade of the L-type VACC by dihydropyridines (DHP), such as isradipine, prevented a Ca^{2+} toxicity induced by an Aβ oligomer in hippocampal neurons from an animal AD model [2]. DHP also induced the autophagy without causing toxic effects in human neuroglioma H4 cells [29]. DHP also acts as a potent activator of an anti-aging neuroprotective protein, sirtuin 1 [30], which appears to regulate the autophagy function [31]. Studies using transgenic animal AD models have shown that the treatment with isradipine was well-tolerated and prevented a neuronal hyperphosphorylation of a microtubule-associated Tau protein, and yet improved the autophagy function in the brain [2]. Nilvadipine, an isradipine analogous, improved the cognitive functions in animals treated with human $A\beta_{1-42}$ [32, 33]. Other isradipine analogous, such as nitrendipine and cilnidipine, promoted an $A\beta_{1-42}$ clearance across the blood-brain barrier in wild type mice [32, 33]. Nilvadipine and nitrendipine ameliorated the Aβ clearance, and an explorative activity in a transgenic animal AD model [32, 33]. These findings clearly support that the treatment with L-type CCB can disrupt the pathology of AD due to their neuroprotective properties.

In fact, the pharmacological modulation of the neuronal Ca^{2+} homeostasis by the use of L-type CCB could open a large avenue to the development of novel therapeutic strategies to attenuate the neurodegenerative process in AD, and other neurodegenerative diseases. More recently, we have proposed that the combined use of the L-type CCB with other neuroprotective drugs such as phosphodiesterases (PDE) inhibitors, or the use of hybrid compounds having the moieties of L-type CCB and AChE inhibitor such as tacripirines, could be effective in the AD pharmacotherapy [34, 35]. Thus, a better understanding of these pharmacological neuroprotective strategies will be critical for designing new assays with appropriate drug doses in any future clinical trials for the AD pharmacotherapy.

PHARMACOLOGICAL MODULATION OF THE CA^{2+}/CAMP SIGNALLING AS A POTENTIAL NEUROPROTECTIVE STRATEGY FOR THE AD THERAPY

In addition to a deregulation of the neuronal Ca^{2+} homeostasis, an age-related deregulation of the synthesis, execution, and/or degradation of cyclic nucleotide signalling has been involved in the cognitive deficit in AD and other neurodegenerative diseases [36]. This deregulation includes an abnormal activity of adenylyl cyclase (AC), cyclic adenosine monophosphate (cAMP), cAMP-dependent protein kinase (PKA), cAMP response element binding protein (CREB), exchange protein activated by cAMP (Epac), hyperpolarization-activated cyclic nucleotide-gated ion channels (HCNs), soluble and particulate guanylyl cyclase, cyclic guanosine monophosphate (cGMP), cGMP-dependent protein kinase (PKG) and phosphodiesterases (PDE) [36, 37]. The PDE are enzymes responsible for the breakdown of cyclic nucleotides, cAMP and cGMP. Crucial regulators of the levels of cyclic nucleotide signalling, these second messengers relay and amplify the incoming signals at the receptors on the cell surface, then making them important elements in the signal transduction cascades, and essential in the cellular signalling in a variety of cell functions, including the neurotransmitter release, the neuroplasticity and the neuroprotection [38]. CREB is a transcription factor associated with a memory and a synaptic plasticity, and its signalling is essential for long-lasting changes in a synaptic plasticity that mediates the conversion of a short-term memory to a long-term memory [38]. The Aβ peptide alters a hippocampal-dependent synaptic plasticity and memory, then mediating a synapse loss through the CREB signalling pathway [37]. Synaptic efficacy mediating a memory storage requires the activation of specific gene expression programs regulated, among others, by CREB [37]. In response to signals at the cell surface, CREB is phosphorylated in the nucleus by various protein kinases *via* secondary messengers such as cAMP and/or Ca^{2+} for regulating specific genes [38 - 40]. CREB signalling has been recently involved in several brain pathological conditions, including the cognitive deficit and neurodegenerative disorders [41].

Over the past decades, researchers have become more interested in the role of the cAMP/PKA/CREB signalling in AD, and other neurodegenerative diseases. The most reproducible findings associated to a deregulation in the cAMP/PKA/CREB signalling in AD include: 1) a reduced AC activity in the hippocampus and specific cortical regions, 2) a reduced expression/activity of PKA in the temporal cortex and hippocampus, 3) a reduced phosphorylation of CREB in the hippocampus, 4) a reduced expression/activity of the PDE4 family and 5) beneficial effects of selective PDE4 inhibitors [41]. Thus, the development of novel neuroprotective pharmacological strategies based on the cAMP/PKA/CREB signalling could produce important advances for the AD therapy.

The PDE4 are vital controllers of the cAMP abundance in the central nervous system through their capacity to modulate the PKA activity, the CREB phosphorylation, and other important issues of the signalling pathways. By preventing the cAMP breakdown, PDE4 inhibitors can enhance an intracellular signal transduction, and increase the CREB phosphorylation and transcription of proteins related to a synaptic plasticity, and an associated memory formation [41]. PDE4 inhibitors have received increasing attention as antidepressant and cognition-enhancers in neurological/psychiatric disorders related to a cognitive deficit [42]. Rolipram, a selective PDE4 inhibitor, was the first compound found to effectively restore a cognitive deficit in AD models. Other PDE4 inhibitors, such as HT-0712, roflumilast and BPN14770 were also able to restore a cognitive deficit in AD models [41, 42]. These findings consistently suggest that the pharmacological modulation of the cAMP/PKA/CREB signalling by an inhibition of the PDE4 restores the cognitive deficit in AD [43 - 45].

Recently, we discovered that the mutual use of L-type CCB (in low concentration) and PDE4 inhibitor rolipram significantly increased the synaptic neurotransmission due to an increment in the neurotransmitter release, then preventing a neuronal death [44, 45]. As the AC activity is finely regulated by Ca^{2+}, the reduction of $[Ca^{2+}]_c$ due to a partial blockade of the L-type VACC by CCB (in low concentration) results in an increase of AC activity, and consequently the elevation of the cytosolic cAMP concentration ($[cAMP]_c$), that stimulates the PKA activity in neurons [2 - 6]. In the activated state, PKA increments the activity of RyR-regulated ER Ca^{2+} channels, forming Ca^{2+} microdomains that facilitate the traffic and docking of secretory vesicles in the neuronal membrane [2 - 6]. This neuronal response stimulates the Ca^{2+}-mediated fusion of a vesicle secretory in the plasma membrane, increasing the exocytosis of these vesicles, and consequently the synaptic neurotransmission [2 - 6]. We observed that this increment in the neurotransmitter release was reproduced by other drugs that produce an increment of $[cAMP]_c$ (cAMP-enhancers), such as AC activators (forskolin), and it was abolished by AC inhibitors (SQ 22536), confirming the participation of a functional interaction between the intracellular signalling pathways mediated by Ca^{2+} and cAMP, named by us as Ca^{2+}/cAMP signalling interaction. Thus, these findings could subsidize the development of a new therapeutic goal to rise the synaptic transmission in the neurodegenerative diseases related to a drastic deficit in the synaptic transmission, such as in AD [2 - 6, 44 - 46].

It is well established that the increase of [cAMP]c induced by PDE4 inhibition enhances a CREB phosphorylation, and transcription of proteins related to a synaptic plasticity and a neuronal survival, producing a neuroprotection [44, 45]. We have anticipated that a neuronal death resultant of a cytosolic Ca^{2+} overload related to the neurodegenerative disorders could be reduced, or prevented, in response to a stimulus of the neuronal survival pathways facilitated by the cAMP/PKA/CREB signalling by means through the pharmacological manipulation of the Ca^{2+}/cAMP signalling interaction [2-6, 44, 45, (Fig. **2**)].

Thus, we have proposed that the pharmacological manipulation of the neuronal Ca^{2+}/cAMP signalling by the mutual use of the L-type CCB and cAMP-enhancers, such as PDE4 inhibitors, could be used in the AD pharmacotherapy to prevent a neuronal death caused by a cytosolic Ca^{2+} overload due to a stimulation of cellular survival pathways regulated by the cAMP/PKA/CREB signalling pathway, and additionally to attenuate a deficit of cognition due to a rise in the central cholinergic neurotransmission caused by an increase in the ACh release from the cholinergic neurons [2-6, 44, 45, (Table **1**)].

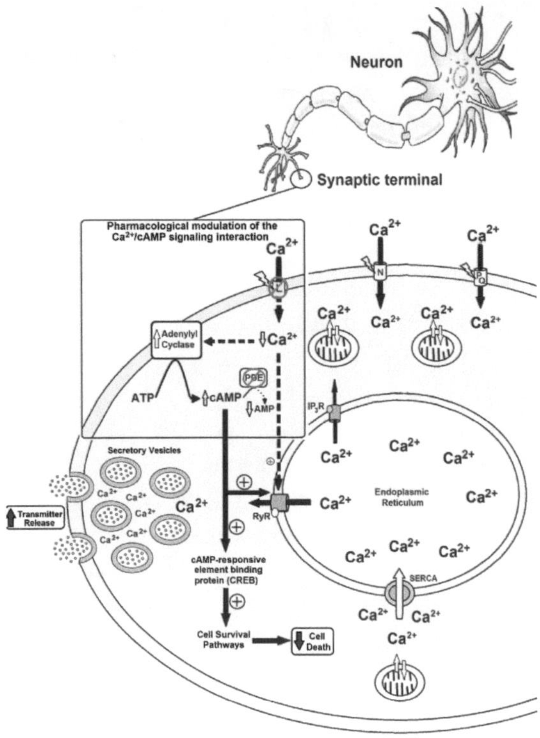

Fig. (2). Increase of the neurotransmission and neuroprotection due to the pharmacological manipulation of the Ca^{2+}/cAMP signalling interaction. The reduction by L-type CCB of the Ca^{2+} influx through the L-type voltage-activated Ca^{2+} channels (VACC) enhances the adenylyl cyclase (AC) activity, and consequently $[cAMP]_c$. These CCB-effects can be potentiated by the cAMP-enhancer compounds (like PDE inhibitors). Combined use of the CCBs with the cAMP-enhancer compounds could attenuate the degeneration, and death, of the motor neurons triggered mainly by a cytosolic Ca^{2+} overload (neuroprotector effect). Additionally, this pharmacological strategy could attenuate the deficit in the motor neurotransmission. Our studies suggest that this pharmacological strategy based in the modulation by drugs of the Ca^{2+}/cAMP signalling interaction could be useful to attenuate the neurological/psychiatric diseases. PDE - Phosphodiesterases, RyR - Ryanodine receptors, IP_3R - IP_3 receptors, SERCA - Sarcoendoplasmic reticulum Ca^{2+}-ATPase.

Table 1. CCB and cAMP-enhancer compounds.

Ca^{2+} Channel Blockers (CCB)	cAMP-enhancer Compounds
1. Verapamil	1. Rolipram
2. Nifedipine	2. 3-isobutyl-1-methylxanthine (IBMX)
3. Diltiazem	3. Forskolin
4. Isradipine	4.Aminophylline
5. Amlodipine	5. Theophylline
6. Nicardipine	6. Paraxanthine

Thus, the discovery of our group of the role of the Ca^{2+}/cAMP signalling interaction in the synaptic transmission and neuroprotection, and its pharmacological manipulation, may open an extraordinary pathway for the development of a new therapeutic goal for the neurodegenerative disorders such as AD.

CONCLUSIONS

In this chapter, I have discussed the future perspectives for the pharmacotherapy of AD by the pharmacological manipulation of the neuronal Ca^{2+}/cAMP signalling interaction endorsed by the mutual use of the L-type CCB (used in the antihypertensive therapy) and cAMP-enhancers (used in the antidepressant therapy). This new pharmacological strategy for the AD therapy could efficiently reduce, or prevent, a neuronal dysfunction and death by two main mechanisms: (1) an attenuation of a cytosolic Ca^{2+} overload and (2) an enhancement of cellular survival pathways facilitated by the cAMP/PKA/CREB signalling pathways. In addition, this new pharmacological strategy could attenuate or prevent a deficit of cognition due to a rise in the central cholinergic neurotransmission caused by an increase in the ACh release from the cholinergic neurons. Thus, the pharmacological manipulation of the neuronal Ca^{2+}/cAMP signalling interaction could be a new therapeutic goal to slow or prevent the progression of AD.

SUMMARY POINTS

- This chapter discusses the classical and the novel concepts for the Alzheimer´s disease pharmacotherapy, including the manipulation by medicines of the interaction between Ca^{2+} and cAMP signalling.
- The interaction between Ca^{2+} and cAMP signalling is a fundamental cellular process presented in several cells and tissues, characterized by an efficient interaction between Ca^{2+} and cAMP signalling pathways.
- The increase of the cAMP concentration induced by a PDE4 inhibition enhances the CREB phosphorylation, then proteins associated to the plasticity of the synapses are up-regulated, thus achieving a neuronal survival and producing a neuroprotection.
- A cytosolic Ca^{2+} overload is highly associated to the neurodegenerative disorders, then the attenuation of this overload could be a new therapeutic target. A stimulation of the neuronal survival pathways mediated by the cAMP/PKA/CREB could be associated with an attenuation of the Ca^{2+} overload.

ABBREVIATIONS

Aβ amyloid peptide

AC Adenylyl cyclase

ACh	Acetylcholine
AChE	Acetylcholinesterase
nAChR	Nicotinic cholinergic receptors
AD	Alzheimer's disease
APP	Amyloid precursor protein
BACE 1	Beta secretase 1
$[Ca^{2+}]_c$	Cytosolic Ca^{2+} concentration
CaV 1.2	L-type voltage-activated Ca^{2+} channels
cAMP	Cyclic adenosine monophosphate
$[cAMP]_c$	Cytosolic cAMP concentration
CCB	Ca^{2+}channel blockers
cGMP	Cyclic guanosine monophosphate
CREB	cAMP response element binding protein
DHP	Dihydropyridine
EphB2	Ephrin type-B receptor 2
Epac	Exchange protein activated by cAMP
ER	Endoplasmic reticulum
GC	Guanylyl cyclase
HCN	Hyperpolarization-activated cyclic nucleotide-gated ion channels
IP3	Inositol trisphosphate
IP3R	Inositol trisphosphate receptors
MCU	Mitochondrial Ca^{2+} uniporter
mNCX	Mitochondrial Na^+/ Ca^{2+}-ATPase (mNCX)
NMDA	N-methyl-D-aspartate
PDE	Phosphodiesterases
PKA	cAMP-dependent protein kinase
PKG	cGMP-dependent protein kinase
PLSCR1	Ca^{2+}-sensitive phospholipid scrambalase 1
PTP	Permeability transition pore
RyR	Ryanodine receptors
TRP	Transient receptor potential channels
VACC	Voltage-activated Ca^{2+} channels

CONSENT FOR PUBLICATION

Not applicable.

CONFLICT OF INTEREST

The author declares no conflict of interest, financial or otherwise.

ACKNOWLEDGEMENTS

Declared none

REFERENCES

[1] Mohamed T, Shakeri A, Rao PP. Amyloid cascade in Alzheimer's disease: Recent advances in medicinal chemistry. Eur J Med Chem 2016; 113: 258-72. [http://dx.doi.org/10.1016/j.ejmech.2016.02.049] [PMID: 26945113]

[2] Bergantin LB, Caricati-Neto A. Challenges for the pharmacological treatment of neurological and psychiatric disorders: Implications of the Ca($^{2+}$)/cAMP intracellular signalling interaction. Eur J Pharmacol 2016; 788: 255-60. [http://dx.doi.org/10.1016/j.ejphar.2016.06.034] [PMID: 27349146]

[3] Caricati-Neto A, García AG, Bergantin LB. Pharmacological implications of the Ca(2+)/cAMP signaling interaction: from risk for antihypertensive therapy to potential beneficial for neurological and psychiatric disorders. Pharmacol Res Perspect 2015; 3(5): e00181. [http://dx.doi.org/10.1002/prp2.181] [PMID: 26516591]

[4] Bergantin LB. Neurodegenerative diseases: where to go from now? thought provoking through Ca^{2+}/cAMP signaling interaction. Brain Disord Ther 2017; 6: e125. [http://dx.doi.org/10.4172/2168-975X.1000e125]

[5] Bergantin LB. Neurological disorders: is there a horizon? emerging ideas from the interaction between Ca^{2+} and camp signaling pathways. J Neurol Disord 2017; 5: e124. [http://dx.doi.org/10.4172/2329-6895.1000e124]

[6] Bergantin LB. Dysregulation of Intracellular Ca^{2+} and Camp Signalling: Plausible Targets for Neurological Disorders. J Neurol Disord 2018; 6: e125. [http://dx.doi.org/10.4172/2329-6895.1000e125]

[7] Bradley Yat-Wah Man, Ho-Man Chan, Chung-Hang Leung *et al.*. Group 9 metal-based inhibitors of β-amyloid (1–40) fibrillation as potential therapeutic agents for Alzheimer's disease. Chem Sci (Camb) 2011; 2: 917-21. [http://dx.doi.org/10.1039/c0sc00636j]

[8] Ma DL, Chan DS, Ma VP, Leung KH, Zhong HJ, Leung CH. Current advancements in Aβ luminescent probes and inhibitors of Aβ aggregation. Curr Alzheimer Res 2012; 9(7): 830-43. [http://dx.doi.org/10.2174/156720512802455377] [PMID: 22631884]

[9] Baranello RJ, Bharani KL, Padmaraju V, *et al.* Amyloid-beta protein clearance and degradation (ABCD) pathways and their role in Alzheimer's disease. Curr Alzheimer Res 2015; 12(1): 32-46. [http://dx.doi.org/10.2174/1567205012666141218140953] [PMID: 25523424]

[10] Bergantin LB, Caricati-Neto A. Emerging Concepts for Neuroscience Field from Ca^{2+}/cAMP Signalling Interaction. J Neurol Exp Neurosci 2017; 3(1): 29-32. [http://dx.doi.org/10.17756/jnen.2017-024]

[11] Maroto M, de Diego AM, Albiñana E, *et al.* Multi-target novel neuroprotective compound ITH33/IQM9.21 inhibits calcium entry, calcium signals and exocytosis. Cell Calcium 2011; 50(4): 359-69. [http://dx.doi.org/10.1016/j.ceca.2011.06.006] [PMID: 21839513]

[12] Caricati-Neto A, D'angelo LC, Reuter H, Hyppolito Jurkiewicz N, Garcia AG, Jurkiewicz A. Enhancement of purinergic neurotransmission by galantamine and other acetylcholinesterase inhibitors

in the rat vas deferens. Eur J Pharmacol 2004; 503(1-3): 191-201.
[http://dx.doi.org/10.1016/j.ejphar.2004.09.034] [PMID: 15496314]

[13] Berridge MJ. Dysregulation of neural calcium signaling in Alzheimer disease, bipolar disorder and schizophrenia. Prion 2013; 7(1): 2-13.
[http://dx.doi.org/10.4161/pri.21767] [PMID: 22895098]

[14] Neher E, Zucker RS. Multiple calcium-dependent processes related to secretion in bovine chromaffin cells. Neuron 1993; 10(1): 21-30.
[http://dx.doi.org/10.1016/0896-6273(93)90238-M] [PMID: 8427700]

[15] Caricati-Neto A, Padín JF, Silva-Junior ED, *et al.* Novel features on the regulation by mitochondria of calcium and secretion transients in chromaffin cells challenged with acetylcholine at 37°C. Physiol Rep 2013; 1(7): e00182.
[http://dx.doi.org/10.1002/phy2.182] [PMID: 24744861]

[16] Bezprozvanny I, Mattson MP. Neuronal calcium mishandling and the pathogenesis of Alzheimer's disease. Trends Neurosci 2008; 31(9): 454-63.
[http://dx.doi.org/10.1016/j.tins.2008.06.005] [PMID: 18675468]

[17] Forette F, Seux ML, Staessen JA, *et al.* Prevention of dementia in randomised double-blind placebo-controlled Systolic Hypertension in Europe (Syst-Eur) trial. Lancet 1998; 352(9137): 1347-51.
[http://dx.doi.org/10.1016/S0140-6736(98)03086-4] [PMID: 9802273]

[18] Forette F, Seux ML, Staessen JA, *et al.* The prevention of dementia with antihypertensive treatment: new evidence from the Systolic Hypertension in Europe (Syst-Eur) study. Arch Intern Med 2002; 162(18): 2046-52.
[http://dx.doi.org/10.1001/archinte.162.18.2046] [PMID: 12374512]

[19] Fritze J, Walden J. Clinical findings with nimodipine in dementia: test of the calcium hypothesis. J Neural Transm Suppl 1995; 46: 439-53.
[PMID: 8821080]

[20] Hanon O, Pequignot R, Seux ML, *et al.* Relationship between antihypertensive drug therapy and cognitive function in elderly hypertensive patients with memory complaints. JHypertens 2006; 24(10): 2101-7.
[http://dx.doi.org/10.1097/01.hjh.0000244961.69985.05] [PMID: 16957572]

[21] Paran E, Anson O, Lowenthal DT. Cognitive function and antihypertensive treatment in the elderly: a 6-year follow-up study. Am J Ther 2010; 17(4): 358-64.
[PMID: 20019592]

[22] Peters R, Booth A, Peters J. A systematic review of calcium channel blocker use and cognitive decline/dementia in the elderly. J Hypertens 2014; 32(10): 1945-57.
[http://dx.doi.org/10.1097/HJH.0000000000000273] [PMID: 25068540]

[23] Rouch L, Cestac P, Hanon O, *et al.* Antihypertensive drugs, prevention of cognitive decline and dementia: a systematic review of observational studies, randomized controlled trials and meta-analyses, with discussion of potential mechanisms. CNS Drugs 2015; 29(2): 113-30.
[http://dx.doi.org/10.1007/s40263-015-0230-6] [PMID: 25700645]

[24] Tollefson GD. Short-term effects of the calcium channel blocker nimodipine (Bay-e-9736) in the management of primary degenerative dementia. Biol Psychiatry 1990; 27(10): 1133-42.
[http://dx.doi.org/10.1016/0006-3223(90)90050-C] [PMID: 2187540]

[25] Trompet S, Westendorp RG, Kamper AM, de Craen AJ. Use of calcium antagonists and cognitive decline in old age. The Leiden 85-plus study. Neurobiol Aging 2008; 29(2): 306-8.
[http://dx.doi.org/10.1016/j.neurobiolaging.2006.10.006] [PMID: 17101196]

[26] Wu CL, Wen SH. A 10-year follow-up study of the association between calcium channel blocker use and the risk of dementia in elderly hypertensive patients. Medicine (Baltimore) 2016; 95(32): e4593.
[http://dx.doi.org/10.1097/MD.0000000000004593] [PMID: 27512890]

[27] Yasar S, Corrada M, Brookmeyer R, Kawas C. Calcium channel blockers and risk of AD: the Baltimore Longitudinal Study of Aging. Neurobiol Aging 2005; 26(2): 157-63. [http://dx.doi.org/10.1016/j.neurobiolaging.2004.03.009] [PMID: 15582745]

[28] Nimmrich V, Eckert A. Calcium channel blockers and dementia. Br J Pharmacol 2013; 169(6): 1203-10. [http://dx.doi.org/10.1111/bph.12240] [PMID: 23638877]

[29] Zhang L, Yu J, Pan H, *et al.* Small molecule regulators of autophagy identified by an image-based high-throughput screen. Proc Natl Acad Sci USA 2007; 104(48): 19023-8. [http://dx.doi.org/10.1073/pnas.0709695104] [PMID: 18024584]

[30] Mai A, Valente S, Meade S, *et al.* Study of 1,4-dihydropyridine structural scaffold: discovery of novel sirtuin activators and inhibitors. J Med Chem 2009; 52(17): 5496-504. [http://dx.doi.org/10.1021/jm9008289] [PMID: 19663498]

[31] Lee IH, Cao L, Mostoslavsky R, *et al.* A role for the NAD-dependent deacetylase Sirt1 in the regulation of autophagy. Proc Natl Acad Sci USA 2008; 105(9): 3374-9. [http://dx.doi.org/10.1073/pnas.0712145105] [PMID: 18296641]

[32] Bachmeier C, Beaulieu-Abdelahad D, Mullan M, Paris D. Selective dihydropyiridine compounds facilitate the clearance of β-amyloid across the blood-brain barrier. Eur J Pharmacol 2011; 659(2-3): 124-9. [http://dx.doi.org/10.1016/j.ejphar.2011.03.048] [PMID: 21497592]

[33] Paris D, Bachmeier C, Patel N, *et al.* Selective antihypertensive dihydropyridines lower Aβ accumulation by targeting both the production and the clearance of Aβ across the blood-brain barrier. Mol Med 2011; 17(3-4): 149-62. [http://dx.doi.org/10.2119/molmed.2010.00180] [PMID: 21170472]

[34] Caricati-Neto A, Bergantin LB. New therapeutic strategy for the neurodegenerative diseases: pharmacological modulation of Ca^{2+}/camp signaling interaction. Int Arch Clin Pharmacol 2018; 4(15).

[35] Caricati-Neto A, Bergantin LB. Perspectives of the pharmacological modulation of Ca^{2+}/cAMP signaling interaction as a new neuroprotector therapeutic strategy for amyotrophic lateral sclerosis (ALS). Biomed J Sci Tec Res 2017; 1: 1. [http://dx.doi.org/10.26717/BJSTR.2017.01.000131]

[36] Kelly MP. Cyclic nucleotide signaling changes associated with normal aging and age-related diseases of the brain. Cell Signal 2018; 42: 281-91. [http://dx.doi.org/10.1016/j.cellsig.2017.11.004] [PMID: 29175000]

[37] Prickaerts J, Heckman PRA, Blokland A. Investigational phosphodiesterase inhibitors in phase I and phase II clinical trials for Alzheimer's disease. Expert Opin Investig Drugs 2017; 26(9): 1033-48. [http://dx.doi.org/10.1080/13543784.2017.1364360] [PMID: 28772081]

[38] Caricati-Neto A, Bergantin LB. The passion of a scientific discovery: the "calcium paradox" due to Ca^{2+}/camp interaction. J Syst Integr Neurosci 2017; 3 [http://dx.doi.org/10.15761/JSIN.1000186]

[39] Sommer N, Löschmann PA, Northoff GH, *et al.* The antidepressant rolipram suppresses cytokine production and prevents autoimmune encephalomyelitis. Nat Med 1995; 1(3): 244-8. [http://dx.doi.org/10.1038/nm0395-244] [PMID: 7585041]

[40] Xiao L, O'Callaghan JP, O'Donnell JM. Effects of repeated treatment with phosphodiesterase-4 inhibitors on cAMP signaling, hippocampal cell proliferation, and behavior in the forced-swim test. J Pharmacol Exp Ther 2011; 338(2): 641-7. [http://dx.doi.org/10.1124/jpet.111.179358] [PMID: 21566211]

[41] Zamponi GW. Targeting voltage-gated calcium channels in neurological and psychiatric diseases. Nat Rev Drug Discov 2016; 15(1): 19-34. [http://dx.doi.org/10.1038/nrd.2015.5] [PMID: 26542451]

[42] Bergantin LB. Revisiting the clinical link between alzheimer's disease and depression through the Ca^{2+}/camp signalling interaction. Brain Disord Ther 2018; 7: e127.
[http://dx.doi.org/10.4172/2168-975X.1000e127]

[43] Uddin MS, Stachowiak A, Mamun AA, *et al.* Autophagy and Alzheimer's Disease: From Molecular Mechanisms to Therapeutic Implications. Front Aging Neurosci 2018; 10: 04.
[http://dx.doi.org/10.3389/fnagi.2018.00004] [PMID: 29441009]

[44] Neto AC, Bergantin LB. New therapeutic perspectives for the cognitive deficit in alzheimer's disease: pharmacological modulation of Ca^{2+}/cAMP signaling interaction. Int J Cogn Behav 2017; 1(1): 1-6.

[45] Caricati-Neto A, Bergantin LB. Pharmacological modulation of neural Ca^{2+}/camp signaling interaction as therapeutic goal for treatment of Alzheimer´s disease. J Syst Integr Neurosci 2017.
[http://dx.doi.org/10.15761/JSIN.1000185]

[46] Liu CG, Wang JL, Li L, Wang PC. MicroRNA-384 regulates both amyloid precursor protein and β-secretase expression and is a potential biomarker for Alzheimer's disease. Int J Mol Med 2014; 34(1): 160-6.
[http://dx.doi.org/10.3892/ijmm.2014.1780] [PMID: 24827165]

158 *Frontiers in Clinical Drug Research - Alzheimer Disorders*, 2018, *Vol. 7*, 158-213

CHAPTER 6

Alzheimer's Disease: An Approach for Non-Pharmacological Therapies

M.G.V. Gottlieb[1,*], V.E. Closs[2], V.M. Junges[3], A. von Gunten[4], Z.C.L. Lindôso[5], J.P. Rocha[1], B.J.P. Lopes Filho[1], C.R. Oliveira[6] and **F. Loureiro[1]**

[1] *Graduate Program in Biomedical Gerontology (GERONBIO), School of Medicine, Pontifícia Universidade Católica do Rio Grande do Sul. Porto Alegre, RS, Brazil*

[2] *Study Group on Cardiometabolic Risk, Aging And Nutrition (GERICEN), Institute of Geriatrics and Gerontology (IGG), Pontifícia Universidade Católica do Rio Grande do Sul. Porto Alegre, RS, Brazil*

[3] *Integrated Center for Obesity Treatment (CINTRO), Porto Alegre, RS, Brazil*

[4] *Department of Psychiatry, University Hospital Lausanne, Lausanne, Switzerland*

[5] *Federal University of Pelotas, Pelotas-RS, Brazil*

[6] *Psychology Graduate Program, Faculdade Meridional Imed. Passo Fundo, RS, Brazil*

Abstract: The increase in life expectancy and lifestyle changes, such as inadequate diets, sedentarism and social inequality have contributed to an increase in neuropsychiatric disorders, such as Alzheimer's disease (AD). AD has a multifactorial origin, with a chronic and progressive nature, leading to cognitive and functional decline, including the gradual loss of autonomy, independence and social function, severely impairing the quality of life of both patient and family. The disease onset and progression become a burden on the family and caregivers, requiring an interdisciplinary and multidisciplinary approach. AD demands continuous assistance and increasing burdens during treatment. Health professionals, such as nutritionists, physical educators, physiotherapists and occupational therapists, neuropsychologists and speech therapists, offer complimentary therapies, becoming essential for the prevention of a quick decline in quality of life, and allowing patients with AD to remain functional and cognitively active for longer. In this setting, the contributions and actions of various health professionals play a major role in managing AD, and health actions directed at the elderly should have the prime objective of keeping the person within their community, together with their families, in the most dignified and comfortable manner possible. Their transfer to long-stay institutions (asylums, hospitals, retirement homes and the like) should only be considered when all other actions have failed. In this scenario, this chapter aims to address the role of different non-pharmacological therapies administered by a multi-professional health team to

[*] **Corresponding author Maria Gabriela Valle Gottlieb:** Graduate Program in Biomedical Gerontology (GERONBIO), School of Medicine, Pontifícia Universidade Católica do Rio Grande do Sul. Porto Alegre, RS, Brazil; Tel: 555133536096; Email: maria.gottlieb@pucrs.br.

Atta-ur-Rahman (Ed.)

delay the deterioration of cognition, autonomy, functionality and independence, maintaining an acceptable quality of life for the elderly with AD.

Keywords: Aging, Alzheimer's Disease, Dementia, Disability, Elderly, Interventions, Neuropsychologists, Non-Pharmacological Therapies, Nutrition, Occupational Therapy, Physiotherapy, Physical Educators, Quality of Life, Speech Therapy.

INTRODUCTION

Alzheimer's disease (AD) is a neurodegenerative disorder of insidious onset and progressive course, eventually evolving into a dementia syndrome. Dementia is a syndrome of cognitive decline, which, by definition, hampers the activities of daily living of those affected. A number of diseases in addition to AD can lead to dementia, more often than not neurodegenerative, vascular and of mixed disorders, but more rarely other conditions can be involved. The estimation of prevalence of AD is challenging, as is the case with all dementias. AD is considered the most common dementia, accounting for 50%-75% of the total [1]. Some 30%–40% of those aged 85 years old or more and about half of the elderly aged 90 years have dementia, and even more so beyond this age [2, 3], many of them having AD. However, the diagnosis may at times be difficult, *e.g.* in the very old as the inter-individual variability increases with age; in other words, distinguishing normality from pathological cognitive decline becomes more difficult as people grow older [4]. Features from AD and vascular dementia or other brain pathologies often coexist [5]. AD, among other dementias, has become one of the most frequent clinical conditions in the elderly in high-, middle- and low-income countries, secondary to the more general increase in human life expectancy [6 - 8].

AD affects the very essence of our personhood and may cause enormous suffering and disability for those having the disease. Dementia also changes the lives of family members and caregivers, bringing with it an enormous physical and psychological cost, with many caregivers having excess morbidity and mortality as compared to those who do not have the responsibility of caring for a person with dementia [9, 10].

Although most dementias have no cure and no disease-modifying treatments are available, we can do much to alleviate both the person affected and their caregivers, to improve their quality of life. An adequate response to the needs of people with dementia and their families usually requires a combination of medical, psychological, physical, occupational and social care interventions, depending, among other factors, on the stage of the disease. Primary care is an essential component of the care provided to people with dementia, from early primary prevention, early detection, and treatment in the most advanced stages of the illness [11].

ALZHEIMER'S DISEASE AND THE CONVENTIONAL PHARMACOLOGICAL THERAPY

Alzheimer's Disease

AD is of complex, heterogeneous and of ultimately unknown origin, which cannot be explained in a monocausal, mechanistic and linear way. AD is a clinical syndrome defined by a typical clinical constellation likely to be secondary to AD neuropathological features including neurofibrillary tangles and senile plaques, but also neuronal and synaptic loss. The typical clinical AD syndrome corresponds to an initially insidious and consequently progressive cognitive decline that affects first memory, and later executive functions, language, and visuospatial skills [12].

Despite the presence of these identifiable clinical features, polymorbidity with advancing age increases the likelihood of a patient to have two or more conditions, each of which may contribute to their cognitive decline [13]. So, clinically, in order to diagnose any comorbidity and for reasons of differential diagnosis a physical examination and a series of paraclinical investigations are usually required.

Conclusive diagnoses of the disease are not available. The use of diagnostic neuroimaging, usually Magnetic Resonance Imaging (MRI), helps exclude primary disorders of dementia, but this assessment is clearly not available in low- and middle-income countries. More recently, AD biomarkers in the cerebrospinal liquid have become available in some places, and dosing these biomarkers allows going some way in improving the accuracy of AD diagnosis [clear decrease of Amyloid-β of 42 amino acids (Aβ1-42) and increase of T-τ and Phosphorylated τ181 protein (P-τ181P) in typical AD] [14, 15]. In patients with neuropathologically confirmed AD, neuropsychological, functional and behavioral assessment are necessary for the definition of pharmacological and non-pharmacological treatment and intervention to be adopted (Fig. **1**).

The neuropsychological assessment quantifies the extent of impairment for each cognitive domain, including executive functioning and attention, memory, language, and visuo-spatial capacities. Its usefulness lies in the profiling of the cognitive impairment that may add considerably to the differential diagnosis of a dementia syndrome. At least as importantly, it lays the grounds for possible therapeutic interventions based on neuropsychological methods.

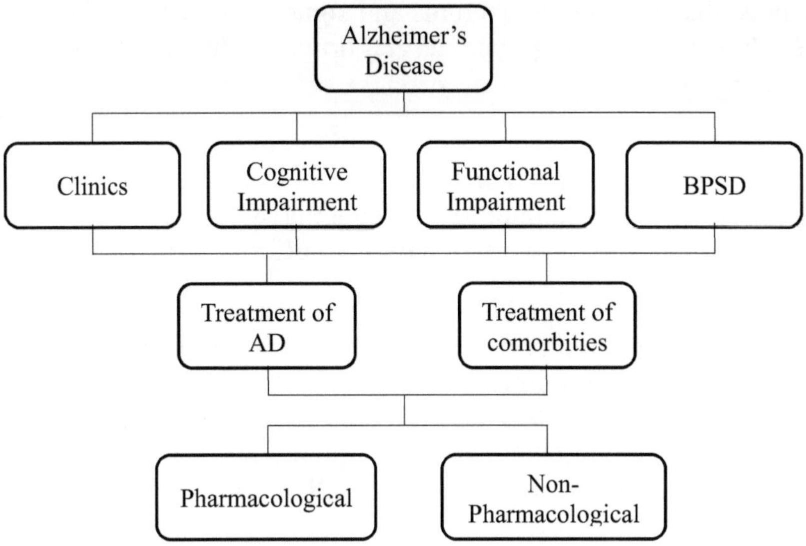

Fig. (1). Semiology and treatment of Alzheimer's disease.
Notes: BPSD: Behavioral and Psychological Symptoms of Dementia; AD: Alzheimer's Disease.

Cognitive deficits end up causing functional impairment that follows a typical pattern in pure cases [16]. The assessment of this temporal pattern i) allows for functional staging of disease progression, ii) has some predictive power of what lies ahead for patient and caregiver once the patient has reached a given stage, and iii) suggests the presence of some new or different condition if the disease progression fails to follow the predicted course.

With regards to BPSD, the psychopathological investigation is paramount in every patient independently of the dementia stage. The semiology of BPSD is extremely rich and includes many features of affective, psychotic and behavioral disturbances [17 - 19]. Considering BPSD as the result of stressors combined with variable degrees of vulnerability a host of psychological and systemic factors (personality, environmental elements both physical and emotional, psychiatric diseases) may contribute to the occurrence of BPSD, and even be a risk factor for cognitive decline and AD [10, 19 - 24].

In other hand, despite mountains of money spent and ongoing efforts, there is still no disease-modifying treatment of AD [25]. There are, however, some disease-specific treatments in the form of the different procognitive or anti-dementia drugs that have been approved for the treatment of AD and Lewi Body (LB) disorders. Although there is a huge literature on these drugs, they are sometimes controversially discussed with national agency and expert recommendations that may come to different conclusions. However, more often than not, it is accepted or recomended that cognitive symptoms and signs of AD can or should be treated using the cholinergic and glutamatergic drugs available as disease-specific treatments [26 - 33].

We may also consider the treatment of specific comorbidities as disease-specific treatments of the dementia syndromes. Surely, the diagnosis and subsequent treatment of diseases concomitant to the dementia syndrome are among the more important approaches when caring for a person suffering from dementia.

In many countries, the Acetylcholinesterase inhibitors (AChEI) and memantine are authorized for the treatment of cognitive signs of AD. The conditions under which and by whom they are prescribed may differ between countries and it is advisable to refer to the national legislation. Usually, the AChEI can be used in the beginning to moderate stages of AD although some efficacy has also been shown for more severe dementia stages [34 - 49]. Some controversy related to this treatment may stem from the observation that telling a responder from a non-responder is difficult as their beneficial clinical effects are often not immediately perceptible, the overall modest efficacy in most cases, their uselessness in MCI, the impossibility to predict which patients will respond, the occurrence of adverse events, and the difficulty to define when to stop the drug [50, 51].

Drugs approved by the U.S. Food and Drug Administration (FDA), while there is no cure for AD, are to treat its symptoms, and the most frequent side effects related to the treatment are nausea, vomiting, loss of appetite, increased frequency of bowel movements, constipation, headache, confusion and dizziness [52]. There are criticisms as to the cost benefit of these medications and in relation to limitations in the methodology of clinical trials and on subtle bias in the way the data are presented, especially in trials sponsored by pharmaceutical companies, where the benefits could been inflated [53].

Surely, clinicians should avoid as much as possible the frequently prescribed anti-cholinergic or anti-muscarinic drugs that counter the procholinergic effect of the AChEIs [36]. Clearly, the prescription of anti-dementia drugs requires a psychosocial set-up that guarantees the correct intake and its follow-up in patients having trouble to do so themselves in consequence of their cognitive or functional impairment.

Symptomatic biological treatments are needed at times, especially to treat disruptive BPSD. These treatments may include mainly psychoactive medication, and possibly light therapy, neuromodulation and others [54 - 63]. The use of many recommended drugs may correspond to their off-label use in numerous countries and it is the sole responsibility of the prescribing physician depending on the national legislation [64]. Overall, the cornerstone of treating patients with dementia lies in the use of psychosocial support and help that may be complemented by drug treatments as in the case of BPSD.

Over the last decades, in turn, there are many symptomatic and useful non-pharmacological treatment approaches that have been developed. These treatments may target cognitive or functional signs and symptoms of dementia and they are often highly efficient in the treatment of the different forms of BPSD.

In this context, this chapter aims to address the role of different non-pharmacological therapies administered by neuropsychologists, physiotherapists, physical educators, nutritionists, and speech and language therapists to delay the deterioration of cognition, autonomy, functionality, independence and of the adequate quality of life of elders with AD.

NEUROPSYCHOLOGIST ASSESSMENT AND INTERVENTION

Cognition and AD

Impairments to the memory and/or other cognitive functions are an inevitable part of the process of senescence, particularly where you have a mild neurocognitive disorder - significant dysfunction in cognition but in a manner that is yet to impair patient functionality. However, in AD, the patient is affected by multiple deficits, which occur gradually and heterogeneously, varying between individuals [65]. Bertolucci *et al.* propose that the appearance of AD follows four distinct phases, as shown in Table **1**.

Table 1. Phases and Characteristics of Alzheimer's Disease [66].

Phase	Characteristics
Normal aging	No symptoms or signs of the disease.
Preclinical phase	No cognitive complaint and objective assessment indicates no change in performance. Diagnosis should come from an examination of cerebrospinal fluid or diagnostic imaging.
Prodromal phase	Progressive cognitive complaints, especially regarding memory. Such complaints appear, even, in objective evaluation, but without impact on functional capacity.
AD Dementia	Presence of difficulties in functional capacity, which progress with time. From this stage, the disease follows its typical progression.

It is through memory that we are able to store and access our experiences, and what we learn and develop, in addition to forming our own identity as an individual. The principle symptom of AD relates to memory impairment, making it difficult to access the information acquired throughout life, sometimes rendering the content inaccessible. The ability to recognize and recall memories is compromised, affecting learning, memorization and orientation in time and space. The individual begins to forget the names of people, objects, and even their own personal history, family and friends, in a loss that is chronologically inverse to acquisition - most current memories to the oldest ones [67 - 69].

The first symptoms of AD tend to be declines in recent memory, disorientation as to time and space, momentarily forgetting some words and difficulty in making decisions, besides irritability and aggressiveness. These symptoms develop over time, and in the intermediate phase of the disease, motor disturbances begin to emerge, as well as sleep disruption and possible hallucinations. Also present may be speech disorders, resulting in language that is more disconnected and less understandable [70 - 72].

The advanced stages of AD, however, are more critical, bringing prominent impairment to cognitive and motor aspects due to the progression of neural degeneration, and requiring special care from family members and monitoring by specialized caregivers. All previously developed symptoms are exacerbated, affecting even aspects like personal hygiene (urinary and fecal incontinence are common), and apraxia begins to appear, namely, disorders that impair the performance of certain gestures and manipulation of objects. The most characteristic forms of apraxia in AD are ideational apraxia (limitations in handling and manipulation of objects) and dressing apraxia (inability to put on clothes independently). In the terminal stages of AD, the progression of symptoms is enormous, restricting the patient to bed for long periods, which can lead to the appearance of pressure ulcers and bedsores. Feeding ability is prejudiced and cannot be done without assistance, often being performed using a feeding tube [66, 69 - 71].

Neuropsychological Assessment in Alzheimer's Disease

The first step in cases of suspected AD is an assessment of the functional capacity of the individual. Losses will usually be identified in more complex activities, evolving to more routine activities. Once the suspicion is confirmed, a differential diagnosis of AD can be made through the use of a variety of methods, such as screening instruments, more complex neuropsychological batteries and brief cognitive assessment instruments, as well as subjective scales [66].

Neuropsychological evaluation is a procedure that investigates the quality of cognitive functions, like memory, attention, language, executive functions and praxis. It assists in the primary differentiation of clinical conditions such as dementia, mild neurocognitive disorder, psychiatric disorders and focal neuropsychological conditions. Evaluation is performed through the application of objective tests, as well as subjective scales, seeking to reveal the functional performance of the patient through quantifying altered cognitive functions and comparing them with the mean or average performance [73].

Some tests are recommended in the literature for the initial AD screening, such as the Mini-Mental State Examination (MMSE) [74], Pfeffer Functional Activities Scale [75], and the Clock Drawing Test (CDT) [68]. The MMSE is widely used as a population screening method to identify cognitive dysfunction, and is also indicated as an initial evaluation for AD [76 - 78]. The Pfeffer Functional Activities Scale and CDT are other tests that are very much used for screening within clinical evaluation and research protocols, demonstrating satisfactory results, according to the review presented by Hamdan (2008) [68]. However, screening tests may not show alterations in highly intellectual people due to their cognitive reserve capacity - brain capacity that reduces the impact of neurodegenerative processes [79, 80]. It is even common for an individual to perform adequately in the MMSE but be deficient in the CDT due to the different demands of the tasks, which is why it is important to use complementary evaluation methods [66].

Consequently, memory evaluation is very important because impairments in this function are the most common in AD. Tests like word lists or images that deal with memory recall can be used. More complex lists and tasks involving the participation of executive functions are also recommended, as they involve the creation of memory strategies, as well as problem-solving, decision-making and cognitive flexibility. Language is also compromised, as evidenced by the difficulty in finding words and reduction in expressive vocabulary, as well as attentional processes and visuomotor and visuospatial capacities, requiring a battery of neuropsychological tests to be well thought out and aligned with questionnaires for the subjective complaints of the patient and family/caregivers [66, 68]. In addition to the previously mentioned tests, some of the most recommended exams are the Rey Auditory Verbal Learning Test [81], Logical Memory subtest of the Wechsler Memory Scale, Random Letter Test, Digit Extension Test, Trail Test, Boston Diagnostic Aphasia Examination Battery, Boston Naming Test, and the Semantic Verbal Fluency Test (animals/minute). The complexity and time of evaluation for these are variable [82].

Strategies of Cognitive Stimulation

There is a constant search for treatments that will decrease the progression of symptoms typical of AD, including neuropsychological rehabilitation techniques. Among the various intervention activities, valid strategies for AD non-pharmacological treatment options include reality orientation (RO) techniques, mnemonic strategy training, facilitation of learning, compensatory strategies and environmental adaptation [83 - 85].

Although there is the need for general cognitive stimulation, many significant improvements are identified when specific skill training occurs within the context in which the skill will be used, involving multiple sensory and cognitive systems in the acquisition of information. In this way, the patient can easily recall a memory or word, for example, because they were active in its creation when performing tasks involving verbal, visual, kinesthetic and motor records (procedural and implicit memory) [86, 87].

Effective strategies in the patient's environment are fundamental for their cognitive stimulation, such as environment signs, clear or non-verbal language, use of figures, photos, music and other stimuli, facilitating the recall of memories. RO, as well as reminiscence therapy, are techniques that make use of such resources. Compensatory strategies, like the use of notebook agendas, alarm clocks/alarms, are also important as they can help with memory impairment by temporarily bypassing the problem, especially in the early stages of AD [83].

Families/caregivers also merit attention in relation to the creation of strategies, since they are active in maintaining the quality of life of patients with AD. The family should be helped to deal with the occupational and emotional stress of the situation by providing appropriate information in relation to the disease and the resources available for its treatment [88].

OCCUPATIONAL THERAPY ASSESSMENT AND INTERVENTION

In order to better understand how the Occupational Therapist (OT) works with the elderly with AD, it is necessary to describe the central aspects that encompass the work of this professional that allows them to more appropriately manage and guide the caregiver and family of the elderly person. It is important to understand from the outset that the main focus of the intervention of this professional is to keep the individual with AD as autonomous and independent as possible for the longest period of time, and this is what maintains their social participation.

Every human being in their daily existence needs to enter into activities that allow them to live their day-to-day life. These occupations are part of different contexts, such as health, education, culture and social. In these contexts, the demands that are needed for the individual to have a routine relate to productivity, leisure and self-care. These are the aspects considered of paramount importance for daily life and social participation.

The term Occupation is any activity performed in an individual's daily life. This is confirmed when Dickie (2011) [89] states that “to read an article, wash hands, throw a discus, walk through a colorful market in a strange country, tell a story..." are examples of occupations that are a part of people's daily lives. Obviously, the occupations in which the individual will engage depend on their interests and, therefore, are never the same. There is a "variety of activities that people perform every day, they practice lifelong occupation, perhaps without even knowing it" [89].

The American Occupational Therapy Association (AOTA) (2015) classifies Occupations as follows: Activities of Daily Living (ADL), Instrumental Activities of Daily Living (IADL), rest and sleep, education, work, play, leisure, and social participation. These areas are considered essential for a dignified life. The AOTA considers that occupations are equally fundamental in the identity and sense of competence of a person [90].

The terms productivity, leisure, and self-care are well-defined terms in the Canadian Model of Occupational Performance, one of the several models that underlie occupational therapy practice and brings the definition of the term Occupational Performance (OP). Productivity encompasses occupations that aim at economic preservation, home maintenance, voluntary work and personal development. The term Leisure are occupations in which the individual performs when they are free from the obligation to be productive, and Self-care are occupations that a person performs to maintain personal care, functional mobility and functioning in the community. With regard to OP, it is defined as the interaction between the individual and the occupation (and all aspects that refer to them), and the environment where the occupation occurs [91].

AD, as a progressive neurodegenerative disease, brings negative repercussions in the life of the elderly person and interferes directly in their occupations and, consequently, in their social participation. The importance of occupational therapy is given by the fact that this professional deal specifically with the Human Occupation and all aspects related to it, as previously described. The work of this professional is another one for the list of non-pharmacological interventions that needs to be part of the team assisting the elderly with AD. Pharmacological treatment of AD does not present the same efficacy when it becomes the only means of treatment and its management becomes more complicated. Therefore, the involvement of a multi- and interdisciplinary team that act in a non-pharmacological way is of paramount importance [92].

In the symptomatic period, AD is divided into three phases that present specific characteristics. In each one, it is possible to perceive cognitive, functional and behavioral changes on the part of the individual. In Table **2**, it is possible to observe the alterations related to these phases and, in a general way, the form in which the OT intervenes. It is important to herein emphasize that the occupational therapist uses specific therapeutic activities and techniques that will permit the achievement of adequate performance of the elderly in their occupations.

Table **2** demonstrates the degree to which the activities of the elderly person become more compromised as AD progresses. For example, one may consider a trip to the supermarket (IADL); shopping in general (IADL); meal preparation (IADL); self-care activities (ADL), such as bathing, dressing, toilet use; craft activities (or any other *hobbies*), use of public transport (IADL); rest and sleep (older people sleep for shorter periods of time, can wander at night and wake up more frequently). These and other situations can have a limiting effect on the elderly. It should be recognized that failure to adequately perform one task might compromise the performance of another (or other) activity. For example, an elderly person who does not sleep well may end up being negatively affected in day-to-day tasks due to tiredness and despondency as a result of non-restorative sleep (the role of the OT in being fully aware of the quality of sleep of the elderly person must be emphasized) [93]. In this respect, management is aimed at guiding and training the occupational therapist in the application of the ADL and IADL for the monitoring of sleep, cognitive and physical rehabilitation, and environmental adaptations. In addition, the OT should guide the family and caregiver so the tasks of the elderly person can be adapted to each phase of AD.

The cognitive intervention performed by the OT is mainly applied in the initial and intermediate phases of AD, when the elderly person is still with remaining capacities and the possibility to learn with regard to the cognitive skills needed to perform their activities. Therapeutic activities should be fragmented, simplified into small and routine tasks (the caregiver and/or family are also encouraged to stimulate the elderly person under the guidance of the OT). This is why it is so important that the professional conduct the activity analysis (described in Table **2**). It is also essential for the OT to correlate the cognitive loss and decline of functional abilities in order to make their intervention appropriate [95].

Table 2. Phases of alzheimer's disease and the occupational therapy intervention.
Source: Adapted from Bernardo (2018) [93], Grilo (2009) [94] and ABRAZ (2017) [70].

AD Phase	Overview of the Occupational Therapy Intervention
Initial Phase (average duration of 2 to 3 years)	The OT should evaluate and intervene in the following situations: 1- cognitive alterations such as memory, concentration, attention, temporal and spatial orientation; 2- behavioral symptoms like apathy, irritability and disinterest in routine activities that used to be pleasurable; 3 - ADL and IADL *, specifically in the basic activities of each one. It should be noted in the ADL that sexual activity should also be the focus of attention.

(Table 2) cont.....

AD Phase	Overview of the Occupational Therapy Intervention
Intermediate Phase (average duration of 2 to 10 years)	The OT should evaluate and intervene in the following situations: 1- worsening of cognitive alterations; 2- worsening of spatial and temporal orientation; 3- changes in language and communication (tendency to constantly question on the part of the elderly person, aphasia); 4- gnostic alterations (difficulties in recognizing images or objects); 5- praxis alterations (mainly: ideational apraxia where a person can name objects but is unable to use them correctly, bringing limitations to voluntary movements; ideomotor apraxia where a person retains the semantic knowledge but is unable to perform the activity at the right time, and constructional apraxia leading to difficulties in organizing complex acts within a given space); 6 - mobility; 7- ADL and IADL; 8- neuropsychiatric disorders.
Advanced Phase (average duration of 8 to 12 years)	The OT must evaluate and intervene in the following situations: 1 - the elderly person is totally dependent for carrying out activities; 2- guidance to the caregiver **; 3- family orientation **.
NOTE: All the situations described should also be considered in the activity analysis process performed by the professional after establishment of the patient/client therapeutic plan. Activity Analysis: occupational therapy procedure necessary to adapt the activity to the current situation of the patient/client. * ADL: Activities of Daily Living, IADL: Instrumental Activities of Daily Living. ** Considered to be transversal in OT intervention, becoming necessary at all stages of the disease.	

The Compensatory Cognitive Approach is one of the models applicable to patients with AD. This model targets people with cognitive incapacity and focuses on the acquisition of processing strategies in which patients/clients use their resources to achieve a successful occupational performance. Initially the focus is on the current cognitive abilities of the person, which will be used to improve the broader aspects of function, enabling them to carry out their occupations, albeit with limitations [96]. The general guidance from the OT to the caregiver and/or family is that they have the patience to wait for the response of the elderly person when they are stimulated, and to also keep them focused until the activity ends. Cognitive activities performed without the presence of the OT should be of short duration (20 minutes would seems like an acceptable time) to avoid fatiguing the individual. It is important to emphasize that the OT should always be consulted for adequacy of cognitive stimulation, and it is up to this professional to guide caregivers and family members on how to perform tasks together with the older person (family and caregivers become treatment collaborators). Therefore, the OT is essential for the care of the patient.

The environment, whether physical or social, is also the focus of OT intervention. These adaptations are needed, among other things, to enable the elderly to continue performing their daily activities. Family members and caregivers must be attentive and consult the OT accordingly. In the physical environment itself, Bernardo (2018) [93] suggests visual cues; signs containing directions; drawings on labels, cabinets, drawers; indicators of paths within the house (arrows, images), as possible alternatives for the elderly to remain active in their residence. The author reinforces that these suggestions can be adapted for long-term residential institutions. Assistive technology can also be great collaborator in adapting not only the physical environment but also the personal objects of the elderly (toothbrush, comb, nail clipper, books, among others). The environment of the elderly person should not be totally modified, just as their routine must also be maintained to avoid deterioration in their clinical situation and behavior.

The environment from the social point of view is also part of the OT responsibility, as it will help the elderly to maintain the social relationships that were established in their lives. In this moment, the OT uses educational strategies aimed at the patient, the caregiver and family in order to make them understand the importance of keeping the person in social relationships that are pleasurable to them [93]. It should also be emphasized that the leisure activities of the elderly with AD is an occupation that should not be disregarded, and the OT also acts in this sense. While the elderly person is still in a position to leave the home, the family should motivate them to do so (leisure pursuits can be done inside and outside the home). Adjustments that might become necessary should be evaluated, monitored and guided by the OT.

Therefore, the physical and social environments are interconnected and contribute to maintaining important occupations for the elderly person, and consequently their social participation inside and outside of their own home. Family members and caregivers should be prepared to deal with all the needs of the relative with AD, but they also merit the assistance and attention of the OT.

PHYSICAL EDUCATOR ASSESSMENT AND INTERVENTION

The rate of onset of AD symptoms is influenced by patient lifestyle, including the level of physical activity, which is indicated as a protective factor, by decreasing the predisposition to develop dysfunction in cognitive abilities [97 - 99], besides influencing factors such as inflammatory processes [100] and maintenance of functional capacity [101]. It is even suggested that physical inactivity could be one of the main risk factors for the development of AD [102]. Physical training programs could bring beneficial results to the quality of life of people with AD, providing greater autonomy and functional independence [103].

Physical Exercise and Cognition in AD

The level of physical activity is important for the improvement and maintenance of cognitive abilities throughout the aging process [165], acting as a neuroprotective factor for AD [104 - 107], both in neurotrophic aspects of neuronal growth [108] and in alterations in brain metabolism [109] and cognitive reserve capacity [79, 80]. The performance of physical exercise, that is to say, a planned and guided physical activity, is highly related to the preserved ability to learn new tasks, improving and protecting brain function, as the cognitively active elderly are more likely to maintain their cognitive abilities [110, 111].

Even though it is characterized as a disease that affects cognitive abilities, the progression of AD symptoms influences the decline of factors related to physical-motor skills. As AD progresses, impairing cognition, there is clear interference in the functional capacity of the patient, which affects the performance of ADL and more complex daily activities [112 - 115]. The study by Lira and Santos (2012) [76] evaluated the relationship between cognitive function (by MMSE) and functional capacity, more specifically the reaction time, muscle strength and balance (by the Timed Up and Go Test – TUG) of 30 elderly people, demonstrating that the lower the cognitive performance of a patient with AD, the lower their functional capacity. This is very important, as such skills are essential for the maintenance of the health of the individual [116, 117], including those who develop AD [117].

Several studies point to significant improvements in cognition after the performance of physical training. Aerobic exercises are widely studied and seem to have a beneficial effect on cognitive abilities, especially in relation to executive functions and memory [107, 113, 118 - 120], as they promote neurogenesis, angiogenesis and stimulate synaptic plasticity, as well as contribute to the cognitive reserve [121, 122]. The study of Frederiksen (2015) [123] demonstrated that aerobic exercises in a population of 282 elderly people, lasting over a period of three years, promoted improvements in executive functions and processing speed.

Anaerobic exercises, such as resistance training, can also bring benefits to cognition [124], provided they are performed at moderate to high intensity, but not mild [125]. Resistance exercises commonly show significant improvements in overall cognitive functioning, memory, executive functions, attention and processing speed [126], which are essential aspects to be worked on with AD patients. In a recent study, Garcia *et al.* (2017) [127] compared the effects of anaerobic exercises in an animal model of AD using 80 rodents. Their adopted protocol included the periodic performance of a resistance training, which consisted of carrying a weight attached to the tail of the animal when climbing a stairway. A progression in load was included, ranging from 25% to 100% of the maximum load supported by the animal. At the end of the experiment, the sample showed significant improvements, attenuating object recognition memory deficits.

Multimodal exercise (combination of different physical abilities, such as strength, balance, agility…) and those with a dual task (focus divided between two skills) have been the subject of research on the cognition of elderly people with AD, showing itself to be potentially more effective for cognitive stimulation due to the complexity of performance [128, 129]. Ferreira (2017) [130] conducted a 12-week multimodal training program with 19 elderly patients with AD in the mild and moderate phases. After the intervention period, the participants presented improvements in frontal cognitive functions (abstract reasoning, mental flexibility, programming, inhibitory control). The training sessions included activities of aerobic capacity, muscular strength, agility and balance, mixed in different ways for each encounter, according to a pre-established schedule.

Intervention Strategies for Patients with AD

A physical training program brings many benefits for AD patients, but there is still no certainty as to the amount of stimulus needed to produce these responses. In order for there to be health benefits for the elderly with AD, it is essential that the chosen exercise programs has an impact on several parameters, whether physical, motor or physiological, in order to stimulate the abilities of the patient [131, 132]. Although the majority of the benefits of physical exercise appear after a few months, it is common for compromised populations, such as in the case of AD, to present significant improvements in a short period of time [133].

As previously mentioned, multimodal (or multicomponent) training has been recommended, as it stimulates various abilities of the individual, favoring their overall development and autonomy [134 - 136]. It is important that this training be varied and that it encompasses the needs of the patient, in order to foster their participation and engagement. Table **3** presents a possible model of an intervention protocol.

Physical exercise, especially strength training, can play an essential role for the patient, aiding in the modulation of inflammatory processes. Physical exercise performance causes an increase in muscle tissue, which can stimulate endocrinal aspects in the production and regulation of cytokines and myosins that fight the inflammatory process [137, 138], as occurs with interleukin-6 (IL-6), a multifunctional protein that can act as a pro- and anti-inflammatory agent. Studies have demonstrated that exercise performed on a regular basis is associated with decreased levels of IL-6 [139, 140]. This happens as the levels of IL-6 increase acutely during the performance of exercise, stimulating the synthesis of the cytokine Interleukin 10 (IL-10) to balance the body, which acts as an anti-inflammatory agent and inhibits the production of Tumor Necrosis Factor-α (TNF-α) [141, 142]. Therefore, the performance of regular physical exercise, guided and monitored by qualified professionals, can comprehensively contribute to slowing the progression of AD.

Table 3. Example of multimodal intervention for patients with alzheimer's disease.

Stage	Activities*	Duration
Warm-up	Light exercises involving joint mobility and warm-up of structures. Ex: light walk or jog; varied joint movements.	5 minutes
Main part	Choose two or three of the activities below for each session, following a previously agreed plan. The intensity and difficulty of the tasks vary according to the person. It is important that activities are stimulating and combine tasks. a) *Aerobic capacity*: walking, running; b) *Muscular strength*: resistance training with elastic bands, weights or own weight; c) *Balance*: movement with obstacles and/or markings on the ground (level of difficulty varied); d) *Agility*: movement between cones (speed increasing gradually); e) *Power*: sprint and plyometric exercise; f) *Coordination*: maintain a balloon in the air, with light strokes (one, two or three).	50 minutes
Cool-down	Guided stretching and breathing activities	5 minutes

*Prior assessment of the patient's stage of Alzheimer's disease required for the planning of physical activities.

Physical exercise has been adopted as a non-pharmacological treatment of AD, but there are few studies related to its effects on the elderly who are at an advanced stage of the disease, as these patients present severe cognitive and motor impairment, making evaluation and the development of a research and intervention protocol difficult. It is, however, important to emphasize that physical intervention may be possible even in patients with advanced AD, subject to meticulous management and medical supervision, as with an accentuated cognitive decline and progression of symptoms the risk of injuries and falls increases, demanding a redoubling of attention. It is work that requires collaboration between family members, caregivers and professionals of physical education and physiotherapy in order to maintain strict control of the elderly persons' routine, so that all activities are carried out as planned. In this way, the interventions can take place safely and bring the maximum benefits possible.

PHYSIOTHERAPIST ASSESSMENT AND INTERVENTION

The physiotherapist seeks to preserve functional independence as much as possible in order to provide conditions for a good quality of life. During the progression of dementia, this health professional should reassess the techniques used to preserve full mobility of joints, cardiovascular and respiratory functions, kinesthetic, sensory and pain-related proprioception, as close to normality as possible. In the more advanced phase of the disease, when the individual develops apraxia, maintenance of joint mobility, cardiovascular and proprioceptive responses will facilitate positional changes for patients restricted to bed for long periods, bed-to-chair transfers, and other care.

Physiotherapeutic assessment, however, is not restricted to the evaluation of body functions only. It also involves a broader examination of situations that might compromise functionality. Therefore, the physiotherapist assesses the current history of the disease, cognitive function, comorbidities, level of physical activity, falls risk, environmental restrictions, and the level of knowledge of the caregiver, in addition to the physical and functional evaluation [143].

In general, training activities involve more extensive and functional movements, which train praxias through imitating everyday situations such as combing hair, taking food to the mouth and clothes dressing, which are stimulated by simple and short commands, demonstrations of activity, and tactile stimuli, among others, all adapted to the current physical and cognitive condition of the patient [143].

The physiotherapist stimulates functional skills aimed at delaying functional decline, encourages, and guides caregivers and family members to adopt this behavior with the patient. Depending on the need, the physiotherapist can guide active exercises, assisting in mobilization or passively moving the patient's joints. Muscle stretching, flexibility exercises, coordination, balance training, muscle strengthening, thermal or electrical analgesia resources, functional electrical stimulation, exercises to improve neuro-proprioception, aerobic training, gait training with auxiliary devices, upper respiratory tract and pulmonary secretion hygiene, are some of the many activities the physiotherapist is able to perform in order to add to the non-pharmaceutical treatment of AD.

The physiotherapist is part of a multi-professional team and must communicate with all members of the group. For example, among the many possible situations, the physiotherapist works together with: a) the nutritionist to ensure the necessary nutritional support for the therapeutic physical exercise; b) the pharmacist, investigating medications that may increase the risk of postural hypotension, falls and cardiovascular and proprioceptive alterations, among others; c) the psychologist, understanding the mental health of the patient, which will impact on the motivation needed for the patient to become the protagonist of their own treatment; d) the occupational therapist, the best time for physiotherapy, the need for environmental adaptations and gait devices and assistive technologies; e) the physical educator, the functional components to be improved for the maintenance of regular physical activity; the caregiver and family members, the identification of signs and symptoms suggestive of alteration of the clinical status, care with movements and postural changes and transfers, among others; f) and with the doctor, to understand the current clinical situation of the patient, the prognosis and any other important information; the nurse, for adaptations that facilitate the care, in the presence of pressure sores or the need for mobilization in the bed, among other situations.

The techniques used in therapy vary according to the stage of the patient within the progression of AD. In mild to moderate phases there are many resources that can be chosen to stimulate the motivation of the patient in their own treatment. Techniques such as dual-task exercise and game therapy have been described in studies with patients with mild to moderate AD [144].

An intervention involving multitasking or multidomain training has been widely used in physiotherapeutic practice, consisting of doing cognitive and physical training simultaneously. Although there is not yet strong scientific evidence of the benefits of this technique for patients with AD, there are studies that show positive cognitive outcomes. In a study involving patients with mild to moderate AD, the individuals were submitted to one-hour sessions of dual-task training, three times weekly for sixteen weeks. Tasks included motor activities, such as gait training, balance and agility, associated with cognitive tasks, such as, saying the names of animals, people or fruits with certain characteristics, for example. The results demonstrated a positive impact on the evaluation of frontal cortex cognitive function, but no significant gains in the components of ambulation [145].

The cognitive benefits of an intervention involving multiple domains are greater in patients with AD in the initial phase rather than those with moderate to advanced disease, and in patients with non-dementia cognitive impairment. This was observed in a 12-week multidisciplinary intervention, which offered two weekly sessions of six hours each, involving recreational activities, verbal and written expression, physiotherapy and physical training. The intervention also reduced depressive symptoms for all groups [3, 146], which can improve motivational gain and adherence to treatment in a broader evaluation of the results, since depression challenges rehabilitation [143].

The use of technological resources, such as games, has been a leisure option that assists physical and cognitive training [144] through different devices, including virtual reality, computer games and games involving physical exercises. A systematic review study observed that training periods ranged from 30 minutes to an hour (3 to 5 times a week, in general for 8 weeks duration, which were organized into three phases, warm-up, training and cool-down, involving aerobic exercise, muscle strengthening, balance training and multitasking, supervised by physiotherapists, physical educators, psychologists and formerly trained caregivers) using videogames with an interface for reading patient gestures represented in a virtual in-game character found cognitive, emotional and functional gains in patients with dementia, although the results cannot be broadly extrapolated as the sample sizes are limited [147].

In later stages of the disease, when it becomes more difficult to interact with the patient, the physiotherapist minimizes the harmful effects of bed restriction through passive mobilization, bed-to-chair transfers, and bronchial hygiene techniques, among other activities. The effects of immobility syndrome resulting from prolonged bed rest increase the risk of musculoskeletal weakness and atrophy, pressure sores, atelectasis, systemic inflammation, joint contractions, thromboembolic diseases, insulin resistance and microvascular dysfunction [148]. Furthermore, in relation to the neurological state of the patient, immobility may be associated with a decrease in neurotrophic factors, reducing the capacity for neurogenesis and further aggravating cognition [149]. Both immobility and dementia are isolated risk factors for aspiration pneumonia [150].

Throughout the therapeutic process, the learning capacity of the patient deteriorates and determines the choice of therapeutic techniques. The physiotherapist uses several strategies to improve motor learning. Some simple and applicable examples [151]:

1. To use movements that simulate everyday activities to strengthen muscles, such as sitting and standing from a chair to strengthen muscles of the lower limbs, or moving cans with weights on a table or placing them on a higher shelf, for upper limbs. These strategies also deal with implied memory resources facilitating the exercise.
2. It can sometimes be interesting to do training for a functional task in steps, for example, to prepare a cup of coffee in an electric coffeemaker, first selecting the type of coffee and then how to use the coffeemaker in the same training session. Thus, as each step is learned, another step is added.
3. To stimulate tasks necessary to the patient that will simulate their daily life. This is important because the training results follow the principle of specificity.
4. To provide significant challenges during training. For example, in balance training it will be important to promote situations of imminent instability to allow self-perception of the real possibility of postural correction by the patient.

Another important aspect of the contributions of physiotherapy refers to the prevention of falls, which are a frequent cause of hospitalization in patients with AD [152]. As it is a geriatric syndrome with a variety of causes, treatment should be individualized, and the researches so far have not been able to determine the techniques that best prevent this event. Even the response to a one-year functional training program with one-hour sessions held twice a week, offering aerobic, muscle strengthening and dual-task activities, showed different outcomes among participants with moderate and severe AD. The group of patients comprising the most severe cases was observed to be the one with the lowest risk for falls after treatment, while those with moderate impairment had greater functional gains than their controls [153]. Therefore, it is important to emphasize that the intervention of the physiotherapist at any stage of AD is essential in an attempt to postpone the rapid advance in loss of independence and functionality of the patient.

NUTRITIONAL ASSESSMENT AND INTERVENTION

In addition to the patient with AD presenting all the cognitive and motor changes already mentioned above, the patient also develops a visual and tactile agnosia for food, and it does not make sense to consume something that is not identified as food. With the passage of time and progress of the disease, apraxia occurs for eating and swallowing. In the physiological alterations in swallowing there is a reduction in tongue lateralization, a delay in the pharyngeal phase, bilateral pharyngeal weakness, and reduced mobility of the base of the tongue and jaw, which may increase the swallow time to more than 3 minutes. In the most advanced phase of the disease the use of a nasoenteral catheter is likely to be required. The difficulties for food intake can lead to malnutrition and weight loss, further aggravating the health of the individual. The loss of muscle mass increases the functional dependency of the patient, meaning there is a higher chance of pressure sores (due to reduced mobility), infection and death [154].

Patients should receive a well-balanced diet rich in protein and fiber, adequate in calories depending on height and body weight, avoiding loss or gain of weight, and aiming for an ideal healthy weight according to height and age. Many patients develop a preference for frequent sweets and treats, and this is an issue that requires attention, as food consumption should take into account other diseases that might need diet modification, such as diabetes, obesity or hypertension. The safest consistency for patient feeding is semi-solid, with the consistency of a puree [155]. Liquid foods can increase the risk of lung aspiration and, therefore, even the consumption of water should be monitored to avoid dehydration and choking. The problem of the prostate causing discomfort is common in elderly men, as it results in a frequent and urgent need for urination, especially in cold weather. Even when there is a reduction in fluid intake, many times there is also a decreased sensation of thirst, which together with the anxiety in relation to incontinence and toilet use, many lead to dehydration and cognitive and physical impairment, or an increased risk of mortality [156]. When there are signs of urinary incontinence, the possibility of urinary tract infection or damage to the urinary tract should be investigated [155, 156].

In the natural course of AD, damage to the brain regions involved in appetite control and food intake (hypothalamus and temporal cortex) causes anorexia, which may occur in the preclinical phase of the disease. With cognitive impairment, the patient may simply forget to eat. Apraxia and impairment of executive functions may reduce the ability to use utensils and also to prepare meals. Aphasia and communication problems affect the ability to ask for food and communicate hunger. Impaired decision-making may delay food choice and reduce its consumption. This can appear in the initial phases of the disease when the severity is mild to moderate. With the psychological symptoms of the individual altered, apathy appears and is associated with less interest in food. Sadness and depressive symptoms are associated with anorexia in the mild to moderate phases of disease progression. Behavioral symptoms such as agitation, aggression and hostility lead to tiredness and aversion to eating, and these behaviors could interfere with family members and caregivers who may not be motivated to provide food and/or accompany meals. Personality changes can alter attitudes toward food and food preferences, which might make it difficult to understand and recognize the demands of the patient when the disease is in an advanced or severe stage. These changes can begin very early in the course of the disease, even before the diagnostic clinical procedure [157].

The natural aging process brings with it some inevitable consequences, such as olfactory dysfunction, which is also frequently associated with numerous neurodegenerative diseases. Olfactory dysfunction has strong practical implications for daily activities, since the sense of smell is very relevant and throughout evolution has had a protective role in human survival (for example, smell of gas; rotten or spoiled food) [158]. Olfactory dysfunction affects the palate and may reduce appetite, and is a natural process that occurs during aging [159], however, loss of smell is more visible in AD and may already be present in the preclinical phase and worsen with disease severity [157].

Disorders of taste and smell can cause food aversion and affect the capacity of adequate nutrition. This can result in reduced strength, muscle mass, function, and quality of life. It can also affect the ability to differentiate intensities and/or concentrations of specific flavors, which may result in increased salt and sugar intake, jeopardizing the treatment of chronic diseases, such as heart failure and diabetes. This can be a challenge in elderly patients who are particularly frail, use polypharmacy and have multiple comorbidities [157]. The most pronounced increase in detection threshold has been observed for sour taste and bitter tastes, but the perception of salty, sweet and umami tastes also seems to diminish with age [157].

Another perception effected is the somatosensory system (pain, heat and mechanosensory sensations), involving detection by many sensory receptors that are decreased in the elderly. These sensory receptors are contained in ciliary neurons, specialized in detecting changes in environmental conditions and participating in behavioral decisions, ranging from food choice to avoidance of risky situations, such as very hot foods or the smell of smoke or burning objects [160].

Oral and dental health is essential for maintaining health and well-being. Tooth loss, dental or gum disease, poorly fitting prostheses, ulcers and infections have an impact on the chewing process and can cause pain that interferes with food intake, as well as leading to infections and periodontitis [157]. With these deficiencies, there is a loss in the quality of food, as there is a limitation in chewing leading to inefficient preparation of the food bolus and fatigue during feeding [161]. These issues are a normal part of aging and can negatively impact on nutrition when dental care is compromised, together with the progress of dementia symptoms [157]. The oral cavity, from a psychosomatic point of view, can be considered an organ of extreme importance for the individual. It is there where the vegetative and psychological are intersected, as it assures biologic functions, communication through the articulation of words and speech, and the beginning of feeding, gestures or kisses [161].

The tongue plays a key role in generating pressures for the transport of liquids and food through the mouth until swallowing happens [162]. The tongue is part of the chewing process and when not functioning properly, it is a risk factor for patients with AD and their overall systemic health, such as physical and mental impairment and mortality. The decrease in oral food intake reduces motivation and one more skill of daily life [163]. Aging leads to a decrease in tongue pressure and also to motor function of the lips. It is possible that the swallow function decreases in older individuals when the meal is slower, especially at the end of chewing, with early fatigue occurring [164]. Many studies on the effect of aging on esophageal motor function show that peristaltic function worsens with age and in addition, the esophagus becomes stiffer. There is greater rigidity and peristalsis deteriorates, with a decline in esophageal function after the age of 40 years [165, 166].

Aging of the gastric mucosa and its greater susceptibility to injury include partial atrophy of the gastric glands and impaired mucosa defense (bicarbonate and prostaglandin production are decreased and reduced sensory innervation). There is also a vulnerability to damage that can be caused by many agents, such as ethanol, aspirin and other Nonsteroidal Anti-inflammatory Drugs (NSAIDs). This can impair the healing of the lesion and reduce the efficacy of ulcer healing drugs. Gastric aging is a clinically important topic, due to the increase in life expectancy of populations. Older patients are at increased risk of developing gastroduodenal ulcers and gastrointestinal complications (for example, gastric injury caused or induced by the use of NSAIDs). The increased vulnerability of the gastric mucosa to lesions can be reversed or reduced with medication use [167].

Alterations in the intestinal function with aging have consequences for esophageal, gastric, and colonic motility. Elderly people are susceptible to malnutrition, postprandial hypotension, dysphagia, constipation, and fecal incontinence. There is a decrease in the number of cells in the nerves of the myenteric plexus, which impairs digestive absorption and the surface area of the small intestine, due to the alterations and activity of the villi, which may lead to less absorption of nutrients [157]. In addition, there is an increase in energy expenditure at rest, as a central hypermetabolism occurs, secondary to the alterations of the hypothalamus and temporal cortex, with greater basal expenditure in all phases of dementia, beginning in the preclinical phase. Motor disturbances, such as wandering increase the average level of physical activity and energy expenditure, usually occurring in the most severe phase [157]. Sleep disturbances also add to the extra energy expenditure, as the increase in the number of waking hours means the patient has less rest time. This can occur initially in the mild to moderate phases of the disease but becomes more intense in the severe phase. Behavioral symptoms, like agitation, excess activity and body movements, mean increased energy expenditure, and may occur in the early to severe phases [157].

In addition, studies have shown increased levels of proinflammatory cytokines such as interleukin 1 and 6 and TNF-α, both in patients with cognitive decline and with AD [168 - 174] which contributes to a catabolic musculoskeletal state, leading to loss of muscle mass, that also begins in the preclinical phase and is aggravated by the increased inflammatory response in damaged regions of the brain. The impaired intestinal immune system resulting from aging, including the mucosal layer of the gastrointestinal tract, may significantly contribute to the increase in incidence and severity of infections [175]. Disorders such as fecal incontinence, chronic constipation, evacuation dyssynergia and fecal impaction are very prevalent in the elderly with AD [176]. They affect quality of life in an important way, represent a burden on patient health care, and can turn into a chronic disease with severe complications (impaction and intestinal perforation). There is social stigma and emotional distress, which motivates dependency, among other health problems [177].

It can also cause problems in relation to social factors, as in most cultures, eating is a social activity from which people with AD can be excluded, particularly when they develop food dependency (need to be fed). Isolation and poverty have important implications for the acquisition, availability of food and nutritional quality. The social context is a major factor at any stage of the disease, including the preclinical phase when subtle changes in personality and mild cognitive impairment may not be perceived by friends and family, but might affect quality of life, and social and economic activities, negatively impacting on the nutritional status of the elderly with AD [157].

The influence of nutritional aspects in the aging process and in dementia has been studied, from its protective participation to its possible action in the delay of the dysfunctions and degenerative alterations inherent to aging [178, 179].

Nutritional intervention, besides being a noninvasive and less expensive treatment with no or minimal side effects, has been described as an important adjuvant therapy in the delay of cognitive decline [180].

Adequate nutrition is directly linked to the quality of life and health maintenance of patients with AD, and nutritional therapy introduced early has a positive impact on their treatment [181]. In addition, the establishment of a healthy lifestyle with a multifactorial approach during middle age can minimize the risk of AD [180].

Food as a Protective Factor Against AD

It is believed that feeding care during all stages of life may prevent cognitive impairments [182], and changes in diet may possibly protect the brain, and prevent, delay or minimize damages caused by AD [183, 184].

As a result of the 2013 International Conference on Nutrition and the Brain, guidelines on a healthy diet for the prevention of AD were defined [185]. It is advised to give preference to vegetables, legumes, fruits and whole grains, as well as decrease the consumption of meat and dairy products, seeking a better consumption of vitamins E and B12, and avoiding the need for supplementation. A reduction in the intake of saturated fats and trans fats is also suggested [185].

An important path among the nutritional aspects studied in the prevention of AD is the Mediterranean Diet, which includes fruits, vegetables, olive oil, fish and moderate wine consumption, providing vitamins, polyphenols and unsaturated fatty acids. The positive aspects related to this diet are its possible reduction in oxidative stress, the inflammatory response through reduced expression and lower production of proinflammatory cytokines, and the action of polyphenols and unsaturated fatty acids in the vascular endothelium. The diet can also improve cardiovascular risk factors, such as dyslipidemia, hypertension and metabolic syndrome [186, 187]. Thus, dietary components with antioxidant, anti-inflammatory and insulin action can participate in a nutritional preventive strategy for the healthy aging of the brain [188].

Better adherence to the Mediterranean diet ensures greater intake of antioxidants and bioactive substances, such as polyphenols, which in addition to being present in fruits, legumes and cereals, are also found in beverages like wine, tea and coffee [188]. The moderate consumption of coffee or caffeine-rich drinks was associated with the reduction of cognitive decline [189 - 191] and data suggests that quercetin is the principle neuroprotective component for AD found in coffee [192]. A meta-analysis of the dose-response, including nine cohort studies, indicates a reduced risk of the incidence of cognitive disorders when consuming one to two cups of coffee daily [193]. In relation to alcohol, studies have for some time related its moderate consumption with reduced risk of AD and dementia in general [194 - 196].

Carotenoids, also found in fruits, legumes and vegetables, are associated with lower risk of AD [197, 198].

The relationship between the consumption of food with vitamins and/or serum blood levels of vitamins (E, D, B and Folate) and cognition was revised in 2017 [184], and vitamin D was cited in several studies as inversely associated with AD [197 - 199]. A meta-analysis of dose response evaluating the status of vitamin D and AD demonstrated that a higher serum level of 25-hydroxyvitamin D [25(OH)D] was associated with lower risk of dementia and AD, but with no conclusive evidence on serum levels of 25(OH)D>35ng/ml [200]. A higher intake of vitamin B12 was negatively associated with Aß, a marker of AD [197]. Having an adequate micronutrient status can moderate the decline in brain integrity [201], which explains the importance of sufficient intake of food sources of vitamins and minerals.

In relation to vitamin supplementation, epidemiological studies suggest that increased intake of antioxidants, vitamins, B6, B12 and folic acid, is associated with a lower risk of AD, however, randomized clinical trials of vitamins E, B12, B6, C, D and folic acid supplements have not demonstrated any cognitive benefits [185, 202]. Therefore, exploration of the preventive potential attributed to the use of selenium or zinc supplementation for the protection of the brain is not supported by scientific evidence [188, 203 - 205]. Vitamin and mineral supplementation is only indicated when micronutrient deficiency is found [205].

Nutritional Strategy in Modulating AD Mechanisms and Vulnerabilities

The rate and severity of AD can be attenuated by adequate healthy nutrition and, if necessary, by appropriate dietary supplementation. The principle nutrients involved in this strategy are described below [182].

- Polyunsaturated fatty acid (PUFA): present in diets rich in fish, olive oil, nuts and vegetables. Docosahexaenoic acid (DHA) is necessary in the development and functions of the brain [206]. PUFAs are involved in the primary prevention and developmental delay of AD [207]; they seem to improve the relationship between omega6/omega3 [208]; DHA and PUFAs have an antioxidant role and are involved in the regulation of neurotransmitters, neuronal modulation and neuroinflammation [188, 209], which may indicate new therapeutic approaches in degenerative diseases, such as AD [206, 210].
- Amino Acids: Tyrosine consumption (present in high-protein foods like meat, fish, dairy products, nuts, seeds and beans) increases the synthesis of catecholamines (dopamine and noradrenaline), especially dopamine, which is decreased in aging [211, 212]. Phenylalanine, a precursor of tyrosine, can be synthesized by intestinal microbiota and changes in its composition may be associated with AD [213]. The consumption of tryptophan (present in protein foods) influences the synthesis of serotonin, which plays an important role in numerous neurocognitive functions, and therefore the serotonergic system represents a very potent therapeutic target for the treatment of AD [214].
- Polyphenols: microorganisms that are abundant in plant-based food, especially fruits and fruit products. They have been associated with a reduction in the incidence of AD [188] and the most important potential benefit relates to an increased blood flow in the brain [215]. They are involved in processes that maintain the number and quality of synaptic connections in key regions of the brain, and have the potential to prevent the progression of neurodegenerative diseases [216, 217].
- Intervention with nutrient combinations: There is evidence indicating the benefit of a combination of foods and nutrients, which in certain quantities can act synergistically and provide greater health benefits than those conferred by their individual components [184]. The ingestion of natural foods, avoiding industrialized products in a varied diet, may exert more positive effects than the intake of a specific isolated nutrient, due to the greater bioavailability and biochemical synergy between the various constituents [184, 218].

Data from a recent review that more broadly considered dietary factors related to cognitive decline and AD, in other words, evaluating food behavior, food or food groups, and micro and macronutrients, pointed to the following recommendations [184].

- Mediterranean Diet: the most evaluated dietary pattern, which accumulates scientific evidence supporting its protective role against cognitive decline and dementia, and the complete adherence to this diet interferes positively in the risk and development of AD [219].
- Dietary Approach to Stop Hypertension (DASH) and the Mediterranean-DASH diet Intervention for Neurodegenerative Delay (MIND): associated with lower rates of cognitive decline and significant reduction in the development of AD [220, 221].
- Consumption of eggs and red meat: these foods have been partially reconsidered, although there is still a negative correlation between cognitive functions and saturated fatty acids [184].
- High consumption of fish and intake of monounsaturated fatty acids (MUFAs) and PUFAs, particularly w-3 PUFA: they present a protective effect against AD [222].

Nutritional Management - Actions, Therapies and Interventions - to Postpone the Functional and Nutritional Decline of the Elderly with AD

Feeding difficulties suffered by AD patients vary depending on the degree of disease [223], and its management should always be individualized according to the characteristics of the elderly person and disease phase [224]. In order to provide an appropriate diet, given the individual's circumstances, a periodic evaluation of their nutritional status (at least monthly, when there are no complications) is recommended, and to follow weight changes and the quality and quantity of their food [181].

Initial or Mild Disease Phase

In the initial phase of AD, the nutritional approach is centered on two important points, namely, the correct guidance for patients and caregivers about procedures in relation to the prevention of weight loss and reduction of synaptic loss [225].

Management of the nutritional state is required to assess any changes in body weight [181, 224] and in relation to synaptic loss. The importance of the nutritional strategy in modulating mechanisms and vulnerabilities in AD is essential in the development of the disease, as knowledge of its pathophysiology evolves [184, 226]. In this phase, patients can feed themselves independently and important nutritional modifications are not identified. The patient is still able to understand their disease and participate in decisions related to food intake, but significant loss of memory is the factor that interferes most in this initial period [224].

The elderly should be stimulated to feed themselves independently, creating conditions that facilitate the process - sliced foods, suitable position and adequate environment conditions - and allow the elderly individuals to take the time to feed themselves, calmly and in a quiet and suitable place [224].

Weight Loss in AD

The elderly with AD present significant weight loss [205, 227] and there are numerous hypotheses that explain the loss in these cases: medial temporal cortex atrophy and high energy expenditure, leading to reduced muscle mass, organic deficiencies, low energy intake, catabolism, loss of independence and functional dependence, as well as risks of falls, pressure sores and infections [181, 227].

Weight loss is associated with regular infections, a marked increase in energy requirements due to the frequent wandering that characterizes these patients, and inadequate food intake (refusal or forgetfulness, difficulty eating or inability to demonstrate desires). The constant movement requires an additional increase, on average, of 1600 kcal/day, in comparison to sedentary patients [223].

In addition, patients often become angry and throw away food, eat poor quality food, non-food substances, or only their favorite type of food. The delay in feeding begins to be noticed and signs of dysphagia are already observed [223].

Nutritional Management

It is essential that the caregiver does not assume the person who does not eat, does not want to eat. The patient may not recognize food (agnosia), may literally not be able to feed themselves (apraxia), and may also find it difficult to focus on the task and should be gently encouraged to continue [157]. The appetite should be stimulated through adoption of the below strategies [205, 223, 228].

- Healthy and balanced nutrition.
- Frequent snacks and small meals.
- Food offered at different times of the day.
- Food preferences of the patient respected.
- New foods introduced that have not been tried before.
- Soft foods.
- Care taken that food is at the right temperature.
- Foods with high caloric density.
- Nutritional supplements.
- Additional powdered milk in pureed food, porridges and creams.
- Use the moment as an opportunity for social activity and stimulation.
- Ask the patient to assist in food preparation.
- Avoid problems related to coordination, adapting the type of food and utensils

used.

- Make the environment of the meals more appropriate.

Moderate Disease Phase

Significant behavioral changes can occur in the moderate phase of AD, which affect feeding and often result in an insufficient supply of nutrients to maintain nutritional status [225, 228]. In addition to deterioration of the memory, the patient has problems in using utensils and equipment [224]. Distraction, passivity, refusal of food, difficulty in chewing or swallowing food, and delay in the conduct of meals are some of the symptoms that become routine in the daily life of the patient [229]. The morphological deficiencies of parts of the brain involved in the control of eating behavior caused by the disease, adverse effects of medications in the gastrointestinal tract, such as nausea, vomiting, diarrhea, loss of taste, smell and appetite all add up [230]. The risk of malnutrition increases and care is aimed at preventing nutritional and functional loss [224].

This new reality requires greater supervision and increases the work of caregivers, representing a more onerous task [231]. At this stage, the caregiver should be equipped and guided to use specific strategies to circumvent these new symptoms, seeking to keep the patient engaged in the family and social environments [232]. All these guidelines directed at caregivers aim to avoid weight loss, which is maintained in all phases of the disease [225]. A good relationship between the caregiver and patient seems to help with these difficulties [233].

Nutritional Management

Appropriate nutritional management for behavioral change and new disease symptoms should ensure [205, 225]:

- Healthy and balanced nutrition.
- Offering known foods and patient preferred foods [205, 224].
- Offering small portions of densely energetic foods throughout the day (interval of 2 to 3 hours) [224, 234].
- Improving meal presentation, making them colorful and varied, seeking to motivate ingestion [224].
- Promote the patient's adequate body position at mealtime, keeping them as seated as possible [224].
- Choose suitable unbreakable utensils (dishes, cutlery, non-spill cups, straws) that are stable on the table, allowing the patient to feed whilst avoiding accidents [224].
- Prepare the environment in a way that there are no elements that may distract or confuse the patient during meals [224].

- Improve consistency of the food by avoiding dry and raw foods [224].
- Constantly offer liquids to prevent dehydration [224].
- For patients with apraxia, finger foods are an option, as the use of their hands may be an alternative to overcome the difficulty of bringing cutlery to the mouth [235].
- For visual agnosia, verbal and gestural guidance are helpful procedures [236].
- There is a possible indication for use of oral nutritional supplementation when there is weight loss [225].
- Pay attention for signs of sarcopenia [237, 238].
- Adequately provide protein (1.5 g/kg of body weight/day) to keep a positive nitrogen balance and maintenance of muscle mass [225, 239].
- Provide sufficient caloric intake and adequate macronutrient ratios [184, 240, 241].
- The necessary and recommended guideline requirements are often only achievable through the use of dietary supplements added to a patient's usual diet [227, 242].
- Pay attention for signs of dysphagia [205]. Modification of dietary consistency should occur after evaluation by a speech and language therapist, and should consider the need for thickeners to increase the viscosity of liquids [181, 227].
- Observe for other potential causes of malnutrition, such as problems of swallowing, chewing and xerostomia, or side effects of medications [205].

Severe Disease Phase

Severe anatomical and physiological changes are present at this most advanced stage [181]. The elderly may be confined to a bed or wheelchair and need 24-hour care, having difficulty feeding themselves and ingesting fluids. At this point in the disease, oral feeding is normally impaired, there are problems with comprehension, a refusal to eat, motor limitations, the presence of dysphagia and a risk of aspiration pneumonia, leading to a necessity for use of enteral feeding in order to guarantee the required nutritional intake [205, 224].

The detection of dysphagia is a multidisciplinary task, involving a speech and language therapist, nutritionist, medical doctor and nurse, and the major consequences of dysphagia include malnutrition and dehydration, when there is a lack of adequate management [205].

Nutritional Management

In this phase, each decision should contemplate the specific characteristics of the patient, with respect to general disease prognosis and patient preferences, considering [205, 225]:

- Adequate management of dysphagia [205].
- Corrections for weight loss (indication of oral nutrient supplementation) [205].
- Refusal or inability to feed and possible need for enteral nutrition [205].
- When there is an indication for tube feeding (whether or not related to dementia), it should be initiated regardless of the presence of early, mild or moderate dementia. This procedure should only be performed to overcome a crisis situation, with marked insufficiency of oral intake, and when there are no other means of providing the nutritional needs of the patient [268], and any advance healthcare directive should be considered [243].
- Awareness of the risk of pulmonary aspiration [205, 224].
- When tube feeding is contraindicated or not tolerated, the alternative for appropriate nutrition and fluid administration is by the parenteral route, which should be for a limited period to overcome a critical situation, or in the terminal phase [205].

In AD the individual moves from a position of independence, progressing to a frail state, and finally becoming deficient and dependent. In this trajectory, nutritional support and care should be an integral part of the dementia management and must play a fundamental role in the preservation of functions and in postponing the transition to each evolutionary stage of the disease. In all phases, the decision for or against nutritional interventions must be made on an individual basis, after a detailed evaluation of the benefits and consequences, always taking into account the will of the patient and their advance directives [205].

SPEECH ASSESSMENT AND INTERVENTION

AD progresses in three different phases, with memory loss for recent events observed in the first, together with language alterations, such as empty talk, poverty of ideas, anomie and difficulty in creating a list of words. It is in the second phase of the disease that language deterioration becomes more apparent, where the patient presents paraphasic speech and altered comprehension. In the final phase, all cognitive functions are severely compromised and verbal communication is expressed with echolalia and palilalia, culminating in mutism. In this context, the role of the speech and language therapist is essential and should focus on the preservation of communication, speech, and reading, chewing and swallowing of the patient [244]. However, swallowing disorders in patients with AD are closely related to high morbidity and mortality due to malnutrition and pneumonia, which requires maximum attention [245].

Dysphagia

Dysphagia is the term used to describe any difficulty in swallowing that occurs in the food route from the mouth to the stomach, regardless of its etiology [246]. An individual with this symptom presents impairment in food consumption, leading to weight loss, dehydration and malnutrition. Aspiration pneumonia has been described as the leading cause of death in patients with dysphagia due to AD [245].

Some of the main alterations in the swallow process observed in patients with dementia are: stationary food in the mouth, difficulty in chewing, coughing and gagging. Factors contributing to these changes in dysphagia due to AD relate to their cognitive and sensory nature, such as the inability to visually recognize food, tactile agnosia and oral apraxia. The difficulty in feeding tends to be progressive, beginning with subclinical dysphagia and evolving to a continual inability to swallow [247].

Langmore *et al.* (2002) described that patients with functional impairment, with dependency in daily life and institutionalized activities have a higher risk of aspiration pneumonia [248].

The average survival after AD diagnosis is very varied and can reach more than ten years of evolution. One-third of individuals live the majority of their time in the advanced phase of the disease. There appears to be no evidence in the scientific literature of a relationship between the disease stage and severity or nature of dysphagia.

Clinical Signs

In order to detect dysphagia, patient and caregiver complaints should be taken into account and a clinical evaluation of swallowing should be carried out, observing clinical signs suggestive of food aspiration in the airways. Changes in vocal quality, the presence of coughing, more frequent clearing of the throat, and food residues in the oral cavity are considered signs of dysphagia. The reliability of the clinical evaluation of swallowing can increase if aspects such as the presence of preserved voluntary cough, dysarthria and respiratory pattern before and after the meal are observed [249]. In the case of doubt related to the occurrence of a laryngotracheal aspiration, an objective instrumental evaluation should be performed, such as videofluoroscopy swallowing study or videoendoscopy.

The apraxia of swallowing, the main symptom of dysphagia in dementia, jeopardizes the onset of the oral phase. The patient retains food in the mouth, being unable to transfer the food to the pharyngeal phase. In addition, patients with AD develop tactile-oral agnosia and do not recognize food in the mouth. Some patients may take 3 to 4 minutes to initiate the swallow process. Changes in laryngeal and tongue mobility are also observed in this population [249].

Management

The clinical management of dysphagia and prevention of the incidence of pneumonia in dementia are determinants for the prognosis, especially in the advanced phase of disease evolution, and in cases of hospitalization and long-stay institutionalization. The type of approach adopted for dysphagia management should be in line with the recommended palliative care indicated for the treatment of neurodegenerative conditions. For this population, multiple strategies are needed, such as adaptations in food and the environment, as well as an educative approach to caregivers in relation to the physiological mechanisms of swallowing and airway protection. Some crucial approaches in the management of dysphagia are now presented.

Modification in Consistency and Volume of Food

It is possible with the use of instrumental diagnostic techniques to verify the changes that occur in the swallow physiology with the introduction of modifications in the consistency and volume of food and liquids. The therapeutic effect of these strategies is presented in Table **4** [246, 249, 250]. The use of industrialized or homemade thickeners is indicated to provide an increased viscosity in food, and especially in liquids.

Table 4. The effects of increased volume and consistency on bolus feeding.

Strategy	**Effects**
Increase in consistency and volume	Decreases the oropharyngeal transit time.
Increase in volume	Initiates the anterior movement of the tongue base earlier.
Increase in volume	Increases palate elevation time.
Increase in volume	Decreases the delay in pharyngeal response time.
Increase in consistency and volume	Increases duration and hyolaryngeal excursion.
Increase in volume	Increases duration and extent of upper esophageal opening.
Increase in consistency and volume	Increases the period of swallow apnea.
Increase in consistency and volume	Increases oropharyngeal pressure.
Increase in consistency	Increases amplitude and duration of hypopharyngeal pressure.

Direct Approaches to the Patient

The environment of the meal has significant implications for the patient with AD, due to their cognitive impairment. It is important to decrease any lack of attention by reducing noise and the presence of many stimuli. The patient should be properly positioned, and preferably seated at a table.

The use of compensatory swallowing techniques redirects the food bolus flow, but does not modify the physiology of swallowing. Among these techniques is the change in patient body position, as presented in Table **5**, which should be accompanied by the monitoring of meals and guidance in relation to respiratory pauses and voluntary cough production [246, 251, 252].

Table 5. Effects of patient posture change on swallowing.

Swallowing Disorders	Posture	Effects
Tip of the tongue	Head up	Facilitates the gravitational drainage of food Reduces the vallecular space
Base of tongue	Head down	Pushes anterior wall of the pharynx, narrowing the airway; Pushes the tongue base and the epiglottis directing food to the pharynx; Increases the vallecular space.
Unilateral pharyngeal weakness	Head rotated to the affected side or Tilted to the good side	Closes the pyriform sinus region of the compromised side, directing food to the good side.
Reduced laryngeal elevation	Head down	Pushes anterior wall of the pharynx, narrowing the airway; Pushes the tongue base and the epiglottis Facilitates laryngeal elevation; Decreases the risk of aspiration after swallowing.

Some direct therapeutic approaches to the patient described by Logemann (1998) [246] can be tested and adapted for patients with AD. The Mendelsohn maneuver, for example, aims to voluntarily maintain laryngeal elevation by promoting greater opening of the upper esophageal sphincter and protecting from laryngotracheal aspiration. The duration time of this elevation is around tenths of seconds; therefore, it is proposed that the perception of larynx elevation by the patient and/or caregiver should be assisted with the use of tactile support.

Another maneuver that may benefit patients with dysphagia is supraglottic swallowing, aimed at early closure of the larynx. The physiology of swallowing is stimulated under verbal command: exhale – apnea - swallow - expiration (or cough). This strategy induces vocal fold closure. The air kept in the lungs allows the expulsion of the residues that remain in the larynx, exhaling or coughing before the resumption of the next inspiration.

It should be emphasized that individuals with dementia who are not able to follow guidance during the maneuvers are not good candidates for these types of strategies. However, caregivers should be trained to supervise meals in order to reduce the prolonged feeding time by providing clues that assist in the coordination of the swallowing sequence -– breathing - swallowing.

Respiratory re-education associated with swallow rehabilitation is also indicated. Blowing into a water bottle focuses the patient's attention and modulates their breath by breathing out for as long as possible. Voluntary breathing control exercises, such as spirometry, can be preventive and promote better coordination of breathing and swallowing.

Techniques that encourage food control in the oral cavity can also be used during mealtimes through the stimulation of caregivers.

The caregiver should guide the patient to:

- Press the lips together to maximize the lip seal.
- Press the tongue against the palate (behind the teeth) in order to increase intra-oral pressure and ejection of the food into the pharynx.
- Perform "dry" swallowing. In between food offerings, offer an empty spoon. This strategy aims to clean the residues in the pharynx.
- Increase the pressure of the spoon against the tongue to increase oral sensory perception.
- Use straws and feeding cup with a spout to control the volume of liquids intake.

Patient autonomy should be guaranteed for as long as possible, offering the possibility of using the hands and touching in the process of feeding themselves. After the meal, the patient should remain in the seated position for approximately 20 minutes and good oral hygiene should be prioritized.

One of the critical aspects involved in the management of dysphagia in AD patients relates to the duration of meals. Exaggerated slowness, taking up to an hour can compromise nutrition. Considering this, food offerings should be smaller and shorter, repeated several times a day. The inclusion of spicy, sweet, savory and sour foods is recommended to maximize sensory input.

Alternative Feeding Route

Most alternative pathways for tube feeding are inserted during acute admission. The most common causes are due to aspiration pneumonia and dysphagia. Many patients need to be transferred to hospital due to complications with the feeding tube [253].

Few studies have evaluated the results of gastric tube use in individuals with dementia. However, some studies have revealed that enteral feeding *via* percutaneous endoscopic gastrostomy in the advanced dementia phase has no benefit in relation to patient survival [254 - 256]. In a review article [256], no evidence was found indicating the use of enteral nutrition as preventing aspiration pneumonia, increasing survival or decreasing the risk of infections. On the other hand, complications are frequently reported, among which are:

- Pain (infection and bleeding related to feeding tube location).
- Gastrointestinal symptoms, diarrhea, constipation, reflux.
- Agitation and restraint of the patient (physical and medical) to avoid the unplanned withdrawal of the feeding tube.
- Pressure sores.
- Pulmonary edema and increased secretion in the upper airways due to fluid overload.

Aspiration pneumonia is the most common complication associated with the use of feeding tubes [256]. Although there is clear evidence that artificial feeding can be harmful in cases of dysphagia due to dementia, this intervention continues to be frequently used. This has a multifactorial cause, however, among those are the difficulty in dealing with the disease prognosis, lack of knowledge about the possible damage from feeding tube use, and the perception that the patient is feeling hungry without the artificial nutrition and that this resource provides good quality of care. In addition, a longer dispensing time for offering food *via* oral intake favors the search for alternative ways of feeding by the caregiver.

A guideline published in 1993 and revised in 2005 by the American Geriatric Society postulates that feeding tubes are not recommended for individuals with advanced dementia, and priority should be given to patient comfort and efforts to maintain careful oral feeding [243]. Above all, it is essential to maintain the independence of the patient for feeding, allowing them to use their hands and touch food when eating, giving small portions of food and liquids several times a day. It is important to position the patient correctly, paying special attention to the posture of the trunk and neck. The environment should be adjusted by eliminating distractions, such as television and noise. Medications can be adjusted to facilitate a state of alertness during feeding. Finally, caregivers should receive guidance for the detection of clinical signs of dysphagia. Nonetheless, when all these alternatives fail, and the patient with advanced AD is no longer able to feed naturally *via* the oral route, the use of tube feeding must be carefully evaluated by the care team, considering, above all, the basic ethical principles of beneficence and non-maleficence, and advance care directives.

CONCLUDING REMARKS

One of the biggest challenges of our time in terms of geriatric health is to be able to offer multidisciplinary and interdisciplinary non-pharmacological intervention programs and comprehensive health care to the elderly with AD, in an attempt to delay deterioration in their cognition, autonomy, independence, functionality and quality of life. This challenge alone is an arduous and extremely complex task involving far more than just teamwork. Beyond this, it requires valuable human resources, physical structures, budgets and a well-managed public health system (with a rigorous control and evaluation system, regional decentralization, and an independent and empowered social audit), which in developing countries such as Brazil still presents enormous impediments. In the case of populations living in poor countries, the interventions made available by the public health system (when they exist) are sparsely offered, fragmented and unstructured. Alternatively, the family must look to private professionals and pay the expenses for the non-pharmacological treatment of the elderly with AD, which has a very high cost. It is very important to highlight that isolated pharmacological treatment of AD has little efficacy in slowing down disease progression, and therefore, non-pharmacological therapies play a leading role in this scenario. Although there is not a vast body of scientific evidence that non-pharmacological treatment is effective and safe in preventing AD progression, it is essential to use the combination of medications and non-pharmacological therapies in this chronic degenerative disease. The association of therapies may increase the chances of older people with AD experiencing a longer active aging process, with independence, functionality, quality of life and dignity in their home with family members. The World Health Organization (WHO) (2005) itself has for two decades advocated that the active aging process should be "a process of optimizing health, participation and safety opportunities with the goal of improving quality of life as people become older" [257, 258]. The Active Aging Policy applies to both individuals and population groups, with the main focus being to help people realize their potential for physical, social and mental well-being over the course of their lives and for these people to participate in society according to their needs, desires and capacities [257, 258]. Allied to this, it provides protection, safety and proper care when needed. The term Active refers to "continuous participation in social, economic, cultural, spiritual, and civil matters, not just the ability to be physically active or part of a workforce." The goals set by the WHO (2005) for the promotion of active aging can be divided based on three pillars: health, participation and safety [257, 258].

With regard to the promotion of health for the elderly, the WHO (2005) advocates to:

1) "prevent and reduce the burden of excess deficiencies, chronic diseases and premature mortality;" 2) "reduce the risk factors associated with major diseases and increase factors that protect health during life;" 3) "develop accessible, affordable, high-quality, age-appropriate for the elderly social and health services

that address the needs and rights of aging men and women;" 4) "provide training and education for formal and informal caregivers" [257, 258].

With regard to the participation of the elderly, the WHO (2005) advocates to:

1) "provide education and lifelong learning opportunities;" 2) "recognize and allow active participation in economic development activities, formal and informal work and voluntary activities, according to their individual needs, preferences and capacities;" 3) "encourage full participation in family and community life" [257, 258].

With regard to the safety of the elderly, the WHO (2005) advocates to:

1) "ensure protection, safety and dignity through the rights and needs of social, financial and physical security;" 2) "reduce inequalities in the right to security and the needs of older women" [257, 258]. Active aging presupposes not only to increase the expectation of a healthy life for all aging people, including the frail and those with AD, but principally aims to keep them participative and, above all, cognitively active. These WHO (2005) [257] prerogatives are corroborated by the National Institute for Health and Clinical Excellence (NICE) [259], which reiterates that "individuals with mild/moderate dementia of all types should have the opportunity to participate in a structured cognitive stimulation program, regardless of whether they use dementia medications, and that can be introduced in non-academic community settings with positive results [260-262]. In this sense, all of us as a civil society have the duty to provide our elderly with AD social and health support.

ABBREVIATIONS

Aβ_{1-42}	amyloid-β of 42 amino acids
AChEI	acetylcholinesterase inhibitor
AD	Alzheimer Disease
ADL	Activities of Daily Living
ALAT	Alanine aminotransferase
AOTA	American Occupational Therapy Association
ApoE	Apolipoprotein E
APP	Amyloid precursor protein
ASAT	Aspartate aminotransferase
BEHAVE	Behavioral Pathology in Alzheimer's Disease Rating Scale
BPSD	Behavioral and psychological symptoms of dementia
CDR	Clinical Dementia Rating

CERAD-BRS	Consortium to Establish a Registry for Alzheimer's Disease-Behavior Rating Scale
CDT	Clock Drawing Test
DASH	Dietary Approaches to Stop Hypertension
DaTscan	123I-ioflupane SPECT
DHA	Docosahexaenoic acid
GDS_1	Geriatric Deterioration Scale
GDS_2	Geriatric Depression Scale
GGT	Gama glutamil transferase
GDS	Global Deterioration Scale
HbA1c	Glycated hemoglobin
IADL	Instrumental Activities of Daily Living
IL	Interleukin
IQ-CODE	Informant Questionnaire on Cognitive Decline in the Elderly
LB	Lewy Bodies
MCI	Mild cognitive impairment
MIND	Mediterranean-DASH diet Intervention for Neurodegenerative Delay
MMSE	Mini-Mental State Exam
MRI	Magnetic resonance imaging
MUFA	Monounsaturated fatty acids
NOSGER	Nurses' Observation Scale for Geriatric Patients
NPI-Q	Neuropsychiatric Inventory Questionnaire
NSAID	Nonsteroidal Anti-inflammatory Drugs
OP	Occupational Performance
OT	Occupational Therapist
PUFA	Polyunsaturated fatty acid
RO	Reality orientation
$P\text{-}\tau_{181P}$	Phosphorylated τ181 protein
PET	Positron emission tomography
PS1	Presenilin 1
PS2	Presenilin 2
SPECT	Single-photon emission computed tomography
T-τ	Total Tau protein
TNF	Tumor Necrosis Factor
TSH	Thyroid-stimulating hormone
TUG	Timed Up and Go

WHO World Health Organization

CONSENT FOR PUBLICATION

Not applicable.

CONFLIT OF INTEREST

The authors declares no conflict of interest, financial or otherwise.

ACKNOWLEDGEMENTS

This study was financed in part by the Coordenação de Aperfeiçoamento de Pessoal de Nivel Superior – Brasil (CAPES) – Finance Code 001. In addition, a special acknowledgement to Dr. Nutritionist Vera Elizabeth Closs for organizing and formatting this chapter.

REFERENCES

[1] Braak H, Del Tredici K. Where, when, and in what form does sporadic Alzheimer's disease begin? Curr Opin Neurol 2012; 25(6): 708-14. [http://dx.doi.org/10.1097/WCO.0b013e32835a3432] [PMID: 23160422]

[2] Büla C, Joray S, Eyer S, Simeono I, Camus V. Vieillissement cérébral pathologique: les pathologies démentielles.Du vieillissement cérébral à la maladie d'Alzheimer: vulnérabilité et plasticité. 2nd ed. Bruxelles: De Boeck 2013; pp. 239-76.

[3] Ramaroson H, Helmer C, Barberger-Gateau P, Letenneur L, Dartigues JF. PAQUID. Prevalence of dementia and Alzheimer's disease among subjects aged 75 years or over: updated results of the PAQUID cohort. Rev Neurol (Paris) 2003; 159(4): 405-11. [PMID: 12773869]

[4] Yates FE. Complexity of a human being: changes with age. Neurobiol Aging 2002; 23(1): 17-9. [http://dx.doi.org/10.1016/S0197-4580(01)00261-5] [PMID: 11755012]

[5] Gold G, Giannakopoulos P, Herrmann FR, Bouras C, Kövari E. Identification of Alzheimer and vascular lesion thresholds for mixed dementia. Brain 2007; 130(Pt 11): 2830-6. [http://dx.doi.org/10.1093/brain/awm228] [PMID: 17878206]

[6] Ballard C, Fossey J, Chithramohan R, *et al.* Quality of care in private sector and NHS facilities for people with dementia: cross sectional survey. BMJ 2001; 323(7310): 426-7. [http://dx.doi.org/10.1136/bmj.323.7310.426] [PMID: 11520838]

[7] Pot AM. Improving nursing home care for dementia: is the environment the answer? Aging Ment Health 2013; 17(7): 785-7. [http://dx.doi.org/10.1080/13607863.2013.828679] [PMID: 23971862]

[8] Alzheimer's Disease International. World Alzheimer Report. Alzheimer's Disease Internationa.l London 2009.

[9] Wimo A. The Global economic impact of dementia World Alzheimer Report. London: Alzheimer's Disease International 2010.

[10] IPA. International Psychogeriatric Association The IPA Complete Guides to Behavioral and Psychological Symptoms of Dementia (BPSD). International Psychogeriatric Association 2018.

[11] Lima CM, Almeida C, Illife S, Rasmussen J. Dementia in primary care mental health.Companion to primary care mental health. London: Wonca and Ratcliff Publishing 2012; pp. 571-607.

[12] von Gunten A, Bouras C, Kövari E, Giannakopoulos P, Hof PR. Neural substrates of cognitive and behavioral deficits in atypical Alzheimer's disease. Brain Res Brain Res Rev 2006; 51(2): 176-211. [http://dx.doi.org/10.1016/j.brainresrev.2005.11.003] [PMID: 16413610]

[13] Weytingh MD, Bossuyt PM, van Crevel H. Reversible dementia: more than 10% or less than 1%? A quantitative review. J Neurol 1995; 242(7): 466-71. [http://dx.doi.org/10.1007/BF00873551] [PMID: 7595679]

[14] Mattsson N, Andreasson U, Persson S, *et al.* The Alzheimer's Association external quality control program for cerebrospinal fluid biomarkers. Alzheimers Dement 2011; 7(4): 386-395.e6. [http://dx.doi.org/10.1016/j.jalz.2011.05.2243] [PMID: 21784349]

[15] Blennow K, Hampel H, Weiner M, Zetterberg H. Cerebrospinal fluid and plasma biomarkers in Alzheimer disease. Nat Rev Neurol 2010; 6(3): 131-44. [http://dx.doi.org/10.1038/nrneurol.2010.4] [PMID: 20157306]

[16] Reisberg B, Ferris SH, de Leon MJ, Crook T. The Global Deterioration Scale for assessment of primary degenerative dementia. Am J Psychiatry 1982; 139(9): 1136-9. [http://dx.doi.org/10.1176/ajp.139.9.1136] [PMID: 7114305]

[17] Aalten P, Verhey FR, Boziki M, *et al.* Consistency of neuropsychiatric syndromes across dementias: results from the European Alzheimer Disease Consortium. Part II. Dement Geriatr Cogn Disord 2008; 25(1): 1-8. [http://dx.doi.org/10.1159/000111082] [PMID: 18025783]

[18] Kales HC, Gitlin LN, Lyketsos CG. Assessment and management of behavioral and psychological symptoms of dementia. BMJ 2015; 350: h369. [http://dx.doi.org/10.1136/bmj.h369] [PMID: 25731881]

[19] Tible OP, Riese F, Savaskan E, von Gunten A. Best practice in the management of behavioural and psychological symptoms of dementia. Ther Adv Neurol Disorder 2017; 10(8): 297-309. [http://dx.doi.org/10.1177/1756285617712979] [PMID: 28781611]

[20] Browne CJ, Shlosberg E. Attachment theory, ageing and dementia: a review of the literature. Aging Ment Health 2006; 10(2): 134-42. [http://dx.doi.org/10.1080/13607860500312118] [PMID: 16517488]

[21] Johansson L, Guo X, Duberstein PR, *et al.* Midlife personality and risk of Alzheimer disease and distress: a 38-year follow-up. Neurology 2014; 83(17): 1538-44. [http://dx.doi.org/10.1212/WNL.0000000000000907] [PMID: 25274849]

[22] Pocnet C, Rossier J, Antonietti JP, von Gunten A. Personality traits and behavioral and psychological symptoms in patients at an early stage of Alzheimer's disease. Int J Geriatr Psychiatry 2013; 28(3): 276-83. [http://dx.doi.org/10.1002/gps.3822] [PMID: 22552913]

[23] Prior J, Abraham R, Nicholas H, *et al.* Are premorbid abnormal personality traits associated with behavioural and psychological symptoms in dementia? Int J Geriatr Psychiatry 2016; 31(9): 1050-5. [http://dx.doi.org/10.1002/gps.4418] [PMID: 26968137]

[24] von Gunten A, Pocnet C, Rossier J. The impact of personality characteristics on the clinical expression in neurodegenerative disorders--a review. Brain Res Bull 2009; 80(4-5): 179-91. [http://dx.doi.org/10.1016/j.brainresbull.2009.07.004] [PMID: 19616079]

[25] Salomone S, Caraci F, Leggio GM, Fedotova J, Drago F. New pharmacological strategies for treatment of Alzheimer's disease: focus on disease modifying drugs. Br J Clin Pharmacol 2012; 73(4): 504-17. [http://dx.doi.org/10.1111/j.1365-2125.2011.04134.x] [PMID: 22035455]

[26] Monsch AU, Büla C, Hermelink M, *et al.* Konsensus 2012 zur Diagnostik und Therapie von Demenzkranken in der Schweiz. Praxis (Bern) 2012; 101(19): 1239-49. [http://dx.doi.org/10.1024/1661-8157/a001085]

[27] Birks J, Grimley Evans J. Ginkgo biloba for cognitive impairment and dementia Cochrane Database Syst Rev 2009; 1

[28] Deutsche Gesellschaft für Psychiatrie. Psychotherapie und Nervenheilkunde (DGPPN) Deutsche Gesellschaft für Neurologie (Hrsg). 1st., Springer-Verlag Diagnose - und Behandlungsleitlinie Demenz 2010.

[29] Hansen RA, Gartlehner G, Webb AP, Morgan LC, Moore CG, Jonas DE. Efficacy and safety of donepezil, galantamine, and rivastigmine for the treatment of Alzheimer's disease: a systematic review and meta-analysis. Clin Interv Aging 2008; 3(2): 211-25. [PMID: 18686744]

[30] Hort J, O'Brien JT, Gainotti G, *et al.* EFNS Scientist Panel on Dementia. EFNS guidelines for the diagnosis and management of Alzheimer's disease. Eur J Neurol 2010; 17(10): 1236-48. [http://dx.doi.org/10.1111/j.1468-1331.2010.03040.x] [PMID: 20831773]

[31] NICE, National Institute for Health and Clinical Excellence. Donepezil, galantamine, rivastigmine and memantine for the treatment of Alzheimer's disease - Review of NICE technology appraisal guidance. London: National Institute for Health and Clinical Excellence 2011.

[32] Rolinski M, Fox C, Maidment I, McShane R. Cholinesterase inhibitors for dementia with Lewy bodies, Parkinson's disease dementia and cognitive impairment in Parkinson's disease. Cochrane Database Syst Rev 2012; (3): CD006504. [PMID: 22419314]

[33] Schneider LS, Dagerman KS, Higgins JP, McShane R. Lack of evidence for the efficacy of memantine in mild Alzheimer disease. Arch Neurol 2011; 68(8): 991-8. [http://dx.doi.org/10.1001/archneurol.2011.69] [PMID: 21482915]

[34] Birks J. Cholinesterase inhibitors for Alzheimer's disease Cochrane Database Syst Rev 2006; 1 [http://dx.doi.org/10.1002/14651858.CD005593]

[35] Winblad B, Kilander L, Eriksson S, *et al.* Severe Alzheimer's Disease Study Group. Donepezil in patients with severe Alzheimer's disease: double-blind, parallel-group, placebo-controlled study. Lancet 2006; 367(9516): 1057-65. [http://dx.doi.org/10.1016/S0140-6736(06)68350-5] [PMID: 16581404]

[36] Birks J, Flicker L. Donepezil for mild cognitive impairment Cochrane Database Syst Rev 2006; 3 [http://dx.doi.org/10.1002/14651858.CD006104]

[37] Black SE, Doody R, Li H, *et al.* Donepezil preserves cognition and global function in patients with severe Alzheimer disease. Neurology 2007; 69(5): 459-69. [http://dx.doi.org/10.1212/01.wnl.0000266627.96040.5a] [PMID: 17664405]

[38] Bullock R, Touchon J, Bergman H, *et al.* Rivastigmine and donepezil treatment in moderate to moderately-severe Alzheimer's disease over a 2-year period. Curr Med Res Opin 2005; 21(8): 1317-27. [http://dx.doi.org/10.1185/030079905X56565] [PMID: 16083542]

[39] Burns A, Bernabei R, Bullock R, *et al.* Safety and efficacy of galantamine (Reminyl) in severe Alzheimer's disease (the SERAD study): a randomised, placebo-controlled, double-blind trial. Lancet Neurol 2009; 8(1): 39-47. [http://dx.doi.org/10.1016/S1474-4422(08)70261-8] [PMID: 19042161]

[40] Howard R, McShane R, Lindesay J, *et al.* Donepezil and Memantine for Moderate-to-Severe Alzheimer's Disease N Engl J Med. 2012; pp. 893-903.

[41] Jones RW, Soininen H, Hager K, *et al.* A multinational, randomised, 12-week study comparing the

effects of donepezil and galantamine in patients with mild to moderate Alzheimer's disease. Int J Geriatr Psychiatry 2004; 19(1): 58-67.
[http://dx.doi.org/10.1002/gps.1038] [PMID: 14716700]

[42] Lopez OL, Becker JT, Wahed AS, *et al.* Long-term effects of the concomitant use of memantine with cholinesterase inhibition in Alzheimer disease. J Neurol Neurosurg Psychiatry 2009; 80(6): 600-7.
[http://dx.doi.org/10.1136/jnnp.2008.158964] [PMID: 19204022]

[43] Mecocci P, Bladström A, Stender K. Effects of memantine on cognition in patients with moderate to severe Alzheimer's disease: post-hoc analyses of ADAS-cog and SIB total and single-item scores from six randomized, double-blind, placebo-controlled studies. Int J Geriatr Psychiatry 2009; 24(5): 532-8.
[http://dx.doi.org/10.1002/gps.2226] [PMID: 19274640]

[44] McShane R, Areosa Sastre A, Minakaran N. Memantine for dementia Cochrane Database Syst Rev 2006; 2
[http://dx.doi.org/10.1002/14651858.CD003154.pub5]

[45] Porsteinsson AP, Grossberg GT, Mintzer J, Olin JT. Memantine MEM-MD-12 Study Group. Memantine treatment in patients with mild to moderate Alzheimer's disease already receiving a cholinesterase inhibitor: a randomized, double-blind, placebo-controlled trial. Curr Alzheimer Res 2008; 5(1): 83-9.
[http://dx.doi.org/10.2174/156720508783884576] [PMID: 18288936]

[46] Porsteinsson AP, Drye LT, Pollock BG, *et al.* CitAD Research Group. Effect of citalopram on agitation in Alzheimer disease: the CitAD randomized clinical trial. JAMA 2014; 311(7): 682-91.
[http://dx.doi.org/10.1001/jama.2014.93] [PMID: 24549548]

[47] Tariot PN, Farlow MR, Grossberg GT, Graham SM, McDonald S, Gergel I. Memantine Study Group. Memantine treatment in patients with moderate to severe Alzheimer disease already receiving donepezil: a randomized controlled trial. JAMA 2004; 291(3): 317-24.
[http://dx.doi.org/10.1001/jama.291.3.317] [PMID: 14734594]

[48] Wilcock G, Howe I, Coles H, *et al.* GAL-GBR-2 Study Group. A long-term comparison of galantamine and donepezil in the treatment of Alzheimer's disease. Drugs Aging 2003; 20(10): 777-89.
[http://dx.doi.org/10.2165/00002512-200320100-00006] [PMID: 12875613]

[49] Wilkinson DG, Passmore AP, Bullock R, *et al.* A multinational, randomised, 12-week, comparative study of donepezil and rivastigmine in patients with mild to moderate Alzheimer's disease. Int J Clin Pract 2002; 56(6): 441-6.
[PMID: 12166542]

[50] Boudreau DM, Yu O, Gray SL, Raebel MA, Johnson J, Larson EB. Concomitant use of cholinesterase inhibitors and anticholinergics: prevalence and outcomes. J Am Geriatr Soc 2011; 59(11): 2069-76.
[http://dx.doi.org/10.1111/j.1532-5415.2011.03654.x] [PMID: 22091958]

[51] Massoud F, Belleville S, Bergman H, *et al.* Mild cognitive impairment and cognitive impairment, no dementia: Part B, therapy. Alzheimers Dement 2007; 3(4): 283-91.
[http://dx.doi.org/10.1016/j.jalz.2007.07.002] [PMID: 19595949]

[52] Alzheimer's Association. 2017. FDA-approved treatments for Alzheimer's. Alzheimer's Association https://www.alz.org/media/Documents/fda-approved-treatments-alzheimers-ts.pdfAvailable from

[53] Casey DA, Antimisiaris D, O'Brien J. Drugs for Alzheimer's disease: are they effective? P&T 2010; 35(4): 208-11.
[PMID: 20498822]

[54] Ballard C, Waite J. The effectiveness of atypical antipsychotics for the treatment of aggression and psychosis in Alzheimer's disease Cochrane Database Syst Rev 2006; 1

[55] Zhou QP, Jung L, Richards KC. The management of sleep and circadian disturbance in patients with dementia. Curr Neurol Neurosci Rep 2012; 12(2): 193-204.

[http://dx.doi.org/10.1007/s11910-012-0249-8] [PMID: 22314860]

[56] Gauthier S, Loft H, Cummings J. Improvement in behavioural symptoms in patients with moderate to severe Alzheimer's disease by memantine: a pooled data analysis. Int J Geriatr Psychiatry 2008; 23(5): 537-45.
[http://dx.doi.org/10.1002/gps.1949] [PMID: 18058838]

[57] Lyketsos CG, DelCampo L, Steinberg M, *et al.* Treating depression in Alzheimer disease: efficacy and safety of sertraline therapy, and the benefits of depression reduction: the DIADS. Arch Gen Psychiatry 2003; 60(7): 737-46.
[http://dx.doi.org/10.1001/archpsyc.60.7.737] [PMID: 12860778]

[58] Maher AR, Maglione M, Bagley S, *et al.* Efficacy and comparative effectiveness of atypical antipsychotic medications for off-label uses in adults: a systematic review and meta-analysis. JAMA 2011; 306(12): 1359-69.
[http://dx.doi.org/10.1001/jama.2011.1360] [PMID: 21954480]

[59] Oudman E. Is electroconvulsive therapy (ECT) effective and safe for treatment of depression in dementia? A short review. J ECT 2012; 28(1): 34-8.
[http://dx.doi.org/10.1097/YCT.0b013e31823a0f5a] [PMID: 22330702]

[60] Savaskan E, Mueller H, Hoerr R, von Gunten A, Gauthier S. Treatment effects of Ginkgo biloba extract EGb 761® on the spectrum of behavioral and psychological symptoms of dementia: meta-analysis of randomized controlled trials. Int Psychogeriatr 2018; 30(3): 285-93.
[http://dx.doi.org/10.1017/S1041610217001892] [PMID: 28931444]

[61] Seitz D, Lawlor B. IPA Complete Guide to Behavioral and Psychological Symptoms of Dementia (BPSD): Module 6, pharmacological treatment. International Psychogeriatric Association 2010.

[62] Schneider LS, Pollock VE, Lyness SA. A metaanalysis of controlled trials of neuroleptic treatment in dementia. J Am Geriatr Soc 1990; 38(5): 553-63.
[http://dx.doi.org/10.1111/j.1532-5415.1990.tb02407.x] [PMID: 1970586]

[63] Wilcock GK, Ballard CG, Cooper JA, Loft H. Memantine for agitation/aggression and psychosis in moderately severe to severe Alzheimer's disease: a pooled analysis of 3 studies. J Clin Psychiatry 2008; 69(3): 341-8.
[http://dx.doi.org/10.4088/JCP.v69n0302] [PMID: 18294023]

[64] Savaskan E, Bopp-Kistler I, Buerge M, *et al.* Recommendations for diagnosis and therapy of behavioral and psychological symptoms in dementia (BPSD) Praxis (Bern 1994) 2014; 103(3): 135-48.

[65] Chaimowicz F. Saúde do Idoso. Belo Horizonte: Editora Coopme 2009.

[66] Bertolucci PHF. Doença de Alzheimer.Neuropsicologia. 2nd ed., Porto Alegre: Artmed 2015.

[67] Dalgalarrondo P. A memória e suas alterações.Psicopatologia e semiologia dos transtornos mentais. 2nd., Porto Alegre: Artmed 2008.

[68] Hamdan AC. Avaliação neuropsicológica na doença de Alzheimer e no comprometimento cognitivo leve. Psicol Argum 2008; 26(54): 183-92.
[http://dx.doi.org/10.7213/psicolargum.v26i54.19649]

[69] Gil R. Neuropsicologia das Demências.Gil R. Neuropsicologia. 2a., São Paulo: Editora Santos 2005.

[70] ABRAZ. Associação Brasileira de Alzheimer Evolução da Doença http://abraz.org.br/sobre-alzheimer/evolucao-da-doen Available from

[71] Sayeg N. Como diagnosticar e tratar Doença de Alzheimer. Grupo Editorial Moreira Jr 2011; 68(12): 46-58.

[72] Mansur LL, Carthery MT, Caramelli P, Nitrini R. Linguagem e cognição na doença de Alzheimer. Psicol Reflex Crit 2005; 18: 300-7.
[http://dx.doi.org/10.1590/S0102-79722005000300002]

[73] Green J. Neuropsychological evaluation of the older adult: A clinician's guidebook. San Diego: Academic Press 2000.

[74] Folstein MF, Folstein SE, McHugh PR. "Mini-mental state". A practical method for grading the cognitive state of patients for the clinician. J Psychiatr Res 1975; 12(3): 189-98. [http://dx.doi.org/10.1016/0022-3956(75)90026-6] [PMID: 1202204]

[75] Pfeffer RI, Kurosaki TT, Harrah CH Jr, Chance JM, Filos S. Measurement of functional activities in older adults in the community. J Gerontol 1982; 37(3): 323-9. [http://dx.doi.org/10.1093/geronj/37.3.323] [PMID: 7069156]

[76] Lira M, Santos e Santos LCC. Correlação entre função cognitiva e capacidade funcional nos indivíduos com doença de Alzheimer. Cad Pós-Grad Dist Desenvol 2012; 12(2): 36-45.

[77] Nitrini R, Caramelli P, Herrera E Jr, Charchat-Fichman H, Porto CS. Performance in Luria's fist-edg--palm test according to educational level. Cogn Behav Neurol 2005; 18(4): 211-4. [http://dx.doi.org/10.1097/01.wnn.0000195292.48422.d5] [PMID: 16340394]

[78] Brucki SMD, Nitrini R, Caramelli P, Bertolucci PHF, Okamoto IH. Sugestões para o uso do mini-exame do estado mental no Brasil. Arq Neuropsiquiatr 2003; 61(3B): 777-81. [http://dx.doi.org/10.1590/S0004-282X2003000500014] [PMID: 14595482]

[79] Rami L, Valls-Pedret C, Bartrés-Faz D, *et al.* [Cognitive reserve questionnaire. Scores obtained in a healthy elderly population and in one with Alzheimer's disease]. Rev Neurol 2011; 52(4): 195-201. [PMID: 21312165]

[80] Stern Y. Cognitive reserve in ageing and Alzheimer's disease. Lancet Neurol 2012; 11(11): 1006-12. [http://dx.doi.org/10.1016/S1474-4422(12)70191-6] [PMID: 23079557]

[81] Rey A. L'Examen Clinique en Psychologie. Paris: Press Universitaire de France 1958.

[82] Nitrini R, Caramelli P, Bottino CMC, Damasceno BP, Brucki SMD, Anghinah R. Academia Brasileira de Neurologia; Recomendações do Departamento Científico de Neurologia Cognitiva e do Envelhecimento da Academia Brasileira de Neurologia. Diagnóstico de doença de Alzheimer no Brasil: avaliação cognitiva e funcional. Arq Neuropsiquiatr 2005; 63(3A): 720-7. [http://dx.doi.org/10.1590/S0004-282X2005000400034] [PMID: 16172733]

[83] Bottino CMC, Carvalho IAM, Alvarez AMMA, *et al.* Reabilitação cognitiva em pacientes com doença de Alzheimer: Relato de trabalho em equipe multidisciplinar. Arq Neuropsiquiatr 2002; 60(1): 70-9. [http://dx.doi.org/10.1590/S0004-282X2002000100013] [PMID: 11965412]

[84] Wilson B. Mnemônica e estratégias de repetição em reabilitação.Reabilitação da memória: integrando teoria e prática Porto Alegre: Artmed. 2011.

[85] Silva LB, Souza MFS. Neuropsychological and cognitive disorders of Alzheimer's disease: psychotherapy and neuropsychological rehabilitation as alternative treatments Pretextos 2018; 3(5)

[86] Butters MA, Soety E, Becker JT. Memory rehabilitation.Handbook of neuropsichology and aging New York. Plenun Press 1997; pp. 515-27. [http://dx.doi.org/10.1007/978-1-4899-1857-4_34]

[87] Glisky EL, Schacter DL. Remediation of organic memory disorder: current status and future prospects. J Head Trauma Rehabil 1986; 1: 54-63. [http://dx.doi.org/10.1097/00001199-198609000-00009]

[88] Miesen BML. Awareness in dementia patients and family grieving: a practical perspective.Care giving in dementia. 2nd ed. London: Routledge 1997; pp. 67-79.

[89] Dickie V. O que é ocupação?EB Crepeau, ES Cohn, BAB Schell. Rio de Janeiro: Guanabara KooganWillard & Spackman Terapia Ocupacional 2011.

[90] Amini DA, Kannenberg K, Bodison S, *et al.* Estrutura da prática da Terapia Ocupacional: dominio & processo. AOTA, American Occupational Therapy Association Rev Ter Ocup Univ São Paulo 26.

2015; 1-49. Ed.Especial

[91] Magalhães LV, Cardoso AA, Magalhães LC. Medida Canadense de Terapia Ocupacional (COPM). Belo Horizonte: Editora UFMG 2009.

[92] Carvalho PDP, Magalhães CMC, Pedroso JS. Tratamentos não farmacológicos que melhoram a qualidade de vida de idosos com doença de Alzheimer: uma revisão sistemática. J Bras Psiquiatr 2016; 65: 334-9. [http://dx.doi.org/10.1590/0047-2085000000142]

[93] Bernardo LD. Trabalhando com Idosos com Demência do Tipo Alzheimer.Terapia Ocupacional e Gerontologia: interlocuções e práticas. Curitiba: Appris Editora 2018.

[94] Grilo PA. Doença de Alzheimer. Lisboa: Coisas de Ler 2009.

[95] Corrêa SES, Silva DB. Abordagem cognitiva na intervenção terapêutica ocupacional com indivíduos com Doença de Alzheimer. Rev Bras Geriatr Gerontol 2009; 12: 463-74. [http://dx.doi.org/10.1590/1809-9823.2009.00012]

[96] Katz N. Introdução à Intervenção Cognitica e à Avaliação Cognitiva Funcional.São Paulo: SantosNeurociência, Reabilitação Cognitiva e Modelos de Intervenção em Terapia Ocupacional 2014.

[97] Coelho FG, Santos-Galduroz RF, Gobbi S, Stella F. [Systematized physical activity and cognitive performance in elderly with Alzheimer's dementia: a systematic review]. Rev Bras Psiquiatr 2009; 31(2): 163-70. [http://dx.doi.org/10.1590/S1516-44462009000200014] [PMID: 19578690]

[98] Kramer AF, Erickson KI, Colcombe SJ. Exercise, cognition, and the aging brain. J Appl Physiol 2006; 101(4): 1237-42. [http://dx.doi.org/10.1152/japplphysiol.00500.2006] [PMID: 16778001]

[99] Yaffe K, Barnes D, Nevitt M, Lui LY, Covinsky K. A prospective study of physical activity and cognitive decline in elderly women: women who walk. Arch Intern Med 2001; 161(14): 1703-8. [http://dx.doi.org/10.1001/archinte.161.14.1703] [PMID: 11485502]

[100] Wilund KR. Is the anti-inflammatory effect of regular exercise responsible for reduced cardiovascular disease? Clin Sci (Lond) 2007; 112(11): 543-55. [http://dx.doi.org/10.1042/CS20060368] [PMID: 17459004]

[101] Nascimento CMC, Ayan C, Cancela JM, *et al.* Exercícios físicos generalizados capacidade funcional e sintomas depressivos em idosos brasileiros. Rev Bras Cineantropom Desempenho Hum 2013; 15: 486-97. [http://dx.doi.org/10.5007/1980-0037.2013v15n4p486]

[102] Barnes DE, Yaffe K. The projected effect of risk factor reduction on Alzheimer's disease prevalence. Lancet Neurol 2011; 10(9): 819-28. [http://dx.doi.org/10.1016/S1474-4422(11)70072-2] [PMID: 21775213]

[103] Alves AWM. Efeitos de um programa de exercício físico na qualidade de vida de uma idosa portadora de Alzheimer. Campina Grande, PB: Universidade Estadual da Paraíba 2016.

[104] Dao AT, Zagaar MA, Salim S, Eriksen JL, Alkadhi KA. Regular exercise prevents non-cognitive disturbances in a rat model of Alzheimer's disease. Int J Neuropsychopharmacol 2014; 17(4): 593-602. [http://dx.doi.org/10.1017/S1461145713001351] [PMID: 24229510]

[105] García-Mesa Y, López-Ramos JC, Giménez-Llort L, *et al.* Physical exercise protects against Alzheimer's disease in 3xTg-AD mice. J Alzheimers Dis 2011; 24(3): 421-54. [http://dx.doi.org/10.3233/JAD-2011-101635] [PMID: 21297257]

[106] Kim BK, Shin MS, Kim CJ, Baek SB, Ko YC, Kim YP. Treadmill exercise improves short-term memory by enhancing neurogenesis in amyloid beta-induced Alzheimer disease rats. J Exerc Rehabil 2014; 10(1): 2-8.

[http://dx.doi.org/10.12965/jer.140086] [PMID: 24678498]

[107] Yu F, Bronas UG, Konety S, *et al.* Effects of aerobic exercise on cognition and hippocampal volume in Alzheimer's disease: study protocol of a randomized controlled trial (The FIT-AD trial). Trials 2014; 15: 394.
[http://dx.doi.org/10.1186/1745-6215-15-394] [PMID: 25304364]

[108] de Almeida AA, Gomes da Silva S, Lopim GM, *et al.* Resistance Exercise Reduces Seizure Occurrence, Attenuates Memory Deficits and Restores BDNF Signaling in Rats with Chronic Epilepsy. Neurochem Res 2017; 42(4): 1230-9.
[http://dx.doi.org/10.1007/s11064-016-2165-9] [PMID: 28078614]

[109] Eggermont L, Swaab D, Luiten P, Scherder E. Exercise, cognition and Alzheimer's disease: more is not necessarily better. Neurosci Biobehav Rev 2006; 30(4): 562-75.
[http://dx.doi.org/10.1016/j.neubiorev.2005.10.004] [PMID: 16359729]

[110] La Rue A. Healthy brain aging: role of cognitive reserve, cognitive stimulation, and cognitive exercises. Clin Geriatr Med 2010; 26(1): 99-111.
[http://dx.doi.org/10.1016/j.cger.2009.11.003] [PMID: 20176296]

[111] Antunes HKM, Santos RF, Cassilhas R, Santos RVT, Bueno OFA, Mello MT. Exercício físico e função cognitiva: uma revisão. Rev Bras Med Esporte 2006; 12: 108-14.
[http://dx.doi.org/10.1590/S1517-86922006000200011]

[112] Castro SD, Silva DJ, Nascimento GC, Cavalcante JE, Lacerda MCC, Tancredi AV. Alteração de equilíbrio na doença de Alzheimer: Um estudo transversal. Rev Neurocienc 2011; 19(3): 441-8.

[113] Hernandez SSS, Coelho FGM, Gobbi S, Stella F. Efeitos de um programa de atividade física nas funções cognitivas, equilíbrio e risco de quedas em idosos com demência de Alzheimer. Braz J Phys Ther 2010; 14: 68-74.
[http://dx.doi.org/10.1590/S1413-35552010000100011]

[114] Shubert TE, Schrodt LA, Mercer VS, Busby-Whitehead J, Giuliani CA. Are scores on balance screening tests associated with mobility in older adults? J Geriatr Phys Ther 2006; 29(1): 35-9.
[http://dx.doi.org/10.1519/00139143-200604000-00007] [PMID: 16630375]

[115] Talmelli LFS, Gratão ACM, Kusumota L, Rodrigues RAP. Nível de independência funcional e déficit cognitivo em idosos com doença de Alzheimer. Rev Esc Enferm USP 2010; 44(4): 933-9.
[http://dx.doi.org/10.1590/S0080-62342010000400011] [PMID: 21337774]

[116] Balsamo S, Willardson JM, Frederico SdeS, *et al.* Effectiveness of exercise on cognitive impairment and Alzheimer's disease. Int J Gen Med 2013; 6: 387-91.
[PMID: 23737675]

[117] Camara FM, Gerez AG, Miranda MLJ, Velardi M. Capacidade funcional do idoso: formas de avaliação e tendências. Acta Fisiatr 2008; 15(4): 249-62.

[118] de Andrade LP, Gobbi LT, Coelho FG, Christofoletti G, Costa JL, Stella F. Benefits of multimodal exercise intervention for postural control and frontal cognitive functions in individuals with Alzheimer's disease: a controlled trial. J Am Geriatr Soc 2013; 61(11): 1919-26.
[http://dx.doi.org/10.1111/jgs.12531] [PMID: 24219193]

[119] Pedroso RV, Coelho FG, Santos-Galduróz RF, Costa JL, Gobbi S, Stella F. Balance, executive functions and falls in elderly with Alzheimer's disease (AD): a longitudinal study. Arch Gerontol Geriatr 2012; 54(2): 348-51.
[http://dx.doi.org/10.1016/j.archger.2011.05.029] [PMID: 21774999]

[120] Rolland Y, Pillard F, Klapouszczak A, *et al.* Exercise program for nursing home residents with Alzheimer's disease: a 1-year randomized, controlled trial. J Am Geriatr Soc 2007; 55(2): 158-65.
[http://dx.doi.org/10.1111/j.1532-5415.2007.01035.x] [PMID: 17302650]

[121] Zheng G, Xia R, Zhou W, Tao J, Chen L. Aerobic exercise ameliorates cognitive function in older adults with mild cognitive impairment: a systematic review and meta-analysis of randomised

controlled trials. Br J Sports Med 2016; 50(23): 1443-50.
[http://dx.doi.org/10.1136/bjsports-2015-095699] [PMID: 27095745]

[122] Coelho FG, Gobbi S, Andreatto CA, Corazza DI, Pedroso RV, Santos-Galduróz RF. Physical exercise modulates peripheral levels of brain-derived neurotrophic factor (BDNF): a systematic review of experimental studies in the elderly. Arch Gerontol Geriatr 2013; 56(1): 10-5.
[http://dx.doi.org/10.1016/j.archger.2012.06.003] [PMID: 22749404]

[123] Frederiksen KS, Verdelho A, Madureira S, *et al.* LADIS Study. Physical activity in the elderly is associated with improved executive function and processing speed: the LADIS Study. Int J Geriatr Psychiatry 2015; 30(7): 744-50.
[http://dx.doi.org/10.1002/gps.4220] [PMID: 25363336]

[124] Perrig-Chiello P, Perrig WJ, Ehrsam R, Staehelin HB, Krings F. The effects of resistance training on well-being and memory in elderly volunteers. Age Ageing 1998; 27(4): 469-75.
[http://dx.doi.org/10.1093/ageing/27.4.469] [PMID: 9884004]

[125] Vital TM, Hernández SSS, Pedroso RV, *et al.* Effects of weight training on cognitive functions in elderly with Alzheimer's disease. Dement Neuropsychol 2012; 6(4): 253-9.
[http://dx.doi.org/10.1590/S1980-57642012DN06040009] [PMID: 29213805]

[126] Lima ALS. Efeito do exercício físico sobre a cognição de idosos com comprometimento cognitivo leve. Campina Grande, PB: Universidade Estadual da Paraíba 2013.

[127] Garcia A, Carpes PBM, Lima MGP, Daré LR, Schimidt HL. Efeitos do exercício físico anaeróbico, enriquecimento ambiental e social sobre a memória na doença de Alzheimer UNIPAMPA 2017.

[128] Farina N, Rusted J, Tabet N. The effect of exercise interventions on cognitive outcome in Alzheimer's disease: a systematic review. Int Psychogeriatr 2014; 26(1): 9-18.
[PMID: 23962667]

[129] Fatori CO, Leite CF, Souza LAPS, Patrizzi LJ. Dupla tarefa e mobilidade funcional de idosos ativos Dual task and functional mobility of active elderly. 2015; pp. 29-37.

[130] Ferreira BN. Efeito do exercício físico multimodal nos biomarcadores inflamatórios, nas funções cognitivas e na força muscular em idosos com doença de Alzheimer. Uberaba, MG: Universidade Federal do Triângulo Mineiro 2017.

[131] Machado FAB. O efeito de um programa de exercício físico multicomponente em idosos com doença de Alzheimer. Porto: Universidade do Porto 2017.

[132] Forbes D, Forbes SC, Blake CM, Thiessen EJ, Forbes S. Exercise programs for people with dementia Cochrane Database Syst Rev 2015; 4
[http://dx.doi.org/10.1002/14651858.CD006489.pub4]

[133] Sampaio A, Marques EA, Mota J, Carvalho J. Effects of a multicomponent exercise program in institutionalized elders with Alzheimer's disease. London: Dementia 2016.

[134] Baker MK, Atlantis E, Fiatarone Singh MA. Multi-modal exercise programs for older adults. Age Ageing 2007; 36(4): 375-81.
[http://dx.doi.org/10.1093/ageing/afm054] [PMID: 17537741]

[135] Carvalho MJMCB. Treino multicomponente: Conceito, fundamentos e diretrizes metodológicas. Porto: Faculdade de Desporto da Universidade do Porto 2012.

[136] Chodzko-Zajko WJ, Proctor DN, Fiatarone Singh MA, *et al.* American College of Sports Medicine. American College of Sports Medicine position stand. Exercise and physical activity for older adults. Med Sci Sports Exerc 2009; 41(7): 1510-30.
[http://dx.doi.org/10.1249/MSS.0b013e3181a0c95c] [PMID: 19516148]

[137] Barbosa AR, Santarém JM, Jacob Filho W, Marucci MFN. Efeitos de um programa de treinamento contra resistência sobre a força muscular de mulheres idosas. Rev Bras Ativ Fisica Saude 2012; 5(3): 12-20.

[138] Mathur N, Pedersen BK. Exercise as a mean to control low-grade systemic inflammation. Mediators Inflamm 2008; 2008: 109502.
[http://dx.doi.org/10.1155/2008/109502] [PMID: 19148295]

[139] Pedersen BK. IL-6 signalling in exercise and disease. Biochem Soc Trans 2007; 35(Pt 5): 1295-7.
[http://dx.doi.org/10.1042/BST0351295] [PMID: 17956334]

[140] Santos MG. Efeitos do exercício físico multimodal nas concentrações plasmáticas de biomarcadores, funções cognitivas e funcionalidade em pacientes com doença de Alzheimer Rio Claro: Universidade Estadual Paulista 2014.

[141] Papini CB, Nakamura PM, Zorzetto LP, Thompson JL, Phillips AC, Kokubun E. The effect of a community-based, primary health care exercise program on inflammatory biomarkers and hormone levels. Mediators Inflamm 2014; 2014: 185707.
[http://dx.doi.org/10.1155/2014/185707] [PMID: 25136143]

[142] Pedersen BK, Fischer CP. Physiological roles of muscle-derived interleukin-6 in response to exercise. Curr Opin Clin Nutr Metab Care 2007; 10(3): 265-71.
[http://dx.doi.org/10.1097/MCO.0b013e3280ebb5b3] [PMID: 17414493]

[143] Avers D, Williams AK. Cognição no idoso.Fisioterapia geriátrica Rio de Janeiro: Guanabara Koogan. 2013; pp. 109-35.

[144] Robert PH, König A, Amieva H, *et al.* Recommendations for the use of Serious Games in people with Alzheimer's Disease, related disorders and frailty. Front Aging Neurosci 2014; 6: 54.
[http://dx.doi.org/10.3389/fnagi.2014.00054] [PMID: 24715864]

[145] Coelho FG, Andrade LP, Pedroso RV, *et al.* Multimodal exercise intervention improves frontal cognitive functions and gait in Alzheimer's disease: a controlled trial. Geriatr Gerontol Int 2013; 13(1): 198-203.
[http://dx.doi.org/10.1111/j.1447-0594.2012.00887.x] [PMID: 22686565]

[146] Santos GD, Nunes PV, Stella F, *et al.* Multidisciplinary rehabilitation program: effects of a multimodal intervention for patients with Alzheimer s disease and cognitive impairment without dementia. Arch Clin Psychiatry 2015; 42: 153-6.
[http://dx.doi.org/10.1590/0101-60830000000066]

[147] van Santen J, Dröes RM, Holstege M, *et al.* Effects of Exergaming in People with Dementia: Results of a Systematic Literature Review. J Alzheimers Dis 2018; 63(2): 741-60.
[http://dx.doi.org/10.3233/JAD-170667] [PMID: 29689716]

[148] Brower RG. Consequences of bed rest. Crit Care Med 2009; 37(10) (Suppl.): S422-8.
[http://dx.doi.org/10.1097/CCM.0b013e3181b6e30a] [PMID: 20046130]

[149] Adami R, Bottai D. Movement impairment: Focus on the brain. J Neurosci Res 2016; 94(4): 310-7.
[http://dx.doi.org/10.1002/jnr.23711] [PMID: 26762181]

[150] Noguchi S, Yatera K, Kato T, *et al.* Impact of the number of aspiration risk factors on mortality and recurrence in community-onset pneumonia. Clin Interv Aging 2017; 12: 2087-94.
[http://dx.doi.org/10.2147/CIA.S150499] [PMID: 29263657]

[151] Ries JD. Rehabilitation for Individuals with Dementia: Facilitating Success. Curr Geriatr Rep 2018; 7(1): 59-70.
[http://dx.doi.org/10.1007/s13670-018-0237-1]

[152] Rudolph JL, Zanin NM, Jones RN, *et al.* Hospitalization in community-dwelling persons with Alzheimer's disease: frequency and causes. J Am Geriatr Soc 2010; 58(8): 1542-8.
[http://dx.doi.org/10.1111/j.1532-5415.2010.02924.x] [PMID: 20553338]

[153] Öhman H, Savikko N, Strandberg T, *et al.* Effects of Exercise on Functional Performance and Fall Rate in Subjects with Mild or Advanced Alzheimer's Disease: Secondary Analyses of a Randomized Controlled Study. Dement Geriatr Cogn Disord 2016; 41(3-4): 233-41.

[http://dx.doi.org/10.1159/000445712] [PMID: 27160164]

[154] Thomaz FS, Viebig RF. Complicações nutricionais relacionadas à Doença de Alzheimer.Nutrição para Doença de Alzheimer. São Paulo: M. Books do Brasil Editora Ltda 2012; pp. 73-84.

[155] WHO. World Health Organization 2001. Regional Office for South-East Asia. Vas CJ, Rajikumar S. Alzheimer's disease: the brain killer. WHO Regional Office for South-East Asia 2001; pp 50 http://www.who.int/iris/handle/10665/204777[cited: 30th Ju 2018] Avaible from

[156] Rémond D, Shahar DR, Gille D, *et al.* Understanding the gastrointestinal tract of the elderly to develop dietary solutions that prevent malnutrition. Oncotarget 2015; 6(16): 13858-98. [http://dx.doi.org/10.18632/oncotarget.4030] [PMID: 26091351]

[157] Prince M, Albanese E, Guerchet M, Prina M. Nutrition and dementia. Alzheimer's Disease International 2014.

[158] Alves J, Petrosyan A, Magalhães R. Olfactory dysfunction in dementia. World J Clin Cases 2014; 2(11): 661-7. [http://dx.doi.org/10.12998/wjcc.v2.i11.661] [PMID: 25405189]

[159] Feng P, Huang L, Wang H. Taste bud homeostasis in health, disease, and aging. Chem Senses 2014; 39(1): 3-16. [http://dx.doi.org/10.1093/chemse/bjt059] [PMID: 24287552]

[160] Riera CE, Dillin A. Emerging Role of Sensory Perception in Aging and Metabolism. Trends Endocrinol Metab 2016; 27(5): 294-303. [http://dx.doi.org/10.1016/j.tem.2016.03.007] [PMID: 27067041]

[161] Braude Cantergi M. Envelhecimento e paciente bariátrico.Fonoaudiologia e cirurgia bariátrica. São José dos Campos, SP: Editora Pulso 2012.

[162] Fei T, Polacco RC, Hori SE, *et al.* Age-related differences in tongue-palate pressures for strength and swallowing tasks. Dysphagia 2013; 28(4): 575-81. [http://dx.doi.org/10.1007/s00455-013-9469-6] [PMID: 23677389]

[163] Kubo KY, Ichihashi Y, Kurata C, *et al.* Masticatory function and cognitive function. Okajimas Folia Anat Jpn 2010; 87(3): 135-40. [http://dx.doi.org/10.2535/ofaj.87.135] [PMID: 21174943]

[164] Hiramatsu T, Kataoka H, Osaki M, Hagino H. Effect of aging on oral and swallowing function after meal consumption. Clin Interv Aging 2015; 10: 229-35. [PMID: 25624755]

[165] Gregersen H, Pedersen J, Drewes AM. Deterioration of muscle function in the human esophagus with age. Dig Dis Sci 2008; 53(12): 3065-70. [http://dx.doi.org/10.1007/s10620-008-0278-y] [PMID: 18461452]

[166] Besanko LK, Burgstad CM, Cock C, Heddle R, Fraser A, Fraser RJ. Changes in esophageal and lower esophageal sphincter motility with healthy aging. J Gastrointestin Liver Dis 2014; 23(3): 243-8. [PMID: 25267950]

[167] Tarnawski AS, Ahluwalia A, Jones MK. Increased susceptibility of aging gastric mucosa to injury: the mechanisms and clinical implications. World J Gastroenterol 2014; 20(16): 4467-82. [http://dx.doi.org/10.3748/wjg.v20.i16.4467] [PMID: 24782600]

[168] Koyama A, Stone K, Yaffe K. Serum oxidized low-density lipoprotein level and risk of cognitive impairment in older women. Neurobiol Aging 2013; 34(2): 634-635.e2. [http://dx.doi.org/10.1016/j.neurobiolaging.2012.02.030] [PMID: 22483339]

[169] Ge X, Xu XY, Feng CH, Wang Y, Li YL, Feng B. Relationships among serum C-reactive protein, receptor for advanced glycation products, metabolic dysfunction, and cognitive impairments. BMC Neurol 2013; 13: 110. [http://dx.doi.org/10.1186/1471-2377-13-110] [PMID: 23978069]

[170] Lyman M, Lloyd DG, Ji X, Vizcaychipi MP, Ma D. Neuroinflammation: the role and consequences. Neurosci Res 2014; 79: 1-12. [http://dx.doi.org/10.1016/j.neures.2013.10.004] [PMID: 24144733]

[171] Yarchoan M, Louneva N, Xie SX, *et al.* Association of plasma C-reactive protein levels with the diagnosis of Alzheimer's disease. J Neurol Sci 2013; 333(1-2): 9-12. [http://dx.doi.org/10.1016/j.jns.2013.05.028] [PMID: 23978419]

[172] Karim S, Hopkins S, Purandare N, *et al.* Peripheral inflammatory markers in amnestic mild cognitive impairment. Int J Geriatr Psychiatry 2014; 29(3): 221-6. [http://dx.doi.org/10.1002/gps.3988] [PMID: 23857873]

[173] Wichmann MA, Cruickshanks KJ, Carlsson CM, *et al.* Long-term systemic inflammation and cognitive impairment in a population-based cohort. J Am Geriatr Soc 2014; 62(9): 1683-91. [http://dx.doi.org/10.1111/jgs.12994] [PMID: 25123210]

[174] Wu Y-Y, Hsu J-L, Wang H-C, Wu S-J, Hong C-J, Cheng IH-J. Alterations of the Neuroinflammatory Markers IL-6 and TRAIL in Alzheimer's Disease. Dement Geriatr Cogn Disord Extra 2015; 5(3): 424-34. [http://dx.doi.org/10.1159/000439214] [PMID: 26675645]

[175] Soenen S, Rayner CK, Jones KL, Horowitz M. The ageing gastrointestinal tract. Curr Opin Clin Nutr Metab Care 2016; 19(1): 12-8. [http://dx.doi.org/10.1097/MCO.0000000000000238] [PMID: 26560524]

[176] Obokhare I. Fecal impaction: a cause for concern? Clin Colon Rectal Surg 2012; 25(1): 53-8. [http://dx.doi.org/10.1055/s-0032-1301760] [PMID: 23449376]

[177] Yu SW, Rao SS. Anorectal physiology and pathophysiology in the elderly. Clin Geriatr Med 2014; 30(1): 95-106. [http://dx.doi.org/10.1016/j.cger.2013.10.003] [PMID: 24267605]

[178] Moriguti JC, Moriguti EKU, Ferriolli E, de Castilho Cação J, Iucif N Jr, Marchini JS. Involuntary weight loss in elderly individuals: assessment and treatment. Sao Paulo Med J 2001; 119(2): 72-7. [http://dx.doi.org/10.1590/S1516-31802001000200007] [PMID: 11276170]

[179] Anastasiou CA, Yannakoulia M, Kosmidis MH, *et al.* Mediterranean diet and cognitive health: Initial results from the Hellenic Longitudinal Investigation of Ageing and Diet. PLoS One 2017; 12(8): e0182048. [http://dx.doi.org/10.1371/journal.pone.0182048] [PMID: 28763509]

[180] Klimova B, Kuca K. Multi-Nutrient Dietary Intervention Approach to the Management of Alzheimer's Disease - A Mini-Review. Curr Alzheimer Res 2016; 13(12): 1312-8. [http://dx.doi.org/10.2174/1567205013666160603000623] [PMID: 27335038]

[181] Pivi GAK, Kato LC, França AP. Condutas dietéticas para idoso com doenças no Sistema Neurocognitivo.Baruer: Manoleratado de Nutrição em Gerontologia 2015.

[182] Miquel S, Champ C, Day J, *et al.* Poor cognitive ageing: Vulnerabilities, mechanisms and the impact of nutritional interventions. Ageing Res Rev 2018; 42: 40-55. [http://dx.doi.org/10.1016/j.arr.2017.12.004] [PMID: 29248758]

[183] Cooper JK. Nutrition and the brain: what advice should we give? Neurobiol Aging 2014; 35 (Suppl. 2): S79-83. [http://dx.doi.org/10.1016/j.neurobiolaging.2014.02.029] [PMID: 24925810]

[184] Solfrizzi V, Custodero C, Lozupone M, *et al.* Relationships of Dietary Patterns, Foods, and Micro- and Macronutrients with Alzheimer's Disease and Late-Life Cognitive Disorders: A Systematic Review. J Alzheimers Dis 2017; 59(3): 815-49. [http://dx.doi.org/10.3233/JAD-170248] [PMID: 28697569]

[18] Barnard ND, Bush AI, Ceccarelli A, *et al.* Dietary and lifestyle guidelines for the prevention of

Alzheimer's disease. Neurobiol Aging 2014; 35 (Suppl. 2): S74-8.
[http://dx.doi.org/10.1016/j.neurobiolaging.2014.03.033] [PMID: 24913896]

[186] Miranda A, Gómez-Gaete C, Mennickent S. [Role of Mediterranean diet on the prevention of Alzheimer disease]. Rev Med Chil 2017; 145(4): 501-7.
[http://dx.doi.org/10.4067/S0034-98872017000400010] [PMID: 28748997]

[187] Aridi YS, Walker JL, Wright ORL. The Association between the Mediterranean Dietary Pattern and Cognitive Health: A Systematic Review. Nutrients 2017; 9(7): E674.
[http://dx.doi.org/10.3390/nu9070674] [PMID: 28657600]

[188] Vauzour D, Camprubi-Robles M, Miquel-Kergoat S, *et al.* Nutrition for the ageing brain: Towards evidence for an optimal diet. Ageing Res Rev 2017; 35: 222-40.
[http://dx.doi.org/10.1016/j.arr.2016.09.010] [PMID: 27713095]

[189] Panza F, Solfrizzi V, Barulli MR, *et al.* Coffee, tea, and caffeine consumption and prevention of late-life cognitive decline and dementia: a systematic review. J Nutr Health Aging 2015; 19(3): 313-28.
[http://dx.doi.org/10.1007/s12603-014-0563-8] [PMID: 25732217]

[190] Santos C, Costa J, Santos J, Vaz-Carneiro A, Lunet N. Caffeine intake and dementia: systematic review and meta-analysis. J Alzheimers Dis 2010; 20 (Suppl. 1): S187-204.
[http://dx.doi.org/10.3233/JAD-2010-091387] [PMID: 20182026]

[191] Liu QP, Wu YF, Cheng HY, *et al.* Habitual coffee consumption and risk of cognitive decline/dementia: A systematic review and meta-analysis of prospective cohort studies. Nutrition 2016; 32(6): 628-36.
[http://dx.doi.org/10.1016/j.nut.2015.11.015] [PMID: 26944757]

[192] Lee M, McGeer EG, McGeer PL. Quercetin, not caffeine, is a major neuroprotective component in coffee. Neurobiol Aging 2016; 46: 113-23.
[http://dx.doi.org/10.1016/j.neurobiolaging.2016.06.015] [PMID: 27479153]

[193] Wu L, Sun D, He Y. Coffee intake and the incident risk of cognitive disorders: A dose-response meta-analysis of nine prospective cohort studies. Clin Nutr 2017; 36(3): 730-6.
[http://dx.doi.org/10.1016/j.clnu.2016.05.015] [PMID: 27288328]

[194] Peters R, Peters J, Warner J, Beckett N, Bulpitt C. Alcohol, dementia and cognitive decline in the elderly: a systematic review. Age Ageing 2008; 37(5): 505-12.
[http://dx.doi.org/10.1093/ageing/afn095] [PMID: 18487267]

[195] Anstey KJ, Mack HA, Cherbuin N. Alcohol consumption as a risk factor for dementia and cognitive decline: meta-analysis of prospective studies. Am J Geriatr Psychiatry 2009; 17(7): 542-55.
[http://dx.doi.org/10.1097/JGP.0b013e3181a2fd07] [PMID: 19546653]

[196] Neafsey EJ, Collins MA. Moderate alcohol consumption and cognitive risk. Neuropsychiatr Dis Treat 2011; 7: 465-84.
[http://dx.doi.org/10.2147/NDT.S23159] [PMID: 21857787]

[197] Mosconi L, Murray J, Davies M, *et al.* Nutrient intake and brain biomarkers of Alzheimer's disease in at-risk cognitively normal individuals: a cross-sectional neuroimaging pilot study. BMJ Open 2014; 4(6): e004850.
[http://dx.doi.org/10.1136/bmjopen-2014-004850] [PMID: 24961717]

[198] Feart C, Letenneur L, Helmer C, *et al.* Plasma Carotenoids Are Inversely Associated With Dementia Risk in an Elderly French Cohort. J Gerontol A Biol Sci Med Sci 2016; 71(5): 683-8.
[http://dx.doi.org/10.1093/gerona/glv135] [PMID: 26286605]

[199] Littlejohns TJ, Henley WE, Lang IA, *et al.* Vitamin D and the risk of dementia and Alzheimer disease. Neurology 2014; 83(10): 920-8.
[http://dx.doi.org/10.1212/WNL.0000000000000755] [PMID: 25098535]

[200] Jayedi A, Rashidy-Pour A, Shab-Bidar S. Vitamin D status and risk of dementia and Alzheimer's disease: A meta-analysis of dose-response. Nutr Neurosci 2018; •••: 1-10.

[http://dx.doi.org/10.1080/1028415X.2018.1436639] [PMID: 29447107]

[201] Dror Y, Stern F, Gomori MJ. Vitamins in the prevention or delay of cognitive disability of aging. Curr Aging Sci 2014; 7(3): 187-213. [http://dx.doi.org/10.2174/1874609808666150201214955] [PMID: 25643069]

[202] Luchsinger JA, Noble JM, Scarmeas N. Diet and Alzheimer's disease. Curr Neurol Neurosci Rep 2007; 7(5): 366-72. [http://dx.doi.org/10.1007/s11910-007-0057-8] [PMID: 17764625]

[203] Loef M, Schrauzer GN, Walach H. Selenium and Alzheimer's disease: a systematic review. J Alzheimers Dis 2011; 26(1): 81-104. [http://dx.doi.org/10.3233/JAD-2011-110414] [PMID: 21593562]

[204] Loef M, von Stillfried N, Walach H. Zinc diet and Alzheimer's disease: a systematic review. Nutr Neurosci 2012; 15(5): 2-12. [http://dx.doi.org/10.1179/1476830512Y.0000000010] [PMID: 22583839]

[205] Volkert D, Chourdakis M, Faxen-Irving G, *et al.* ESPEN guidelines on nutrition in dementia. Clin Nutr 2015; 34(6): 1052-73. [http://dx.doi.org/10.1016/j.clnu.2015.09.004] [PMID: 26522922]

[206] Lo Van A, Sakayori N, Hachem M, *et al.* Mechanisms of DHA transport to the brain and potential therapy to neurodegenerative diseases. Biochimie 2016; 130: 163-7. [http://dx.doi.org/10.1016/j.biochi.2016.07.011] [PMID: 27496085]

[207] Zhang Y, Chen J, Qiu J, Li Y, Wang J, Jiao J. Intakes of fish and polyunsaturated fatty acids and mild-to-severe cognitive impairment risks: a dose-response meta-analysis of 21 cohort studies. Am J Clin Nutr 2016; 103(2): 330-40. [http://dx.doi.org/10.3945/ajcn.115.124081] [PMID: 26718417]

[208] Hooijmans CR, Pasker-de Jong PC, de Vries RB, Ritskes-Hoitinga M. The effects of long-term omega-3 fatty acid supplementation on cognition and Alzheimer's pathology in animal models of Alzheimer's disease: a systematic review and meta-analysis. J Alzheimers Dis 2012; 28(1): 191-209. [http://dx.doi.org/10.3233/JAD-2011-111217] [PMID: 22002791]

[209] Sun GY, Simonyi A, Fritsche KL, *et al.* Docosahexaenoic acid (DHA): An essential nutrient and a nutraceutical for brain health and diseases. Prostaglandins, leukotrienes, and essential fatty acids. Prostaglandins Leukot Essent Fatty Acids In press

[220] Solfrizzi V, Frisardi V, Capurso C, *et al.* Dietary fatty acids in dementia and predementia syndromes: epidemiological evidence and possible underlying mechanisms. Ageing Res Rev 2010; 9(2): 184-99. [http://dx.doi.org/10.1016/j.arr.2009.07.005] [PMID: 19643207]

[211] Bäckman L, Karlsson S, Fischer H, *et al.* Dopamine D(1) receptors and age differences in brain activation during working memory. Neurobiol Aging 2011; 32(10): 1849-56. [http://dx.doi.org/10.1016/j.neurobiolaging.2009.10.018] [PMID: 19962789]

[212] Abdulrahman H, Fletcher PC, Bullmore E, Morcom AM. Dopamine and memory dedifferentiation in aging. Neuroimage 2017; 153: 211-20. [http://dx.doi.org/10.1016/j.neuroimage.2015.03.031] [PMID: 25800211]

[213] Szablewski L. Human Gut Microbiota in Health and Alzheimer's Disease. J Alzheimers Dis 2018; 62(2): 549-60. [http://dx.doi.org/10.3233/JAD-170908] [PMID: 29480188]

[214] Butzlaff M, Ponimaskin E. The role of Serotonin Receptors in Alzheimer's disease. Opera Med Physiol 2016; 2(1): 77-86.

[215] Lamport DJ, Pal D, Moutsiana C, *et al.* The effect of flavanol-rich cocoa on cerebral perfusion in healthy older adults during conscious resting state: a placebo controlled, crossover, acute trial. Psychopharmacology (Berl) 2015; 232(17): 3227-34. [http://dx.doi.org/10.1007/s00213-015-3972-4] [PMID: 26047963]

[216] Williams RJ, Spencer JPE. Flavonoids, cognition, and dementia: actions, mechanisms, and potential therapeutic utility for Alzheimer disease. Free Radic Biol Med 2012; 52(1): 35-45. [http://dx.doi.org/10.1016/j.freeradbiomed.2011.09.010] [PMID: 21982844]

[217] Bakhtiari M, Panahi Y, Ameli J, Darvishi B. Protective effects of flavonoids against Alzheimer's disease-related neural dysfunctions. Biomed Pharmacother 2017; 93: 218-29. [http://dx.doi.org/10.1016/j.biopha.2017.06.010] [PMID: 28641164]

[218] Gu Y, Nieves JW. PhD SY, Luchsinger JA, Scarmeas N. Food combination and Alzheimer disease risk: a protective diet. Arch Neurol 2010; •••: 67.

[219] Solfrizzi V, Panza F. Mediterranean diet and cognitive decline. A lesson from the whole-diet approach: what challenges lie ahead? J Alzheimers Dis 2014; 39(2): 283-6. [http://dx.doi.org/10.3233/JAD-130831] [PMID: 24270209]

[220] Morris MC, Tangney CC, Wang Y, Sacks FM, Bennett DA, Aggarwal NT. MIND diet associated with reduced incidence of Alzheimer's disease. Alzheimers Dement 2015; 11(9): 1007-14. [http://dx.doi.org/10.1016/j.jalz.2014.11.009] [PMID: 25681666]

[221] Smith PJ, Blumenthal JA, Babyak MA, *et al.* Effects of the dietary approaches to stop hypertension diet, exercise, and caloric restriction on neurocognition in overweight adults with high blood pressure. Hypertension 2010; 55(6): 1331-8. [http://dx.doi.org/10.1161/HYPERTENSIONAHA.109.146795] [PMID: 20305128]

[222] Pooler AM, Guez DH, Benedictus R, Wurtman RJ. Uridine enhances neurite outgrowth in nerve growth factor-differentiated pheochromocytoma cells. Neuroscience 2005; •••: 134.

[223] Longo EN, Navarro ET. Enfoque dietético nas doenças do sistema nervoso.Manual Dietoterápico. Porto Alegre: Artmed 2002; pp. 252-3.

[224] Terra NL. A nutrição e as doenças geriátricas. Porto Alegre: EDIPUCRS 2011.

[225] Pivi GAK, Vieira NMA, da Ponte JB, de Moraes DSC, Bertolucci PHF. Nutritional management [for Alzheimer's disease in all stages: mild, moderate, and severe. Nutrire 2017; 42(1): 1. [http://dx.doi.org/10.1186/s41110-016-0025-7]

[226] Miquel S, Champ C, Day J, *et al.* Poor cognitive ageing: Vulnerabilities, mechanisms and the impact of nutritional interventions. Ageing Res Rev 2018; 42: 40-55. [http://dx.doi.org/10.1016/j.arr.2017.12.004] [PMID: 29248758]

[227] Pivi GAK, da Silva RV, Juliano Y, *et al.* A prospective study of nutrition education and oral nutritional supplementation in patients with Alzheimer's disease. Nutr J 2011; 10: 98. [http://dx.doi.org/10.1186/1475-2891-10-98] [PMID: 21943331]

[228] Cipriani G, Carlesi C, Lucetti C, Danti S, Nuti A. Eating Behaviors and Dietary Changes in Patients With Dementia. Am J Alzheimers Dis Other Demen 2016; 31(8): 706-16. [http://dx.doi.org/10.1177/1533317516673155] [PMID: 27756815]

[229] Correia SM. Avaliação fonoaudiológica da deglutição na doença de Alzheimer em fases avançadas Tese de Doutorado. São Paulo: Universidade de São Paulo 2010.

[230] Piovesan R. Tratamento farmacológico dos transtornos nutricionais.Nutrição em Demências. São Paulo: Scio 2013.

[231] Lin LC, Watson R, Wu SC. What is associated with low food intake in older people with dementia? J Clin Nurs 2010; 19(1-2): 53-9. [http://dx.doi.org/10.1111/j.1365-2702.2009.02962.x] [PMID: 20500244]

[232] Yamaguchi K, Hoshiyama M, Takano M. Biological observation during the daytime of elderly patients with advanced dementia cared for with and without artificial nutrition by percutaneous endoscopic gastrostomy. Geriatr Gerontol Int 2011; 11(2): 221-8. [http://dx.doi.org/10.1111/j.1447-0594.2010.00657.x] [PMID: 21050349]

[233] Mamhidir AG, Karlsson I, Norberg A, Mona K. Weight increase in patients with dementia, and alteration in meal routines and meal environment after integrity promoting care. J Clin Nurs 2007; 16(5): 987-96.
[http://dx.doi.org/10.1111/j.1365-2702.2006.01780.x] [PMID: 17462050]

[234] Franco FS, Martinho KO, Martins MV, Montini TA, Tinôco EF, Tinôco ALA. Transtornos cognitivos.Saúde do idoso Epidemiologia, Aspectos Nutricionais e Processos do Envelhecimento. Rio de Janeiro: Editora Rubio 2015; pp. 291-305.

[235] Kikuchi EL, Filho WJ. Tratamento e prevenção de Distúrbios Físicos associados.Demência Abordagem Multidisciplinar. São Paulo: Atheneu 2006.

[236] Remig VM, Romero C. Terapia Nutricional para Distúbios Neurológicos.Alimentos, Nutrição e Dietoterapia. São Paulo: Roca 2005.

[237] Morley JE, Argiles JM, Evans WJ, *et al.* Society for Sarcopenia, Cachexia, and Wasting Disease. Nutritional recommendations for the management of sarcopenia. J Am Med Dir Assoc 2010; 11(6): 391-6.
[http://dx.doi.org/10.1016/j.jamda.2010.04.014] [PMID: 20627179]

[238] Morley JE. Nutrition and Aging Well. J Am Med Dir Assoc 2017; 18(2): 91-4.
[http://dx.doi.org/10.1016/j.jamda.2016.11.014] [PMID: 28126140]

[239] Fernando WMADB, Rainey-Smith SR, Gardener SL, *et al.* AIBL Research Group. Associations of Dietary Protein and Fiber Intake with Brain and Blood Amyloid-β. J Alzheimers Dis 2018; 61(4): 1589-98.
[http://dx.doi.org/10.3233/JAD-170742] [PMID: 29376865]

[240] Studnicki M, Woźniak G, Stępkowski D. The Calculator of Anti-Alzheimer's Diet. Macronutrients. PLoS One 2016; 11(12): e0168385.
[http://dx.doi.org/10.1371/journal.pone.0168385] [PMID: 27992612]

[241] Gardener SL, Rainey-Smith SR, Sohrabi HR, *et al.* AIBL Research Group. Increased Carbohydrate Intake is Associated with Poorer Performance in Verbal Memory and Attention in an APOE Genotype-Dependent Manner. J Alzheimers Dis 2017; 58(1): 193-201.
[http://dx.doi.org/10.3233/JAD-161158] [PMID: 28387666]

[242] Hanson LC, Ersek M, Gilliam R, Carey TS. Oral feeding options for people with dementia: a systematic review. J Am Geriatr Soc 2011; 59(3): 463-72.
[http://dx.doi.org/10.1111/j.1532-5415.2011.03320.x] [PMID: 21391936]

[243] American Geriatrics Society Ethics Committee and Clinical Practice and Models of Care Committee. American Geriatrics Society feeding tubes in advanced dementia position statement. J Am Geriatr Soc 2014; 62(8): 1590-3.
[http://dx.doi.org/10.1111/jgs.12924] [PMID: 25039796]

[244] Teixeira AL, Caramelli P. Neuropsicologia das demências.Neuropsicologia: teoria e prática. Porto Alegre: Artmed 2008.

[245] Brunnström HR, Englund EM. Cause of death in patients with dementia disorders. Eur J Neurol 2009; 16(4): 488-92.
[http://dx.doi.org/10.1111/j.1468-1331.2008.02503.x] [PMID: 19170740]

[246] Logemann JA. Evaluation and treatment of swallowing disorders. 2nd ed., Austin: Pro-Ed 1998.

[247] Easterling CS, Robbins E. Dementia and dysphagia. Geriatr Nurs 2008; 29(4): 275-85.
[http://dx.doi.org/10.1016/j.gerinurse.2007.10.015] [PMID: 18694703]

[248] Langmore SE, Skarupski KA, Park PS, Fries BE. Predictors of aspiration pneumonia in nursing home residents. Dysphagia 2002; 17(4): 298-307.
[http://dx.doi.org/10.1007/s00455-002-0072-5] [PMID: 12355145]

[249] Boccardi V, Ruggiero C, Patriti A, Marano L. Diagnostic Assessment and Management of Dysphagia

in Patients with Alzheimer's Disease. J Alzheimers Dis 2016; 50(4): 947-55.
[http://dx.doi.org/10.3233/JAD-150931] [PMID: 26836016]

[250] Hiss SG, Strauss M, Treole K, Stuart A, Boutilier S. Effects of age, gender, bolus volume, bolus viscosity, and gustation on swallowing apnea onset relative to lingual bolus propulsion onset in normal adults. J Speech Lang Hear Res 2004; 47(3): 572-83.
[http://dx.doi.org/10.1044/1092-4388(2004/044)] [PMID: 15212569]

[251] Chi-Fishman G, Sonies BC. Effects of systematic bolus viscosity and volume changes on hyoid movement kinematics. Dysphagia 2002; 17(4): 278-87.
[http://dx.doi.org/10.1007/s00455-002-0070-7] [PMID: 12355143]

[252] Alagiakrishnan K, Bhanji RA, Kurian M. Evaluation and management of oropharyngeal dysphagia in different types of dementia: a systematic review. Arch Gerontol Geriatr 2013; 56(1): 1-9.
[http://dx.doi.org/10.1016/j.archger.2012.04.011] [PMID: 22608838]

[253] Chen LL, Li H, Lin R, *et al.* Effects of a feeding intervention in patients with Alzheimer's disease and dysphagia. J Clin Nurs 2016; 25(5-6): 699-707.
[http://dx.doi.org/10.1111/jocn.13013] [PMID: 26420351]

[254] Murphy LM, Lipman TO. Percutaneous endoscopic gastrostomy does not prolong survival in patients with dementia. Arch Intern Med 2003; 163(11): 1351-3.
[http://dx.doi.org/10.1001/archinte.163.11.1351] [PMID: 12796072]

[255] Bamia C, Lagiou P, Jenab M, *et al.* Coffee, tea and decaffeinated coffee in relation to hepatocellular carcinoma in a European population: multicentre, prospective cohort study. Int J Cancer 2015; 136(8): 1899-908.
[http://dx.doi.org/10.1002/ijc.29214] [PMID: 25219573]

[256] Finucane TE, Christmas C, Travis K. Tube feeding in patients with advanced dementia: a review of the evidence. JAMA 1999; 282(14): 1365-70.
[http://dx.doi.org/10.1001/jama.282.14.1365] [PMID: 10527184]

[257] WHO. World Health Organization Envelhecimento Ativo: uma política de saúde. Brasília: Organização Pan-Americana da Saúde 2005.

[258] Gottlieb MGV, Lopes Filho BJP, Lindôso ZCL, *et al.* Estimulação cognitiva em idosos: uma proposta interdisciplinar embasada no envelhecimento ativo e na Política Nacional do Idoso.Temas de geriatria e gerontologia. Porto Alegre: EDIPUCRS 2017; pp. 129-50.

[259] NICE. National Institute for Health and Clinical Excellence; Guidance National Collaborating Centre for Mental Health Dementia: a NICE-SCIE Guideline on supporting seople with dementia and their carers in health and social care. Leicester, UK: British Psychological Society 2007.

[260] Berg-Weger M, Tebb S, Henderson-Kalb J, Zubatsky M, Lundy J, Hayden D. Cognitive stimulation therapy: a tool for your practice with persons with dementia? J Am Med Dir Assoc 2015; 16(9): 795-6.
[http://dx.doi.org/10.1016/j.jamda.2015.06.002] [PMID: 26170036]

[261] Loraine J, Taylor S, McAllister M. Cognitive and physical stimulation therapy. J Am Med Dir Assoc 2014; 15(2): 140-1.
[http://dx.doi.org/10.1016/j.jamda.2013.11.016] [PMID: 24461241]

[262] Morley JE, Berg-Weger M, Lundy J.. Editorial: Nonpharmacological Treatment of Cognitive Impairment. J Nutr Health Aging 2018; 22(6): 632-3.

CHAPTER 7

Past and Present Drug Development for Alzheimer's Disease

Pratap Kumar Sahu*, **Prashant Tiwari, Shakti Ketan Prusty** and **Bharat Bhusan Subudhi**

School of Pharmaceutical Sciences, Siksha O Anusandhan Deemed University, Bhubaneswar, Odisha, India-751029

Abstract: Alzheimer's disease (AD) is a progressive and an irreversible chronic neurodegenerative disorder causing dementia. Worldwide, the prevalence of AD is estimated to be 30 million and likely to quadruple in the next 40 years. Thus, the global cost of dementia is estimated to be 1.09% of global GDP (US$ 818 billion). Several factors including age and family history are involved in its etiology and considered as the predisposing factors for AD. The neurochemical basis of AD can be explained by the 'Cholinergic', 'Amyloid plaque' and 'Tauopathy' hypotheses. The 'Cholinergic' hypothesis put forth a relationship between Acetyl choline (ACh) levels to cognitive memory and the other two hypotheses propose an excessive deposition of amyloid plaques extracellularly and accumulation of tau protein intracellularly, eventually causing neuronal death. The cholinergic system is mainly targeted for therapeutic management of AD symptoms. In view of that, acetylcholinesterase inhibitors (AChEI) such as tacrine, donepezil, rivastigmine and galantamine have been used. Memantine, an N –methyl – D - aspartate (NMDA) receptor antagonist inhibiting glutamate mediated exocitotoxicity, is also used to improve dementia symptoms. However, the degree of improvement with this approach has been minimal as no one of these drugs can reverse the course of AD, nor prevent destruction of neurons. Accordingly, amyloid based strategies including 'secretive enzymes modulation', 'amyloid aggregation prevention' and 'amyloid clearance promotion' have been adopted. Inhibition of tau phosphorylation/oligomerization, microtubule stabilization, reduction of stress/inflammation, modulation of neurotransmitters and cellular calcium homeostasis has also been used as strategy to manage AD with varying degree of success.

A high rate of attrition combined with huge cost of new drug development has encouraged drug repurposing strategies. This approach ensures minimal developmental cost and shorter approval time to launch a drug. Moreover, the risk associated with conventional drug discovery is reduced due to existing pharmacokinetic and safety data. Thus, drug repurposing is considered to be a preferred strategy against AD. Modern advances in disease biology of AD have substantially assembled data from

* **Corresponding author Pratap Kumar Sahu:** School of Pharmaceutical Sciences, Siksha O Anusandhan Deemed University, Bhubaneswar, Odisha, India-751029; Tel: 9437035910; Email-pratapsahu@soa.ac.in

Atta-ur-Rahman (Ed.)

pre-clinical, clinical, *in-vitro*, epidemiological, toxicological, and computational sources. Thus, an implementation of systematic approaches using this on hand information with a clear understanding of the network pharmacology can give way the next therapeutic alternative for successful management of AD.

The current chapter describes the scope and limitations of some currently marketed drugs like cholinergic drugs, cyclooxygenase (COX) and lipoxygenase (LOX) inhibitors, renin angiotensin system (RAS) inhibitors, lipid lowering drugs (statins), NMDA receptor antagonists, anti-diabetics, anti-oxidants, vitamin D *etc* in management of AD. Many of them have the potential against AD and some of them are validated pre-clinically and clinically. But none of them has reached the market yet. Drugs targeting neuroinflammation including COX inhibitors, LOX inhibitors and RAS inhibitors can potentially arrest the disease progression in AD. However, their repurposing potential needs to be clinically validated.

Keywords: Acetylcholine Esterase Inhibitors, Anti-Diabetics, Alzheimer's Disease, Amyloid β, Anti-Oxidants, Blood Brain Barrier, Cyclooxygenase, Drug Repurposing, Immunotherapy, Lipoxygenase, N-Methyl-D-Aspartate Receptor, Renin Angiotensin System, Statins.

INTRODUCTION

Alzheimer's disease (AD) is a progressive and irreversible neurodegenerative disease. It is the most common cause of dementia worldwide. This disease is named after Dr. Alois **Alzheimer**. In 1906, a woman with symptoms like memory loss, unpredictable behavior and language problems died. Dr Alzheimer noticed changes in her brain, described these changes and published his findings [1].

The prevalence of AD is estimated to 30 million people worldwide (2011), and is expected to quadruple in 40 years [2]. It will be a global health problem with huge implications for individuals and society by midcentury [3]. The World Alzheimer Report, published under the auspices of Alzheimer Disease International (ADI) has also recognized AD to become a world health problem. Moreover, it is predicted by ADI investigators that dementia prevalence may double every 20 years, to 65·7 million in 2030 and 115·4 million in 2050 [4, 5].

Age is a predisposing factor for AD and countries with higher fraction of old people are expected to show higher prevalence. This is evident from the fact that; the prevalence of dementia rises from 1% at the age of 60 to at least 35% at the age of 90 [6]. Further, it increases from 3.5 per 1000 per year at ages of 65-69 to 72.8 per 1000 per year at ages of 85 to 89 years. Thus the incidences of AD are considered to double in every 5 years of age beyond 65 [7, 8].

The cases of AD in China (Fig. **1**) can be explained by its huge population base and the overall low education level of Chinese people, compared to those in other developed countries [9]. Interestingly using population as the criteria, the cases reported from USA can be considered high whereas those for India are low. This can be partly explained by the fact that many cases of AD in India go unreported, whereas the incidences are well documented in USA [10, 5]. Besides, majority of the population being young in India, AD incidences can be expected to be low. In contrast the incidences reported for Japan are relatively high which can be attributed to its majority of geriatric population [11, 12].

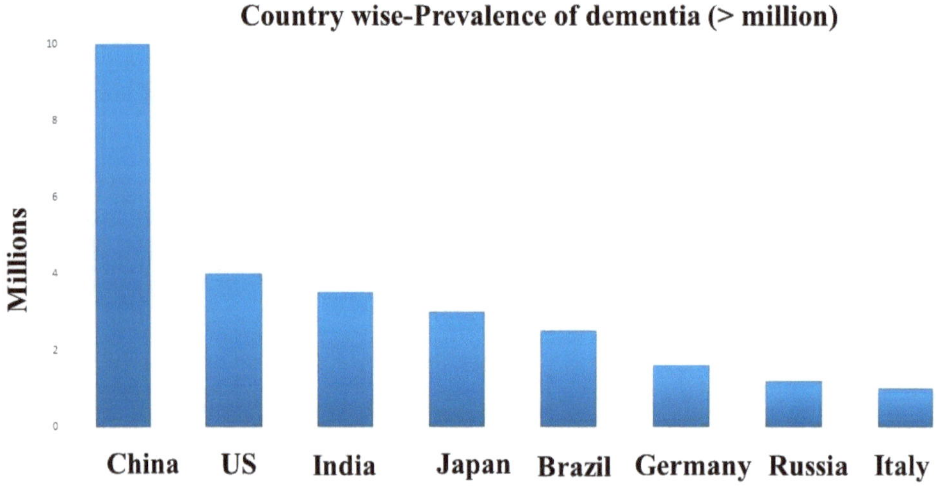

Fig. (1). Country wise prevalence of Alzheimer's disease (Source: World Alzheimer's Report): China has the maximum number of AD patients followed by USA. India has the third highest number of AD patients.

In 2015, the global cost of dementia is 1.09% of global GDP (US$818 billion) which would be the 18th largest economy in the world. By 2018, the global cost of dementia including costs attributed to informal care (40%), direct costs of social care (40%) and the direct costs of medical care (20%) will be more than a trillion US$. The informal care costs (unpaid care provided by family and others) are greatest in the African regions and lowest in developed countries of North America, Western Europe and South America. The social sector costs are lowest in Africa [5].

THERAPEUTIC MANAGEMENT

Although several reasons can be attributed to dementia, most of the patients who develop dementia before 65 years of age and without any specific cause have AD. There are two types of dementia with early onset: *(i)* presenile (before 65 years of age) dementias; and *(ii)* senile (after 65 years of age) dementias [13]. Alzheimer's disease was originally classified as a presenile dementia. However, later in the 1980s, senile dementia of Alzheimer type (SDAT) has also been considered as dementia of Alzheimer's type (DAT) or merely Alzheimer's disease because of presence of same pathological entity.

In addition to rapid progression of cognitive impairment, language problems and visuospatial dysfunctions are commonly associated with onset of AD. In recent years, neurological symptoms including seizures and myoclonic convulsions have been reported to occur infrequently with AD. The etiology of AD onset is not clear. Nevertheless, several risk factors have been linked to AD like age, family history, apolipoprotein (Apo) E4 status, depression, hypertension, diabetes, high cholesterol, atrial fibrillation, low physical and cognitive activity, head injury, and presence of cerebral emboli [14].

The pathogenesis of AD is associated more with genetic factors than with environmental factors [14]. Some types of presenile dementia are linked to chromosome 17. Three genes namely the amyloid precursor gene (APP), and the genes encoding presenilin 1 (PSEN1) and presenilin 2 (PSEN2) on chromosomes 21, 14, and 1 respectively can be linked to familial Alzheimer's disease with early onset [13]. The only gene ApoE (apolipoprotein E) located on chromosome 19 can be linked to late onset AD. The ApoE gene exists in 3 forms like ApoE2, ApoE3, and ApoE4 [15, 16]. Formation of Aβ is facilitated by mutations in APP or presenilin whereas clearance of Aβ is impaired by mutations in ApoE4 gene (Fig. **2**).

Currently, we do not have any therapy to halt disease progression. The therapy is mainly focused on memory-associated brain defects [2]. The neurochemical changes in AD can be explained by three prominent hypotheses [17, 18]. These are the cholinergic, amyloid plaque and tauopathy hypotheses. Based on the cholinergic hypothesis acetyl choline level is directly related to memory. Accordingly, pro-cholinergic effects including acetylcholine esterase (AChE) inhibition and muscarinic M_2 autoreceptor antagonism are supposed to prevent or manage dementia. The amyloid plaque hypotheses involve amyloid peptides produced from its precursor protein [19]. Three proteases/ secretases are involved in the cleavage of amyloid precursor protein (APP). Alpha secretase produces soluble APP which exerts a number of trophic functions whereas beta secretase and gamma secretase generate Aβ peptides like Aβ40 and Aβ42. Aβ42 has a higher tendency to aggregate as amyloid plaques leading to neurodegenerative characteristics of AD [20]. The third hypothesis involves tauopathy. Tau is a normal component of neurons. Its abnormal phosphorylation leads to formation of neurofibrillary tangles associated with AD [21, 22].

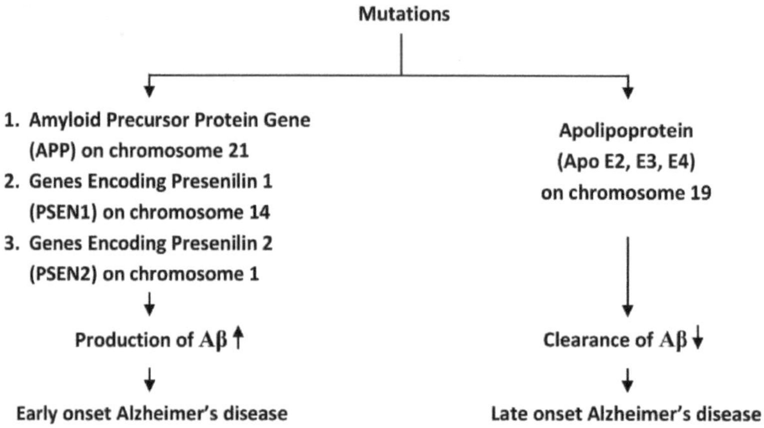

Fig. (2). Genetic link of Alzheimer's disease: The prognosis of AD is correlated to genes and their link with production or clearance of amyloid β (Aβ). The mutation of genes including presenilin 1 (PSEN1) and presenilin 2 (PSEN2) and amyloid precursor protein gene (APP) are responsible for production and accumulation of Amyloid β (Aβ) resulting in early onset of AD. ApoE (apolipoprotein E) gene is responsible for clearance of Aβ. Mutation of ApoE gene can cause late onset AD.

Although these independent hypotheses have been proposed, in several interlinks between them have also been proposed. Both acetylcholinesterase and butyrylcholinesterase (BuChE) have been shown to play important role in Aβ-aggregation during the early stages of senile plaque formation and inhibitors of AChE can potentially increase cholinergic function while reducing the Aβ peptide aggregation [23, 24]. High CSF (cerebrospinal fluid) levels of tau and low CSF levels of amyloid- beta-42 are good predictors for conversion from mild cognitive impairment to AD [25]. Tau-mediated formation of neurofibrillary tangles in AD brains shows better correlation with cognitive impairment than amyloid plaque accumulation [26]. Nonetheless, formation of plaque, neurofibrillary tangles and related neurodegeneration following mutation in transgenic animals has been reproducibly demonstrated in progression of AD [27].

While AD is primarily a neurodegenerative disease process, there are several elements of neuroinflammation that take place at the molecular level [28, 29]. In AD dementia, there are CSF signs of neurodegeneration (increased total tau), synaptic dysfunction (increased neurogranulin), and glial activation (increased YKL-40) [18]. Activation of microglia/astrocytes leads to increased level of chemokines and cytokines in neurons which activates inflammatory process leading to enhancement in intracellular calcium levels, NADPH oxidase (NOX), NF-κB (nuclear factor kappa-light-chain-enhancer of activated B cells) signaling, glutamate uptake (increasing the risk of excitotoxicity) and mitochondrial dysfunction [30 - 32]. Neuroinflammation is also facilitated by oxidative stress [33].

Besides inflammatory process, prostaglandin E2 (PGE2) also modifies synaptic transmission and plasticity of hippocampal neurons leading to loss of memory [33]. Increased activity of choline esterase in CNS is also a contributing factor, as it reduces the level of acetyl choline which impairs the synaptic plasticity in hippocampus [34]. In recent years, involvement of central renin angiotensin system (RAS) in CNS disorder [35] has been increasingly recognized. Considering the key role played by AT1 receptor in inflammation, its contribution to neurodegeneration is considered to be significant (Fig. **3**).

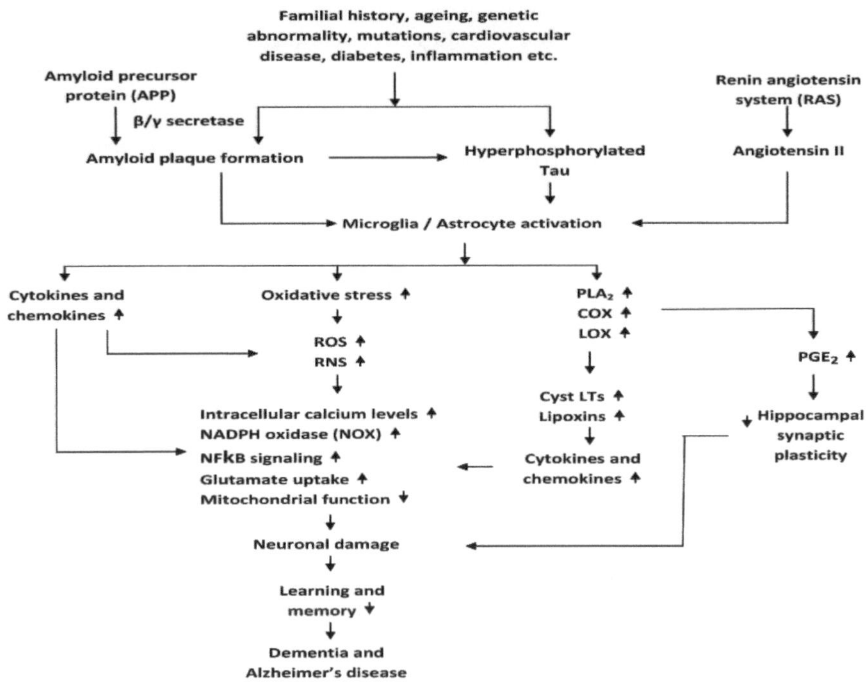

Fig. (3). Role of Inflammation in Neurodegenerative diseases: Risk factors including ageing, genetic abnormality, diabetes *etc* facilitate the formation of amyloid plaque and hyperphosphorylated tau. They activate microglia/astrocytes to generate the inflammatory mediators, to induce oxidative stress, and to reduce hippocampal synaptic plasticity. This leads to neurodegeneration and neurodegenerative diseases like AD. Renin angiotensin system also activates microglia/ astrocytes.

An increased incidence of AD is found in patients with type 2 diabetes mellitus (T2DM). The common factors linking T2DM and AD may be the chronic inflammatory response, oxidative stress, and mitochondrial dysfunction [36]. Similarly, factors like inflammation and oxidative stress may link atherosclerotic disease and AD [37].

To regulate learning and memory processes, the cholinergic system is mainly targeted for therapeutic management of AD. Accordingly acetylcholinesterase inhibitors (AChEIs) including tacrine, donepezil, rivastigmine and galantamine have been used to increase cholinergic transmission by inhibiting acetylcholinesterase (AChE) and butyrylcholinesterase (BuChE) leading to prevention of hydrolysis of acetylcholine. Efficacy of these inhibitors is also partly attributed to their capacity to reduce Aβ deposition [38]. Additionally, independent antioxidant and antiinflammatory actions of these inhibitors also play a role in management of AD [39].

Five drugs are currently approved by the U.S. Food and Drug Administration (FDA) to treat the symptoms of AD (Table **1**). Tacrine (1993) was the first to be approved by US FDA. The success of tacrine is a confirmation of the cholinergic theory of AD. However, it did not get the approval by several regulatory authorities in Europe. It has never been a doctor's choice to prescribe. Its efficacy remains controversial. There was high incidence of adverse events [40].

Table 1. List of U.S. Food and Drug Administration (FDA) approved drugs for AD.

Sl. No.	Drug	Dose	structure	Mechanism	Use	Side effect
1	Tacrine (1993)	10, 20, 30, and 40 mg per day	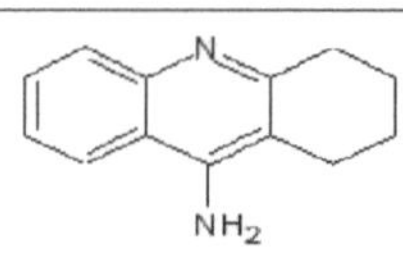	Cholinesterase inhibitor	Mild to moderate	Hepatotoxicity, abdominal pain, skin rash
2	Donepezil (1996)	5, 10 and 23 mg per day	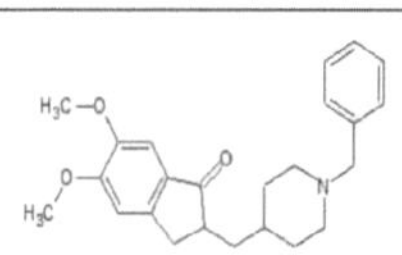	Cholinesterase inhibitor	All stages of Alzheimer's disease	Nausea, vomiting, loss of appetite and increased frequency of bowel movements.
3	Rivastigmine (2000)	6 to 12 mg per day	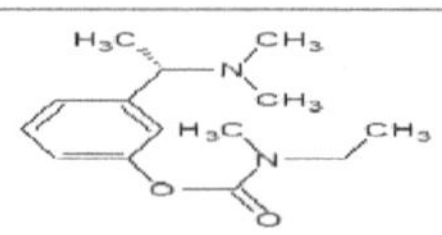	Cholinesterase inhibitor	Mild to moderate	Nausea, vomiting, loss of appetite and increased frequency of bowel movements.
4	Galantamine (2001)	16 to 24 mg per day	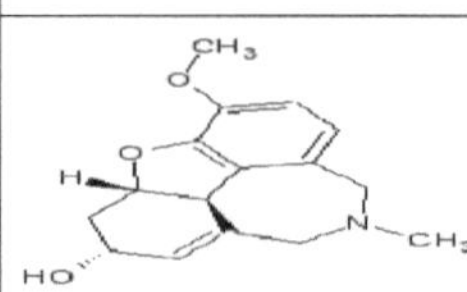	Cholinesterase inhibitor	Mild to moderate	Nausea, vomiting, loss of appetite and increased frequency of bowel movements.
5	Memantine (2003)	5 to 10 mg per day	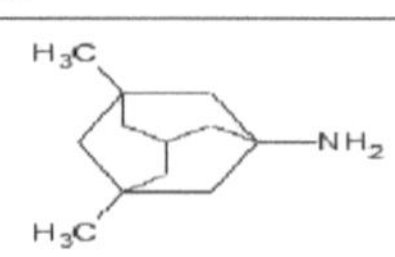	n-Methyl d-Aspartate receptor antagonist	Moderate to severe	Headache, constipation, confusion and dizziness

Source: https://www.alz.org/, https://www.accessdata.fda.gov/.

The other cholinesterase inhibitors approved against AD are donepezil (1996), rivastigmine (2000) and galantamine (2001). These drugs prevent the degradation of acetyl choline in the brain. Unlike these, memantine is an N-methyl-D-aspartate (NMDA) receptor antagonist that inhibits glutamate induced exocitotoxicity in brain leading to protection of neuronal cells and improvement in memory and learning. It was approved in 2002 for treatment of AD by the European Agency for the Evaluation of Medicinal Products (EMEA) and in 2003 by the USA Food and Drug Administration (FDA). Recently a combination of memantine with one of the cholinesterase inhibitors (donepezil) is also approved [41]. However, the degrees of improvement with existing therapy are small and effectiveness is variable. Besides, these drugs are able to neither reverse AD nor stop the underlying destruction of nerve cells. Nonetheless these drugs are used to delay or slow worsening of symptoms [42].

DRUG DISCOVERY PROGRAMME

Unlike cholinergic hypothesis, drugs based on other two hypotheses have not been explored much. Thus amyloid based strategies including secretive enzymes modulation, amyloid aggregation prevention and amyloid clearance promotion have been adopted. Inhibition of tau phosphorylation, tau oligomerization and microtubule stabilization has also been targeted to arrest AD progression. Modulation of neurotransmitters like glutamate, gamma amino butyric acid (GABA), norepinephrine, melatonin and serotonin have also been attempted to manage AD. Alternative and complementary therapeutic concepts including intracellular signaling cascades modulation, oxidative stress reduction, cellular calcium homeostasis, anti-inflammation, lipid modifiers (statins) and epigenetic modifiers have been evaluated against AD to find ideal therapeutic strategy [43]. List of drugs which are under clinical trial are given in (Table **2**).

Table 2. List of drugs under trial for AD with their current clinical trial status and mechanism of action.

Name of Drug	Present Status	Mechanism
1. NMDA receptor antagonists		
AXS-05	In Phase 3 clinical trial	n-Methyl d-Aspartate receptor antagonist
AVP-786	In Phase 3 clinical trial	n-Methyl d-Aspartate receptor antagonist
2. **Cholinergic Drugs**		
Huperzine A	In clinical trial	selective acetylcholinesterase inhibitor
ZT-1 (prodrug of Huperzine A)	In clinical trial	selective acetylcholinesterase inhibitor
Phenserine (derivative of physostigmine)	In clinical trial	acetylcholinesterase inhibitor

(Table 2) cont.....

Name of Drug	Present Status	Mechanism
Ladostigil	In clinical trial	acetylcholin-butyrylcholinesterase inhibitor
AF267B	In clinical trial	M1 selective muscarinic agonist
EVP-6124	In clinical trial	selective agonist of α7 nicotinic acetylcholine receptor
GTS-21	In clinical trial	selective agonist of α7 nicotinic receptor
Memogain (pro-drug of galantamine)	In clinical trial	liberates galantamine; a cholinesterase inhibitor
TAK-071	In Phase 2 clinical trial	Muscarinic M1 receptor modulator
Octohydroaminoacridine succinate	In Phase 3 clinical trial	Acetylcholinesterase inhibitor
CPC-201 (donepezil/Solifenacin combination)	In Phase 2 clinical trial	Cholinesterase inhibitor
Nicotine transdermal	In Phase 2 clinical trial	Nicotinic acetyl choline receptor agonist
3. Amyloid-targeting drugs		
Decreasing Aβ production		
LY2811376	In clinical trial	β-Secretase inhibitor
LY2886721	In clinical trial	β-Secretase inhibitor
MK-8931 (developed by MERCK)	In clinical trial	β-Secretase inhibitor
E2609	In Phase 2 clinical trial	β-Secretase inhibitor
CNP520	In Phase 3 clinical trial	β-Secretase inhibitor
Semagacestat (LY-450139)	Terminated in clinical trial	γ-Secretase inhibitor
Avagacestat (BMS-708163)	In clinical trial	γ-Secretase inhibitor
Begacestat (GSI-953)	In Phase 2 clinical trial	γ-Secretase inhibitor
NIC5-15	In clinical trial	γ-Secretase inhibitor
CHF5074	In clinical trial	γ-Secretase inhibitor
E2012	In clinical trial	γ-Secretase inhibitor
Promoting Aβ clearance		
AN-1752	Terminated in clinical trial	Promoting Aβ clearance
CAD106	In Phase 2 clinical trial	Reduce Aβ accumulation

(Table 2) cont.....

Name of Drug	Present Status	Mechanism
ACI-24	In Phase 2 clinical trial	Promoting Aβ clearance
UB-311	In Phase 2 clinical trial	Promoting Aβ clearance
ACC-001 (Vanutide cridificar)	In clinical trial	Vaccines producing Aβ antibodies
V950 (ISCOMATRIX)	In clinical trial	Vaccines producing Aβ antibodies
Lu AF20513	In clinical trial	Vaccines producing Aβ antibodies
AD02	In clinical trial	Vaccines producing Aβ antibodies
Preventing Aβ aggregation		
Tramiprostate	In clinical trial	Anti-aggregation compound
Scyllo-inositol	In clinical trial	Anti-aggregation compound
Clioquinol	In clinical trial	Anti-aggregation compound
Bexarotene	In clinical trial	Anti-aggregation compound
Epigallocatechin-3-gallate	In clinical trial	Anti-aggregation compound
TTP488 (PF-04494700)	In Phase 2 clinical trial	Antagonizes to the receptor for glycation endproducts
PBT2	In Phase 2 clinical trial	Reduce concentration of Aβ42 by obstructing Aβ oligomerization
ALZT-OP1a + ALZT-OP1b (cromolyn + ibuprofen)	In Phase 3 clinical trial	Anti-amyloid, anti-inflammatory
TTP488 (Azeliragon)	In Phase 3 clinical trial	Anti-amyloid, anti-inflammatory RAGE (receptor for advanced glycation end products) antagonist
4. **AD immunotherapy**		
AAB-001 (Bapineuzumab)	Failed in trial	Humanized monoclonal antibody targeting Aβ
LY-2062430 (Solanezumab)	In Phase 3 clinical trial	Humanized monoclonal antibody targeting Aβ
PF-04360365 (Ponezumab)	In clinical trial	Humanized monoclonal antibody targeting Aβ
GSK-933776	In clinical trial	Humanized inactivated monoclonal antibody targeting Aβ
MABT5102A	In clinical trial	Humanized monoclonal antibody targeting Aβ
Aducanumab	In Phase 3 clinical trial	Humanized monoclonal antibody selectively targets misfolded Aβ peptides
Crenezumab	In Phase 3 clinical trial	Monoclonal antibody

(Table 2) cont.....

Name of Drug	Present Status	Mechanism
Gantenerumab	In Phase 3 clinical trial	Monoclonal antibody
Albumin + Immunoglobulin	In Phase 3 clinical trial	Polyclonal antibody
5. **Neurotransmitter based drugs**		
ITI-007	In Phase 3 clinical trial	Dopamine receptor modulator
Methylphenidate	In Phase 3 clinical trial	Dopamine reuptake inhibitor
Nabilone	In Phase 3 clinical trial	Cannabinoid receptor agonist
Zolpidem	In Phase 3 clinical trial	GABA-A modulator
BI 425809	In Phase 2 clinical trial	Facilitate NMDA receptor activity
Piromelatin	In Phase 2 clinical trial	Melatonin receptor agonist
DAOIB	In Phase 2 clinical trial	NMDA receptor modulator
S47445	In Phase 2 clinical trial	AMPA receptor agonist
Rotigotine	In Phase 2 clinical trial	Dopamine agonist
Lithium	In Phase 2 clinical trial	Ion channel modulator
Idalopirdine	In Phase 2 clinical trial	5HT receptor antagonist
Dronabinol	In Phase 2 clinical trial	Cannabinoid receptor partial agonist
Atomoxetin	In Phase 2 clinical trial	Norepinephrine reuptake inhibitor
6. **Drugs targeting Tau protein**		
LMTX (Leuco-methylthioninium)	In Phase 3 clinical trial	Selective Tau aggregation inhibitor
AADvac1	In preclinical trial	Produce antibodies against Tau protein
ACI-35	In preclinical trial	Produce antibodies against Tau protein
7. **Drugs targeting mitochondrial dysfunction**		

(Table 2) cont.....

Name of Drug	Present Status	Mechanism
Latrepirdine (Dimebon)	Approved	Ameliorate mitochondrial membrane potential and ATP production
MP-101	In Phase 2 clinical trial	Enhances mitochondrial function
8. **PPAR-γ agonists**		
Pioglitazone	In Phase 3 clinical trial	PPAR-γ agonists improving cognition in AD mice
9. **Regenerative drugs**		
hUCB-MSCs	In Phase 2 clinical trial	Stem cell therapy
10. **Neuroprotective drugs**		
AAV2-NGF (CERE-110)	In clinical trial	Delivers NGF in brain
T-817MA	In Phase 2 clinical trial	Produces neuroprotective and neurotrophic effects
DHP1401	In Phase 2 clinical trial	Affects cAMP activity
Deferiprone	In Phase 2 clinical trial	Iron chelating agent
Liraglutide	In Phase 2 clinical trial	Glucagon like peptide 1 receptor agonist
L-Serine	In Phase 2 clinical trial	Stabilize protein misfolding
Riluzole	In Phase 2 clinical trial	Glutamate receptor antagonist
Simvastatin+L-Arginine+Tetrahydrobiopterin	In Phase 2 clinical trial	HMG CoA reductase inhibitor
Telmisartan	In Phase 2 clinical trial	Angiotensin II receptor blocker
Valacyclovir	In Phase 2 clinical trial	Antiviral agent

Source: https://www.alzforum.org/, https://clinicaltrials.gov/

NMDA Receptor Antagonists

Postsynaptic *N*-Methyl-D-aspartate (NMDA) receptor is ionotropic glutamate receptor that mediates excitatory signaling in the presence of glycine and glutamate [44]. This is implicated in neuronal development, synaptic plasticity, learning and memory. Recent findings have suggested interaction of soluble oligomeric Aβ with glutamatergic receptors (NMDA) as one of the etiologic factor of AD. Accordingly NMDA receptor antagonist like Memantine is clinically used for the treatment of AD [45]. In recent years, Dextromethorphan has also been identified as the noncompetitive NMDA receptor antagonist [46] with potential for clinical management of AD.

Cholinergic Drugs

Currently, the major therapeutic strategy to manage AD involves cholinergic drugs. Prompted by their limited clinical success many efforts have been made either to explore new cholinergic drugs or to optimize existing cholinergic drugs to maximize benefits. Huperzine A, isolated from the Chinese herb *Huperzia serrata* (Thunb.) Trev was found to be a relatively selective inhibitor of acetyl cholinesterase (AChE). Although benefits of its selective affinity for AChE over BuChE are not clear, its additional antiinflammatory properties were thought to contribute to its effect against AD [47]. Its prodrug (ZT-1), was used to optimize its bioavailability and is currently under clinical trial [48]. A polyphenolic compound (hopeahainolA) from *Hopea hainanensis* with comparable efficacy to huperzine A is also under investigation against AD [42].

Physostigmine is an AChE inhibitor with limited efficacy and serious side effects [49]. To improve pharmacological properties of Physostigmine a US based biopharmaceutical company Axonyx, developed (-) phenserine as a derivative of physostigmine. In addition to inhibition of AChE, it also possess anti-amyloid activity. Owing to its dual mode of action, it promises to be the more effective therapeutic alternative and is under clinical trial [50].

Memogain (Gln-1062) was developed at Galantos Pharma to improve the brain bioavailability and reduce the peripheral side effects of galantamine. With better hydrophobic properties, it ensured a 10-15-fold higher bioavailability of galantamine in brain with minimal toxicity issues. Currently Canadian company Neurodyn prepares the substance for clinical development [51, 52].

Ladostigil (TV-3326) is a novel multitarget drug candidate developed at Avraham Pharmaceuticals Ltd (Israel). While it reversibly inhibits acetylcholine-butyrylcholinesterase, it irreversibly inhibits monoamine oxidase B in brain. Aditionally it possess neuroprotective properties. Besides it has also been proposed to induce neurogenesis on account of its capacity to promote expression of neurotrophic factors like GDNF (glial cell derived neurotrophic factor) and BDNF (brain derived neurotrophic factor) [53]. Many subsequent cholinesterase inhibitors such as velnacrine, eptastigmine *etc* were not marketed despite of their efficacy because there were safety and patent issues [54].

Direct stimulation of cholinergic receptors is another strategy to improve dementia. NGX267 was developed at TorreyPines Therapeutics, Inc as a selective agonist of M_1 muscarinic acetylcholine receptor. AF102B (cevimeline) is another M_1 agonist developed by Snowbrand Pharmaceuticals. These M1 agonists increase αAPPs, decrease Aβ levels and tau hyper phosphorylation, and block Aβ-induced neurotoxicity *in vitro via* M_1 receptor-mediated modulation of kinases (*e.g.* PKC, MAPK and GSK3β) [55]. Similarly Encenicline (EVP-6124, FORUM Pharmaceuticals, USA) is a selective agonist of the α-7 nicotinic acetylcholine (α7 nACh) receptor and is in Phase III trial for the treatment of cognitive impairment [56]. Another α7 nAChR agonist, ABT-126 [2-(((1R,3R,4S,5S,7S)-1-azaadamantan-4-yl)oxy)-5-phenyl-1,3,4-thiadiazole], developed by AbbVie, USA significantly improved negative symptoms of schizophrenia without ameliorating cognitive deficits in phase II clinical trials [57]. GTS-21 also named DMXB-A, developed by CoMentis is an anabaseine derivative identified as an α7 nAChR agonist and showed promising characteristics during Phase II clinical trial [58].

Amyloid-Targeted Therapies

These drugs can either decrease Aβ production, prevent Aβ aggregation or promote Aβ clearance.

Decreasing Aβ Production

β-Secretase Inhibitors

The first oral non-peptide small molecule that was developed as BACE1 inhibitor [59] was LY2811376 (Cayman chemicals, USA/Canada). Although its pharmacokinetic and pharmacodynamic parameters are satisfactory, its further clinical development was discontinued due to toxicity issues. Nevertheless, encouraged by its potential LY2886721 (Selleckchem, Boston) was developed as the next-generation orally available BACE1 inhibitor. While it overcame some of the limitations of its predecessor, it suffered from hepatotoxicity and discontinued [60, 61]. During the same time MK-8931(Merck Pharmaceuticals Ltd, USA) and E2609 (Forest Biometrics Research Institute, USA) were developed as inhibitor of BACE1. Currently these are under clinical trial for the treatment of AD [62 - 64].

γ-Secretase Inhibitors and Modulators

A thiophenesulfonamide derivative, Begacestat (GSI-953, Sigma aldrich India) and a natural compound NIC5-15 (Pinitol, D-Pinitol, Humanetics Pharmaceuticals Corporation, Edina) were initially reported to inhibit γ-secretase and manage AD. However the results of clinical validation were not good enough for their further trial [65 - 68]. Similarly LY-450139 (Semagacestat, Eli Lilly, USA) and BMS-708163(Avagacestat, Selleckchem, Boston) also failed to offer benefits clinically in spite of their capacity to inhibit γ-secretase [69 - 71]. Nevertheless, few more γ-secretase modulators including CHF5074 (Incorporated, Chiesi Pharmaceuticals Inc, USA) are under trials for management of AD [72, 73].

Promoting Aβ Clearance

Active AD Immunotherapy

Vaccination is a novel strategy to improve immunity and facilitate plaque clearance. With this strategy AN-1792 (Pfizer, USA) was initially tested against AD. However, trial was stopped when side effects observed in about 6% of the participants [74]. With improved safety, a second-generation active immunotherapy vaccine (CAD106) was developed at Novartis Pharmaceuticals Corporation, Switzerland and is currently under clinical trial [75]. This has encouraged development of immunotherapy against AD. While few including ACI-24 (AC Immune SA, Swtzerland) and UB-311(United Neuroscience, Ireland) have been tried without much clinical success [76, 77], few others including ACC-001 (Janssen: Pharmaceutical Companies of Johnson & Johnson, Australia) and LuAF20513 (H. Lundbeck, Otsuka Pharmaceutical Co. Ltd. India) are under clinical trial against AD [78].

Passive AD Immunotherapy

AAB-001 (Bapineuzumab, Janssen, Pfizer) was the first humanized monoclonal antibody tried against AD [79]. Later few other antibodies including Solanezumab (Eli Lilly Pharmaceuticals, Indiana), Ponezumab (Pfizer, New York) targeting the soluble Aβ have been tried with little clinical success [80 - 85]. In animal model, active and passive immunotherapy targeting Aβ has been successful but, in clinical trial encephalitis is occurring in few patients [86]. There is a great need to avoid excessive immune reaction for the success of vaccine therapy in AD patients. Recently to achieve this drive, adjuvant-free vaccine therapies such as DNA vaccines or passive immunization are presently under investigation [87].

Preventing Aβ Aggregation

Orally active Tramiprosate (3-amino-1-propanesulfonic acid, 3APS) slows hippocampal atrophy and improve cognition due to prevention of Aβ aggregation [88 - 90]. However it failed to translate these effects under clinical condition leading to termination of its clinical trials [91]. Similarly trial of an endogenous inositol stereoisomer (Scyllo-inositol) was discontinued due to issues related to its efficacy [92 - 94]. Epigallo-catechin-3-gallate (EGCG), derived from green tea is also shown to inhibit Aβ aggregation [95, 96]. However, when administered orally it has issues related to bioavailability which raises serious questions about its applicability.

Considering the fact that Aβ is co-ordinated to metal ions, use of chelating agent is a strategy to disturb co-ordination leading to lowering of aggregation. PBT1, a metal chelator, employs similar strategy to promote the solubilisation of Aβ. However, the clinical benefits were less than encouraging which led to termination of its phase III trial [97]. Nevertheless, PBT2 was developed as the second-generation metal–protein attenuator (Prana Biotechnology Limited, Florida, United States) [98]. With improved blood brain barrier (BBB) permeability, it obstructed Aβ oligomerization, decreased Aβ and promoted the clearance of Aβ oligomer [99]. Several other molecules have also been reported to prevent aggregation. TTP488/ PF-04494700/ Azeliragon (Pfizer/ TransTech Pharma Inc, USA) is a small T molecule which showed good safety profile and mild to moderate efficacy against AD in clinical condition [100]. Bexarotene, a drug primarily used against cancer was also shown to suppress Aβ 42 deposition by targeting the primary nucleation step in the aggregation [101]. However, its repurposing potential needs to be clinically validated.

Drugs Targeting Tau protein

T-817MA was developed as an orally active neurotrophic agent by Toyama Chemical, Japan. Although its effectiveness in protecting neurons is reported in various cell-based and preclinical models against Aβ-induced neurotoxicity and memory deficits, it is yet to be approved for clinical use [102 - 104]. Inspired by research on tau cleavage generating N-terminally truncated fragments, AADvac1 (Axon peptide 108 conjugated to KLH, Axon Neuroscience SE) was developed as an active vaccine to elicit an immune response against pathologically modified forms of tau protein [105]. To target certain pathological conformers of phosphorylated tau without autoimmune responses, ACI-35 (AC Immune SA, Janssen) was tried as a liposome-based vaccine [106].

In recent years Leuco-methylthioninium (LMTX) has been identified to selectively inhibit Tau aggregation and reduce the Tau pathology in transgenic mouse models [107]. It has been found to be safe and clinically effective in mild or moderate AD [108, 109]. Glycogen synthase kinase 3β (GSK3β) inhibition counteracts Tau protein phosphorylation [110]. Accordingly, NP-031112 (Tideglusib, Zeltia Group, Madrid, Spain) is developed as a GSK3β inhibitor and is under clinical trial against AD [111, 112].

Neurotrophins

Nerve growth factor (NGF) plays an important role in genesis and differentiation of neurons in brain. Cholinergic basal forebrain (CBF) neurons undergo degeneration in AD and are dependent upon NGF and its receptors for their survival [113]. Accordingly, use of NGF is considered as an alternative approach to manage AD. Thus, AAV2-NGF (CERE-110, Sangamo BioSciences, Inc. California, United States) has been developed to deliver NGF [114] in brain. The increase in the production of acetylcholine leading to enhancement of the function of basal forebrain cholinergic neurons, has encouraged its further validation in clinical trials [115].

Drugs Targeting Mitochondrial Dysfunction

Mitochondrial dysfunction is increasingly recognised as a key factor in the development of AD [116]. This is because, mitochondrial dysfunction induces oxidative stress and Tau pathology leading to the process of neurodegeneration in AD [117]. Accordingly molecules modulating this aspect are being investigated against AD. Latrepirdine (Dimebon) which ameliorate mitochondrial membrane potential and ATP production [118] is also reported to modify hippocampal APP/Aβ pathology [119]. Hence, it is considered as a potential candidate for the treatment of AD [120].

REPURPOSING OF DRUGS

Currently drugs are available for symptomatic treatment. These drugs provide short-term benefits, without halting the progression of the disease. Despite of many clinical trials with novel AChEIs, none has been able to reach the market so far [42]. So repurposing of drugs can be a better option to find safer and efficacious drug against AD. Repurposing of drugs means application of a known drug to treat a different disease. Currently it has earned much attention because of many successful drug repositioning cases. Aspirin, sildenafil, thalidomide *etc* are some of the successful examples of repurposing of drug [121]. There are many drugs which have been attempted for repurposing against AD (Table **3**).

Table 3. List of drugs which have been attempted for repurposing against AD with their blood brain barrier (BBB) permeability, primary indication and current status against AD.

Drugs	BBB Permeability	Primary Indication	Current Status Against AD
AChE inhibitors			
Physostigmine	Moderate	Anticholinergic poisoning	Phase 1
Eptastigmine	-	Centrally acting cholinesterase inhibitor	Discontinued
Metrifonate	-	Acetylcholinesterase inhibitor	Discontinued
Muscarinic receptor agonists			

(Table 3) cont.....

Drugs	BBB Permeability	Primary Indication	Current Status Against AD
Cevimeline (AF102B)	Moderate	Selective muscarinic M1 receptor agonist	Discontinued
Milameline	-	Muscarinic receptor agonist	Discontinued
Sabcomeline (SB 202026)	-	Selective muscarinic M1 receptor partial agonist	Discontinued
Talsaclidine	-	Non-selective muscarinic agonist	Discontinued
Xanomeline	Moderate	Non-selective muscarinic agonist	Discontinued
Alvameline (LU 25-109)	-	Selective partial M1 agonist and an M2/M3 antagonist	Discontinued
Drugs inhibiting cyclooxygenase (COX)			
Triflusal	-	Platelet aggregation inhibitor	Phase 2
Flurbiprofen	High	Microglial activation inhibitor	Discontinued
Celecoxib	-	Selective COX-2 inhibitor	Discontinued
Rofecoxib	-	Selective COX-2 inhibitor	Phase 2
Ibuprofen	High	Non-steroidal anti-inflammatory drugs (NSAID)	Phase 4
Aspirin	High	NSAID	Preclinical trial
Naproxen	High	NSAID	Phase 3
Indomethacin	High	NSAID	Phase 3
Drug acting on Renin Angiotensin system			
Captopril	Moderate	Anti hypertensive	Preclinical trial
Perindopril	Moderate	Anti hypertensive	Phase 2
Ramipril	Moderate	Anti hypertensive	Phase 4
Losartan	Poor	Anti hypertensive	Phase 2
Telmisartan	Moderate	Anti hypertensive	Phase 2
Lipid lowering drugs			
Lovastatin	Moderate	Lipid lowering drugs	Phase 4
Simvastatin	Moderate	Lipid lowering drugs	Phase 4
Miscellaneous			
Lithium	Moderate	Psychiatric medication	Phase 2
Minocycline	High	Broad-spectrum tetracycline antibiotic	Phase 2
Exenatide	High	GLP-1 receptor agonist, antidiabetic	Phase 2
Valproic acid	Poor	Antiepileptic	Phase 3
Methylene blue	High	Used to treat methemoglobinemia	Phase 2
Nicotine	Moderate	Parasympathomimetic stimulant	Phase 2

Source: https://www.alzforum.org/, https://clinicaltrials.gov/, https://www.rand.org/

Drugs Acting on COX Pathway

Since neurodegenerative disorders including AD have inflammation as the key etiologic factor, inhibitors of COX may have a role in management of AD. Evidently, many of the epidemiological studies have shown that patient who took NSAIDs had a lower risk of AD (Tuppo EE 2004). Further pre-clinical and clinical evidence also indicate their capacity to reduce Aβ deposition and reduce inflammation in neurons leading to decrease in the risk of developing AD [122]. Accordingly, repositioning of currently available NSAID have the potential to address the unmet challenges of AD. Since salicylates have some successful history of repurposing, few of them have been investigated against AD. Aspirin is the prototype of salicylates that has received wide attention for repurposing. At a daily dosage of 40 mg risk of AD/dementia in type 2 diabetes mellitus patients is decreased [123]. However, in few other cases its efficacy has been found not significant. This questionable efficacy can be explained by the variable brain availability and stability of aspirin. Accordingly, efforts have been made to develop reversible conjugates of Aspirin to improve stability and efficacy. In one of these attempts NOSH-aspirin has been demonstrated with neuroprotective effect in brain in pre-clinical model. Aspirin released from NOSH-aspirin in brain exerts strong antiinflammatory actions. Nitric oxide (NO) and hydrogen sulfide (H_2S) released from NOSH-aspirin remove noxious heavy metal from plaques and increase the oxygen supply to neurons thereby complementing neuroprotective effects in AD [124]. However, these types of modifications need clinical validation. Similarly, triflusal, a salicylic acid derivative which is primarily indicated as platelet aggregation inhibitor has been subjected to trials for repurposing against AD. Its active metabolite, Triflusal-HTB (2-hydroxy-4-trifluoro-methylbenzoic acid) has been reported to account for its effect against CNS inflammation [125, 126]. At a dose of 600 mg once daily it has shown protective effect against AD [127].

Like salicylates, the neuroprotection ability of other NSAIDs have also been suggested. *In vitro* studies have shown their ability to reduce formation of β-amyloid fibrils in the order of ibuprofen > sulindac sulfide > meclofenamic acid sodium salt > aspirin > ketoprofen > flurbiprofen > diclofenac sodium salt > naproxen > indomethacin [128]. Accordingly, drugs like indomethacin, flurbiprofen, naproxen and ibuprofen have been investigated against pre-clinical models of AD [129]. Ibuprofen acts both in COX dependent and independent manner leading to microglial NADPH oxidase (NOX 2) activation, prevention of oxidative damage and plaque clearance in the brain [130]. However, the efficacy in clinical trial was found inconclusive [131].

This may be due to the inconsistent brain availability of ibuprofen. Besides it also suffers from gastrotoxicity and not appropriate for long-term use, as desirable against AD. Thus its repurposing potential against AD needs to be evaluated in terms of its gastrotoxicity and brain access. To bridge this gap, ibuprofen reversible conjugations with glucose and ascorbic acid have been used enabling its higher permeability. Further formulation optimization like nasal delivery has been successfully attempted. While flurbiprofen has similar properties like ibuprofen, its (R) enantiomer (tarenflurbil, flurizan) lacks COX inhibitory property but lowers dementia in terms of its ability to reduce plaque formation. This also has a better safety profile. However, lack of significant efficacy lead to discontinuation of its clinical development by Myriad Genetics, USA. Clinical developments of naproxen and indomethacin have also been discontinued due to fewer benefits against AD than risk. The most contentious issue has been the dose. Since the NSAIDs are known for their gastric and renal toxicity it is not practical to use them for longer period of time at a dose that reduces progression of AD [129 - 133].

Drugs Acting on LOX Pathway

In addition to the COX pathway, the role of LOX pathway is also explored in the context of possible role of inflammation in AD. 5-Lipoxygenase (5LOX) could influence AD by producing pro-inflammatory lipoxins, cysteinyl leukotrienes (Cyst LT) and by an interaction with the gamma-secretase complex [130]. The anti-asthmatic drug Zafirlukast has been repositioned against AD. This is because it is a Cyst LT receptor antagonist. Besides it inhibits microglia activity, decreases the expression of TNF-α, inducible nitric oxide synthase (iNOS) and NO (nitric oxide) release, leading to protection against neuronal degeneration [134]. Its (15 and 30 mg/kg) combination with valdecoxib, a COX 2 inhibitor (5 and 10 mg/kg) has been reported to significantly reverse mito-oxidative damage and decrease neuroinflammation in rats [135]. However, it lacks clinical validation. Montelukast is another drug of this class which have shown potential against AD in pre-clinical model. However, its further clinical translation failed to deliver the desirable efficacy [136].

Drugs Acting on Renin Angiotensin System

Renin Angiotensin system (RAS) is a vital regulator for blood pressure and fluid balance. It comprises of Renin, Angiotensin converting enzyme (ACE), Angiotensin II (Ang-II) and Angiotensin 1 receptor (AT1R) [137 - 139]. The selective binding of Ang-II to AT1R results in broad range of biological activities, impacting several systems including brain, heart, kidney and immune system. However, an abnormality in this RAS affects homeostasis leading to cardiac hypertrophy, hypertension, heart failure and kidney disorders [35, 140]. Angiotensinogen acts as a substrate for RAS pathway. Sequential cleavage to angiotensinogen by ACE and renin leads to generation of Angiotensin-I and Angiotensin-II peptides. These peptides exert their action by acting upon angiotensin receptors like AT1 and AT2 [35].

Ang-II is an important effector of ROS (reactive oxygen species) formation and neuro-inflammation. Ang-II is increasingly being recognized as a major effector of neurodegeneration leading to AD and dementia (Fig. **4**). This is further corroborated by identification of local RAS in brain. Since AD pathogenesis involves inflammatory process, blocking actions of Ang-II can be the key to the neurodegeneration leading to AD [35, 141 - 144].

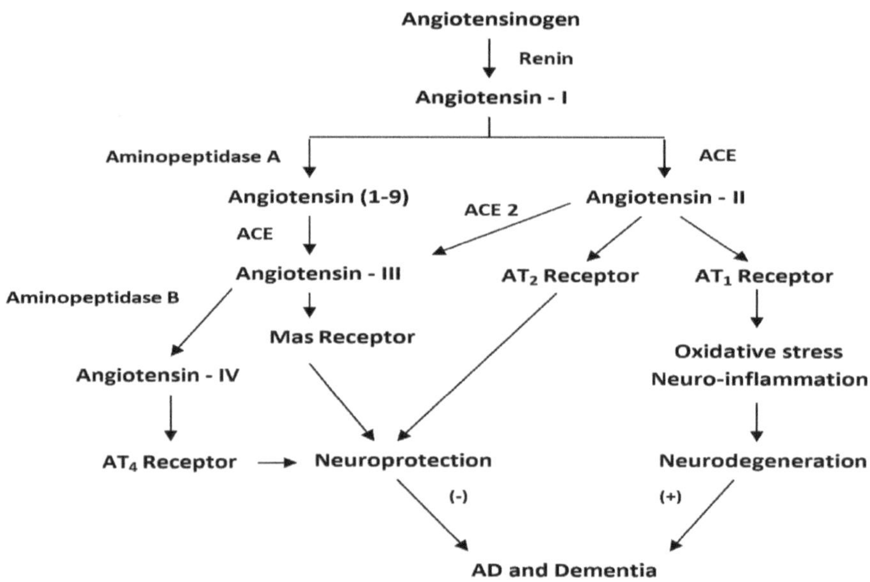

Fig. (4). Role of renin angiotensin system (RAS) in AD. Angiotensinogen acts as a substrate for RAS pathway and by sequential cleavage it generates Angiotensin-I, Angiotensin-II, Angiotensin-III and Angiotensin IV peptides. Angiotensin II causes neurodegeneration (through AT1 receptor) leading to AD and dementia *via* oxidative stress and neuroinflammation. However, Ang-II/AT2 receptor, Ang-III/Mas receptor and Ang-IV/AT4 receptor systems have been reported for cognitive facilitation and neuroprotection.

ACE inhibitors (ACEIs) like Lisinopril attenuate AD due to its antioxidant and anti-inflammatory property [145]. Again, captopril and perindopril have shown neuroprotection against transgenic mice model of AD by decreasing hippocampal ROS formation [146]. Enalapril and lisinopril attenuate cognitive impairment [147]. Accordingly, perindopril improves AD both in clinical and preclinical studies *via* learning and memory function [148]. Similarly, AT1R blockers (ARBs) showed protection against Aβ induced neurodegeneration and brain injury. Valsartan has been reported to act against Aβ-mediated cognitive dysfunction in the Tg 2576 mouse model of AD [149]. Additionally, intranasal injection of losartan showed neuroprotection [150].

Due to the positive results of ACEIs and ARBs with AD patients, further investigation on potential of several angiotensin, including Ang-II/AT1 receptor system must be encouraged. The Ang-II/AT2 receptor and Angiotensin-IV (Ang-IV)/AT4 receptor systems have been reported for cognitive facilitation and are worthy of additional attention [151]. In addition to that, Angiotensin-III (Ang-III)/Mas receptor system has a role in neuroprotection. However, lack of BBB penetration of AT4 receptor agonists and antagonists limits their drug development against neurodegenerative disorders [152 - 154].

Lipid Lowering Drugs

Many biological and epidemiological studies have linked high levels of serum cholesterol with AD. The expression of Alzheimer's pathology is slowed by lowering cholesterol in animal models. There is a possibility that cholesterol lowering drugs might reduce the risk of developing AD [155]. HMG-CoA reductase inhibitors or statins (simvastatin, pravastatin, lovastatin and others) are lipid lowering drugs with proven benefit in vascular disease. They have the ability to activate α-secretase thereby increasing soluble amyloid precursor protein ($sAPP_{\alpha}$) [156]. They also affect cholinergic function, tau phosphorylation, neural oxidative stress, *etc.* [157]. The incidence of AD was significantly lower in statin users. In a 10-year follow-up study, ApoE4-genotyped AD patients treated with statins showed better cognitive function as compared to patients treated with other lipid lowering drug users [158].

Anti-Diabetics

The metabolism of amyloid precursor protein (APP) is modulated by insulin in neurons. Insulin decreases the intracellular accumulation of Aβ peptides [159]. Metformin enhances insulin's effect in reducing Aβ levels [160 - 162]. Long term use of metformin increases the risk of developing AD whereas use of sulfonylureas, thiazolidinediones, or insulin was not associated with risk of developing AD [163]. Natural C-glycosylated derivatives of apigenin like vitexin and isovitexin possess potent anti-diabetic, anti-Alzheimer's disease (anti-AD), and anti-inflammatory activities [164]. Exendin-4 (exenatide), a glucagon-like peptide-1 receptor agonist has shown promising results in protecting nerve cells in the brain from the damaging processes associated with Alzheimer's [165, 166]. Pioglitazone, an insulin sensitizer and peroxisome-proliferator activated receptor γ (PPAR-γ) agonist used as anti-diabetic, is reported to improve cognition in AD mice. However its human trial has yielded mixed results [167].

Antioxidants

Antioxidants like vitamins (E, C and carotenoids) and phytochemicals have been tested for their efficacy in AD. Vit E reduced lipid peroxidation and plaque burden in transgenic AD models but have not shown similar results in clinical trials. Vit E in combination with donepezil and memantine also showed improved efficacy in AD. Flavonoids, carotenoids and other group of antioxidants (rutin, lutein, curcumin and melatonin) are found to be neuroprotective. In experimental setup, antioxidants show promising results but their translation to the clinical trial situation is less successful [43, 168, 169].

Vitamin D

Older adults are vitamin D deficient. The enzyme responsible for synthesizing vitamin D (1α-hydroxylase) and the 1, 25-dihydroxy vitamin D3 receptors are found in human brain. Low serum vitamin D concentrations are associated with AD. Vitamin D stimulates macrophages, which increase the clearance of amyloid plaques. It also reduces amyloid-induced cytotoxicity and apoptosis in primary cortical neurons. Its deficiency leads to increased risk of incident stroke and neurodegeneration [170 - 175]. So there is a possibility of repurposing Vitamin D against AD.

Dextromethorphan

Dextromethorphan exerts its antitussive action by suppression of cough center in CNS. It is a sigma-1 receptor agonist and it also inhibits serotonin and norepinephrine transporters. This is also a low affinity noncompetitive NMDA receptor antagonist. Thus with a long history of clinical application it is considered suitable for repurposing against AD. Its protective effects in dementia are observed at the same clinically validated dose (30-120mg) used to suppress cough. However, it suffers from rapid metabolism to dextrorphan by CYP2D6 and CYP3A4 metabolic enzymes. This limits its bioavailability leading to inconsistent CNS effects. Thus use of inhibitors of these enzymes as co-drug is a viable strategy to repurpose Dextromethorphan against AD [176].

AXS-05 (Axsome therapeutics) is an investigational drug with combination of bupropion and dextromethorphan. Bupropion is a nicotinic acetylcholine receptor antagonist and a dopamine and norepinephrine reuptake inhibitor. It increases the bioavailability of dextromethorphan [177]. AVP-923/Nuedexta is a fixed-dose combination of Dextromethorphan and quinidine developed by Avanir and Concert Pharmaceuticals. AVP-786 is a second-generation version of AVP-923. Quinidine increases the bioavailability of dextromethorphan by slowing its oxidative metabolism by the liver enzyme cytochrome P450-2D6 and by inhibiting the blood-brain barrier protein pump P-glycoprotein [178].

Vitamin B-12

Nutrition is an environmental factor which is related to AD through epigenetic pathways. Vitamin B-12 can alter the one-carbon metabolism and thus interfere in the DNA methylation process. DNA methylation is one of the epigenetics mechanisms of diseases like AD [179]. So Vitamin B-12 can also be repurposed against AD.

MAPK Inhibitor

p38 (mitogen-activated protein kinase) is capable of regulating many events related to AD, such as synaptic dysfunction, tau phosphorylation, neurotoxicity, and neuroinflammation. Thus, the inhibition of p38 MAPK is considered a promising strategy for the treatment of AD. There are several phytoconstituents which can inhibit MAPK. Etazolate, a $GABA_A$ receptor modulator, is a neuroprotective and activates α- secretase, inhibits PDE-4 (phosphodiesterase) activities [180, 181].

Serotonergic Drugs

Serotonergic compounds like monoamine oxidase inhibitors (MAOI) and selective serotonin reuptake inhibitors (SSRI) are under consideration in AD as monotherapy or along with AChEI for their ability to enhance cognition [182]. Lecozotan a $5HT1_A$ antagonist is proved to be safe and effective in Phase I and II clinical trials. Velusetrag, a drug for gastrointestinal disorder has shown efficacy in AD [50]. Idalopirdine (INN) (code name Lu AE58054), a selective $5\text{-}HT_6$ receptor antagonist is under development (phase III clinical trials) by Lundbeck against cognitive deficits associated with AD and schizophrenia [183].

Cannabinoids

Cannabinoids are the active components of marijuana. They affect memory and hippocampal neurotransmission. Synthetic cannabinoids like Nabilone (antiemetic and adjunct analgesic for neuropathic pain) and Dronabinol (appetite stimulant) can be used in cognitive impairment [184]. Dronabinol improved disturbed behavior in a study involving 15 numbers of patients with AD. However, the drug had to be stopped in three patients (one for seizures, and two for infections) [185].

Glycine Transporter Inhibitor

BI 425809 (Boehringer Ingelheim, Germany), a glycine transporter inhibitor has been tried to boost NMDA receptor function and benefit synaptic plasticity and cognition [186]. Similarly, BI 425809 is also under development as a potent and selective GlyT1 inhibitor to improve memory and cognitive function in patients with schizophrenia and AD [187].

Melatonin

Production of melatonin hormone decreases with ageing and may be associated with the progression of AD. Melatonin gives endogenous neuroprotection in neurodegeneration produced by glutamate excitotoxicity and oxidative stress. Neuroprotective functions of melatonin in AD patients (Phase 2) suggest its usefulness as an anti-AD therapy [188, 189].

Tetracyclines

Tetracyclines have been proposed for AD therapy [190]. Tetracycline antibiotics like doxycycline and minocycline have shown the neuroprotective effect in various experimental models of AD [191 - 193]. They also possess anti-amyloidogenic activity [194] and anti-neuroinflammatory effects [195, 196]. So they could be repurposed for use in the treatment of AD.

Lithium

Lithium significantly decreases tau protein concentration in (CSF) [197]. Long-term lithium treatment inhibits tau hyper phosphorylation and slows the progression of cognitive and functional deficits [198]. Side effects with Lithium treatment are mild and reversible in elderly people with AD [199].

Valproic Acid

Valproic acid, an anti-epileptic drug, significantly reduces neuritic plaque formation thereby improving memory in transgenic AD mice. So Valproic acid may be beneficial in the prevention and treatment of AD [200].

Methylene Blue

Various neurotransmitter systems (cholinergic, serotonergic and glutamatergic) are influenced by methylene blue. This is likely to mediate potential beneficial effects of methylene blue against AD [201].

Nicotine

Nicotinic receptor densities are reduced in AD [202]. Nicotine improves learning [203, 204]. Nicotine and nicotinic agents possess neuroprotective effects due to stimulation of $\alpha7$ nicotinic receptors. Additionally, nicotine has been shown to inhibit the deposition of β-amyloid *in vitro* [205].

CONCLUSION

Five drugs are currently approved by the U.S. Food and Drug Administration (FDA) to treat the symptoms of AD. The cholinesterase inhibitors approved against AD are tacrine, donepezil, rivastigmine and galantamine. These drugs prevent the degradation of acetyl choline in the brain. Unlike these, memantine is an N-methyl-D-aspartate (NMDA) receptor antagonist that inhibits glutamate induced exocitotoxicity in brain leading to protection of neuronal cells and improvement in memory and learning. Due to limited success in arresting AD progression with cholinergic drugs, amyloid based strategies including secretive enzymes modulation, amyloid aggregation prevention and amyloid clearance promotion have been adopted. Inhibition of tau phosphorylation, tau oligomerization and microtubule stabilization has also been targeted in recent years.

Because of growing elderly populations and lack of disease-modifying therapeutics, management of AD remains an unmet challenge. The AD drug discovery and development also suffers from lower success rate. This is mainly due to poor translation from pre-clinical to clinical trials and failure to predict safety and efficacy. High rates of attrition combined with huge cost of new drug development have encouraged drug repurposing strategies. This involves low development costs and shorter approval time to launch. The risk associated with conventional drug discovery is also reduced by using existing pharmacokinetic and safety data.

Currently marketed drugs like cholinergic drugs, cyclooxygenase and lipoxygenase inhibitors, renin angiotensin system inhibitors, lipid lowering drugs (statins), NMDA receptor antagonists, anti-diabetics, anti-oxidants, vitamin D *etc* are studied for their efficacy against AD. Many of them have the potential against AD and some of them are validated pre-clinically and clinically. But none of them has reached the market yet. With advances made in disease biology of AD, there is huge data available from pre-clinical, clinical, epidemiological, toxicological, *in vitro* and computational sources. Thus, adoption of systematic approaches using available information with a clear understanding of the network pharmacology can be expected to yield the next therapeutic option for successful management of AD.

CONSENT FOR PUBLICATION

Not applicable.

CONFLICT OF INTEREST

The authors declare no conflict of interest, financial or otherwise.

ACKNOWLEDGEMENTS

The authors wish to thank Regional Medical Research Center (RMRC), Bhubaneswar and Siksha O Anusandhan (Deemed to be University), Bhubaneswar, India for providing library facilities. The authors also thank Mr Tapas Ranjan Satpathy for secretarial assistance.

REFERENCES

[1] Schapira AH. Neurology and Clinical Neuroscience. Elsevier Health Sciences; 2006 Dec 18.

[2] Holtzman DM, Morris JC, Goate AM. Alzheimer's disease: the challenge of the second century. Sci Transl Med 2011; 3(77): 77sr1. [http://dx.doi.org/10.1126/scitranslmed.3002369]

[3] Frozza RL, Lourenco MV, De Felice FG. Challenges for Alzheimer's disease therapy: Insights from novel mechanisms beyond memory defects. Front Neurosci 2018; 12: 37. [http://dx.doi.org/10.3389/fnins.2018.00037]

[4] Dartigues JF. Alzheimer's disease: a global challenge for the 21st century. Lancet Neurol 2009; 8(12): 1082-3. [http://dx.doi.org/10.1016/S1474-4422(09)70298-4]

[5] Prince MJ. World Alzheimer Report 2015: the global impact of dementia: an analysis of prevalence, incidence, cost and trends. Alzheimer's Disease International 2015.

[6] Ferri CP, Prince M, Brayne C, *et al.* Global prevalence of dementia: A Delphi consensus study. Lancet 2005; 366(9503): 2112-7. [http://dx.doi.org/10.1016/S0140-6736(05)67889-0]

[7] Bradley WG, Ed. Neurology in clinical practice: principles of diagnosis and management. Taylor & Francis 2004.

[8] Kasai M, Nakamura K, Meguro K. Alzheimer's disease in Japan and other countries: review of epidemiological studies in the last 10 years. Brain and nerve Shinkei kenkyu no shinpo. 2010; l; 62(7):667-78.

[9] Yu ES, Liu WT, Levy P, *et al.* Cognitive impairment among elderly adults in Shanghai, China. J Gerontol 1989; 44(3): S97-S106. [http://dx.doi.org/10.1093/geronj/44.3.S97]

[10] Barnes LL, Bennett DA. Alzheimer's disease in African Americans: risk factors and challenges for the future. Health Aff 2014; 33(4): 580-6. [http://dx.doi.org/10.1377/hlthaff.2013.1353]

[11] Wakutani Y, Kusumi M, Wada K, *et al.* Longitudinal changes in the prevalence of dementia in a Japanese rural area. Psychogeriatrics 2007; 7(4): 150-4. [http://dx.doi.org/10.1111/j.1479-8301.2007.00203.x]

[12] Prince M, Bryce R, Albanese E, Wimo A, Ribeiro W, Ferri CP. The global prevalence of dementia: a systematic review and metaanalysis. Alzheimers Dement 2013; 9(1): 63. [http://dx.doi.org/10.1016/j.jalz.2012.11.007]

[13] Miyoshi K. What is early onset dementia? Psychogeriatrics 2009; 9(2): 67-72. [http://dx.doi.org/10.1111/j.1479-8301.2009.00274.x]

[14] Hanin I. Alzheimer's and Parkinson's disease: Strategies in Research and Development.Alzheimer's and Parkinson's disease. Boston, MA: Springer 1986; pp. 669-78. [http://dx.doi.org/10.1007/978-1-4613-2179-8_75]

[15] Burns A, Byrne J, Ballard C, Holmes C. Sensory stimulation in dementia: an effective option for managing behavioural problems. BMJ: British Medical Journal 2002; 325(7376): 1312. [http://dx.doi.org/10.1136/bmj.325.7376.1312]

[16] Heneka MT, Carson MJ, El Khoury J, *et al.* Neuroinflammation in Alzheimer's disease. Lancet Neurol 2015; 14(4): 388-405. [http://dx.doi.org/10.1016/S1474-4422(15)70016-5]

[17] Cummings JL, Back C. The cholinergic hypothesis of neuropsychiatric symptoms in Alzheimer's disease. Am J Geriatr Psychiatry 1998; 6(2): S64-78. [http://dx.doi.org/10.1097/00019442-199821001-00009]

[18] Merluzzi AP, Carlsson CM, Johnson SC, *et al.* Neurodegeneration, synaptic dysfunction, and gliosis are phenotypic of Alzheimer dementia. Neurology 2018; 29: 10-212.

[19] Van Nostrand WE, Davis Salinas J, Saporito Irwin SM. Amyloid β Protein Induces the Cerebrovascular Cellular Pathology of Alzheimer's Disease and Related Disordersa. Ann N Y Acad Sci 1996; 777(1): 297-302. [http://dx.doi.org/10.1111/j.1749-6632.1996.tb34436.x]

[20] Hardy J, Selkoe DJ. The amyloid hypothesis of Alzheimer's disease: progress and problems on the road to therapeutics science Science. 2002; 297(5580): 353-6.

[21] Nelson PT, Alafuzoff I, Bigio EH, *et al.* Correlation of Alzheimer disease neuropathologic changes with cognitive status: a review of the literature. J Neuropathol Exp Neurol 2012; 71(5): 362-81. [http://dx.doi.org/10.1097/NEN.0b013e31825018f7]

[22] Chu J, Praticò D. The 5-Lipoxygenase as modulator of Alzheimer's γ-secretase and therapeutic target. Brain Res Bull 2016; 126: 207-12. [http://dx.doi.org/10.1016/j.brainresbull.2016.03.010]

[23] De Ferrari GV, Canales MA, Shin I, Weiner LM, Silman I, Inestrosa NC. A structural motif of acetylcholinesterase that promotes amyloid β-peptide fibril formation. Biochemistry 2001; 40(35): 10447-57. [http://dx.doi.org/10.1021/bi0101392]

[24] Rees T, Hammond PI, Soreq H, Younkin S, Brimijoin S. Acetylcholinesterase promotes beta-amyloid plaques in cerebral cortex. Neurobiol Aging 2003; 24(6): 777-87. [http://dx.doi.org/10.1016/S0197-4580(02)00230-0]

[25] Landau SM, Harvey D, Madison CM, *et al.* Comparing predictors of conversion and decline in mild cognitive impairment. Neurology 2010; 75(3): 230-8. [http://dx.doi.org/10.1212/WNL.0b013e3181e8e8b8]

[26] Jeong S. Molecular and cellular basis of neurodegeneration in Alzheimer's disease. Mol Cells 2017; 40(9): 613.

[27] Weiner MW, Veitch DP, Aisen PS, *et al.* Impact of the Alzheimer's disease neuroimaging initiative, 2004 to 2014. Alzheimers Dement 2015; 11(7): 865-84. [http://dx.doi.org/10.1016/j.jalz.2015.04.005]

[28] Heppner FL, Ransohoff RM, Becher B. Immune attack: the role of inflammation in Alzheimer disease. Nat Rev Neurosci 2015; 16(6): 358. [http://dx.doi.org/10.1038/nrn3880]

[29] Birch AM, Katsouri L, Sastre M. Modulation of inflammation in transgenic models of Alzheimer's disease. J Neuroinflammation 2014; 11(1): 25. [http://dx.doi.org/10.1186/1742-2094-11-25]

[30] Gonzalez-Reyes R, Nava-Mesa M, Vargas-Sanchez K, Ariza-Salamanca D, Mora-Muñoz L. Involvement of astrocytes in Alzheimer′ s disease from a neuroinflammatory and oxidative stress perspective. Front Mol Neurosci 2017; 10: 427. [http://dx.doi.org/10.3389/fnmol.2017.00427]

[31] Moore AH, Bigbee MJ, Boynton GE, *et al.* Non-steroidal anti-inflammatory drugs in Alzheimer's disease and Parkinson's disease: reconsidering the role of neuroinflammation. Pharmaceuticals 2010; 3(6): 1812-41. [http://dx.doi.org/10.3390/ph3061812]

[32] Reddy HP, Reddy PT. Mitochondria as a therapeutic target for aging and neurodegenerative diseases. Curr Alzheimer Res 2011; 8(4): 393-409. [http://dx.doi.org/10.2174/156720511795745401]

[33] Chen C, Magee JC, Bazan NG. Cyclooxygenase-2 regulates prostaglandin E2 signaling in hippocampal long-term synaptic plasticity. J Neurophysiol 2002; 87(6): 2851-7. [http://dx.doi.org/10.1152/jn.2002.87.6.2851]

[34] Mitsushima D, Sano A, Takahashi T. A cholinergic trigger drives learning-induced plasticity at hippocampal synapses. Nat Commun 2013; 4: 2760. [http://dx.doi.org/10.1038/ncomms3760]

[35] Prusty S, Sahu PK, Subudhi BB. Angiotensin mediated oxidative stress and neuroprotective potential of antioxidants and AT1 receptor blockers. Mini Rev Med Chem 2017; 17(6): 518-28. [http://dx.doi.org/10.2174/1389557516666161025094539]

[36] Angiotensin mediated oxidative stress and neuroprotective potential of antioxidants and AT1 receptor blockers. Mini reviews in medicinal chemistry. 2017; 17(6): 518-28.

[37] Rosendorff C, Beeri MS, Silverman JM. Cardiovascular risk factors for Alzheimer's disease. Am J Geriatr Cardiol 2007; 16(3): 143-9. [http://dx.doi.org/10.1111/j.1076-7460.2007.06696.x]

[38] Anand P, Singh B. A review on cholinesterase inhibitors for Alzheimer's disease. Arch Pharm Res 2013; 36(4): 375-99. [http://dx.doi.org/10.1007/s12272-013-0036-3]

[39] Tabet N. Acetylcholinesterase inhibitors for Alzheimer's disease: anti-inflammatories in acetylcholine clothing. Age Ageing 2006; 35(4): 336-8. [http://dx.doi.org/10.1093/ageing/afl027]

[40] Qizilbash N, Birks J, López-Arrieta J, Lewington S, Szeto S. Tacrine for Alzheimer's disease. Cochrane Database Syst Rev 2000; (2): CD000202.

[41] Greig SL. Memantine ER/donepezil: A review in Alzheimer's disease. CNS Drugs 2015; 29(11): 963-70. [http://dx.doi.org/10.1007/s40263-015-0287-2]

[42] Galimberti D, Scarpini E. Old and new acetylcholinesterase inhibitors for Alzheimer's disease. Expert Opin Investig Drugs 2016; 25(10): 1181-7. [http://dx.doi.org/10.1080/13543784.2016.1216972]

[43] Anand R, Gill KD, Mahdi AA. Therapeutics of Alzheimer's disease: Past, present and future. Neuropharmacology 2014; 76: 27-50. [http://dx.doi.org/10.1016/j.neuropharm.2013.07.004]

[44] Yamamoto H, Hagino Y, Kasai S, Ikeda K. Specific roles of NMDA receptor subunits in mental disorders. Curr Mol Med 2015; 15(3): 193-205. [http://dx.doi.org/10.2174/1566524015666150330142807]

[45] Danysz W, Parsons CG. Alzheimer's disease, β amyloid, glutamate, NMDA receptors and memantine–searching for the connections. Br J Pharmacol 2012; 167(2): 324-52.

[http://dx.doi.org/10.1111/j.1476-5381.2012.02057.x]

[46] Strong KL, Jing Y, Prosser AR, Traynelis SF, Liotta DC. NMDA receptor modulators: an updated patent review (2013–2014). Expert Opin Ther Pat 2014; 24(12): 1349-66. [http://dx.doi.org/10.1517/13543776.2014.972938]

[47] Shamsizadeh A, Roohbakhsh A, Ayoobi F, Moghaddamahmadi A. The Role of Natural Products in the Prevention and Treatment of Multiple Sclerosis. InNutrition and Lifestyle in Neurological Autoimmune Diseases 2017; pp. 249-60. [http://dx.doi.org/10.1016/B978-0-12-805298-3.00025-6]

[48] Jia JY, Zhao QH, Liu Y, *et al.* Phase I study on the pharmacokinetics and tolerance of ZT-1, a prodrug of huperzine A, for the treatment of Alzheimer's disease. Acta Pharmacol Sin 2013; 34(7): 976. [http://dx.doi.org/10.1038/aps.2013.7]

[49] Coelho F, Birks J. Physostigmine for Alzheimer's disease. Cochrane Database Syst Rev 2001; (2): CD001499.

[50] Winblad B, Giacobini E, Frolich L, *et al.* Phenserine efficacy in Alzheimer's disease. J Alzheimers Dis 2010; 22(4): 1201-8. [http://dx.doi.org/10.3233/JAD-2010-101311]

[51] Bhattacharya S, Maelicke A, Montag D. Nasal application of the galantamine pro-drug memogain slows down plaque deposition and ameliorates behavior in 5X familial Alzheimer's disease mice. J Alzheimers Dis 2015; 46(1): 123-36. [http://dx.doi.org/10.3233/JAD-142421]

[52] Maelicke A, Hoeffle-Maas A, Ludwig J, *et al.* Memogain is a galantamine pro-drug having dramatically reduced adverse effects and enhanced efficacy. J Mol Neurosci 2010; 40(1-2): 135-7. [http://dx.doi.org/10.1007/s12031-009-9269-5]

[53] Weinreb O, Amit T, Bar-Am O. BH Youdim M. Ladostigil: a novel multimodal neuroprotective drug with cholinesterase and brain-selective monoamine oxidase inhibitory activities for Alzheimer's disease treatment. Curr Drug Targets 2012; 13(4): 483-94. [http://dx.doi.org/10.2174/138945012799499794]

[54] Schneider LS, Mangialasche F, Andreasen N, *et al.* Clinical trials and late stage drug development for A lzheimer's disease: an appraisal from 1984 to 2014. J Intern Med 2014; 275(3): 251-83. [http://dx.doi.org/10.1111/joim.12191]

[55] Fisher A. M1 muscarinic agonists target major hallmarks of Alzheimer's disease–the pivotal role of brain M1 receptors. Neurodegener Dis 2008; 5(3-4): 237-40. [http://dx.doi.org/10.1159/000113712]

[56] Prickaerts J, van Goethem NP, Chesworth R, *et al.* EVP-6124, a novel and selective α7 nicotinic acetylcholine receptor partial agonist, improves memory performance by potentiating the acetylcholine response of α7 nicotinic acetylcholine receptors. Neuropharmacology 2012; 62(2): 1099-110. [http://dx.doi.org/10.1016/j.neuropharm.2011.10.024]

[57] Li Q, Yang H, Chen Y, Sun H. Recent progress in the identification of selective butyrylcholinesterase inhibitors for Alzheimer's disease. Eur J Med Chem 2017; 132: 294-309. [http://dx.doi.org/10.1016/j.ejmech.2017.03.062]

[58] Zawieja P, Kornprobst JM, Métais P. 3 (2, 4 Dimethoxybenzylidene) anabaseine: A promising candidate drug for Alzheimer's disease? Geriatr Gerontol Int 2012; 12(3): 365-71. [http://dx.doi.org/10.1111/j.1447-0594.2011.00827.x]

[59] May PC, Willis BA, Lowe SL, *et al.* The potent BACE1 inhibitor LY2886721 elicits robust central Aβ pharmacodynamic responses in mice, dogs, and humans. J Neurosci 2015; 35(3): 1199-210. [http://dx.doi.org/10.1523/JNEUROSCI.4129-14.2015]

[60] Martenyi F, Dean RA, Lowe S, *et al.* BACE inhibitor LY2886721 safety and central and peripheral PK and PD in healthy subjects (HSs). Alzheimers Dement 2012; 8(4): 583-4.

[http://dx.doi.org/10.1016/j.jalz.2012.05.1588]

[61] Willis B, Martenyi F, Dean R, *et al.* Central BACE1 inhibition by LY2886721 produces opposing effects on APP processing as reflected by cerebrospinal fluid sAPPalpha and sAPPbeta. Alzheimers Dement 2012; 8(4): 582. [http://dx.doi.org/10.1016/j.jalz.2012.05.1584]

[62] Forman M, Palcza J, Tseng J, *et al.* The novel BACE inhibitor MK-8931 dramatically lowers cerebrospinal fluid Aβ peptides in healthy subjects following single-and multiple-dose administration. Alzheimers Dement 2012; 8(4): 704. [http://dx.doi.org/10.1016/j.jalz.2012.05.1900]

[63] Forman M, Kleijn HJ, Dockendorf M, *et al.* The novel BACE inhibitor MK-8931 dramatically lowers CSF beta-amyloid in patients with mild-to-moderate Alzheimer's disease. Alzheimers Dement 2013; 9(4): 139. [http://dx.doi.org/10.1016/j.jalz.2013.04.083]

[64] Bernier F, Sato Y, Matijevic M, *et al.* Clinical study of E2609, a novel BACE1 inhibitor, demonstrates target engagement and inhibition of BACE1 activity in CSF. Alzheimers Dement 2013; 9(4): 886. [http://dx.doi.org/10.1016/j.jalz.2013.08.244]

[65] Martone RL, Zhou H, Atchison K, *et al.* Begacestat (GSI-953): a novel, selective thiophene sulfonamide inhibitor of amyloid precursor protein γ-secretase for the treatment of Alzheimer's disease. J Pharmacol Exp Ther 2009; 331(2): 598-608. [http://dx.doi.org/10.1124/jpet.109.152975]

[66] Hopkins Corey R. ACS chemical neuroscience molecule spotlight on Suvorexant. 2012: 647-648.

[67] Pasinetti G, Rosen Z, Grossman H. Nic5-15: a novel natural gamma-secretase inhibitor that attenuates brain beta-amyloid content and improves cognition. Alzheimers Dement 2009; 5(4): e28. [http://dx.doi.org/10.1016/j.jalz.2009.07.110]

[68] Grossman H, Marzloff G, Luo X, LeRoith D, Sano M, Pasinetti G. NIC5-15 as a treatment for Alzheimer's: safety, pharmacokinetics and clinical variables. Alzheimers Dement 2009; 5(4): 259. [http://dx.doi.org/10.1016/j.jalz.2009.04.287]

[69] Henley DB, May PC, Dean RA, Siemers ER. Development of semagacestat (LY450139), a functional γ-secretase inhibitor, for the treatment of Alzheimer's disease. Expert Opin Pharmacother 2009; 10(10): 1657-64. [http://dx.doi.org/10.1517/14656560903044982]

[70] Blennow K, Zetterberg H, Haass C, Finucane T. Semagacestat's fall: where next for AD therapies. Nat Med 2013; 19(10): 1214-5. [http://dx.doi.org/10.1038/nm.3365]

[71] Doody RS, Raman R, Farlow M, *et al.* Siemers E, Sethuraman G, Mohs R, Semagacestat Study Group. A phase 3 trial of semagacestat for treatment of Alzheimer's disease. N Engl J Med 2013; 369(4): 341-50. [http://dx.doi.org/10.1056/NEJMoa1210951]

[72] Ross J, Sharma S, Winston J, *et al.* CHF5074 reduces biomarkers of neuroinflammation in patients with mild cognitive impairment: a 12-week, double-blind, placebo-controlled study. Curr Alzheimer Res 2013; 10(7): 742-53. [http://dx.doi.org/10.2174/13892037113149990144]

[73] Hashimoto T, Ishibashi A, Hagiwara H, Murata Y, Takenaka O, Miyagawa T. E2012: A novel gamma-secretase modulator-pharmacology part. Alzheimers Dement 2010; 6(4): S242. [http://dx.doi.org/10.1016/j.jalz.2010.05.787]

[74] Holmes C, Boche D, Wilkinson D, *et al.* Long-term effects of Aβ42 immunisation in Alzheimer's disease: follow-up of a randomised, placebo-controlled phase I trial. Lancet 2008; 372(9634): 216-23. [http://dx.doi.org/10.1016/S0140-6736(08)61075-2]

[75] Winblad B, Andreasen N, Minthon L, *et al.* Safety, tolerability, and antibody response of active Aβ immunotherapy with CAD106 in patients with Alzheimer's disease: randomised, double-blind, placebo-controlled, first-in-human study. Lancet Neurol 2012; 11(7): 597-604. [http://dx.doi.org/10.1016/S1474-4422(12)70140-0]

[76] Muhs A, Hickman DT, Pihlgren M, *et al.* Liposomal vaccines with conformation-specific amyloid peptide antigens define immune response and efficacy in APP transgenic mice. Proc Natl Acad Sci USA 2007; 104(23): 9810-5. [http://dx.doi.org/10.1073/pnas.0703137104]

[77] Wang CY, Finstad CL, Walfield AM, *et al.* Site-specific UBITh® amyloid-β vaccine for immunotherapy of Alzheimer's disease. Vaccine 2007; 25(16): 3041-52. [http://dx.doi.org/10.1016/j.vaccine.2007.01.031]

[78] Arai H, Suzuki H, Yoshiyama T. Vanutide cridificar and the QS-21 adjuvant in Japanese subjects with mild to moderate Alzheimer's disease: results from two phase 2 studies. Curr Alzheimer Res 2015; 12(3): 242-54. [http://dx.doi.org/10.2174/1567205012666150302154121]

[79] Bard F, Barbour R, Cannon C, *et al.* Epitope and isotype specificities of antibodies to β-amyloid peptide for protection against Alzheimer's disease-like neuropathology. Proc Natl Acad Sci USA 2003; 100(4): 2023-8. [http://dx.doi.org/10.1073/pnas.0436286100]

[80] Salloway S, Sperling R, Fox NC, *et al.* Two phase 3 trials of bapineuzumab in mild-to-moderate Alzheimer's disease. N Engl J Med 2014; 370(4): 322-33. [http://dx.doi.org/10.1056/NEJMoa1304839]

[81] Samadi H, Sultzer D. Solanezumab for Alzheimer's disease. Expert Opin Biol Ther 2011; 11(6): 787-98. [http://dx.doi.org/10.1517/14712598.2011.578573]

[82] Doody RS, Thomas RG, Farlow M, *et al.* Solanezumab study group. Phase 3 trials of solanezumab for mild-to-moderate Alzheimer's disease. N Engl J Med 2014; 370(4): 311-21. [http://dx.doi.org/10.1056/NEJMoa1312889]

[83] Siemers ER, Sundell KL, Carlson C, *et al.* Phase 3 solanezumab trials: secondary outcomes in mild Alzheimer's disease patients. Alzheimers Dement 2016; 12(2): 110-20. [http://dx.doi.org/10.1016/j.jalz.2015.06.1893]

[84] Freeman GB, Lin JC, Pons J, Raha NM. 39-week toxicity and toxicokinetic study of ponezumab (PF-04360365) in cynomolgus monkeys with 12-week recovery period. J Alzheimers Dis 2012; 28(3): 531-41. [http://dx.doi.org/10.3233/JAD-2011-110869]

[85] Miyoshi I, Fujimoto Y, Yamada M, *et al.* Safety and pharmacokinetics of PF-04360365 following a single-dose intravenous infusion in Japanese subjects with mild-to-moderate Alzheimer's disease: a multicenter, randomized, double-blind, placebo-controlled, dose-escalation study. Int J Clin Pharmacol Ther 2013; 51(12): 911-23. [http://dx.doi.org/10.5414/CP201816]

[86] Wisniewski T, Goni F. Immunotherapy for Alzheimer's disease. Biochem Pharmacol 2014; 88(4): 499-507. [http://dx.doi.org/10.1016/j.bcp.2013.12.020]

[87] Kohyama K, Matsumoto Y. Alzheimer's disease and immunotherapy: what is wrong with clinical trials? ImmunoTargets Ther 2015; 4: 27.

[88] Aisen PS, Gauthier S, Vellas B, *et al.* Alzhemed: a potential treatment for Alzheimer's disease. Curr Alzheimer Res 2007; 4(4): 473-8. [http://dx.doi.org/10.2174/156720507781788882]

[89] Gervais F, Paquette J, Morissette C, *et al.* Targeting soluble Aβ peptide with Tramiprosate for the treatment of brain amyloidosis. Neurobiol Aging 2007; 28(4): 537-47. [http://dx.doi.org/10.1016/j.neurobiolaging.2006.02.015]

[90] Saumier D, Duong A, Haine D, Garceau D, Sampalis J. Domain-specific cognitive effects of tramiprosate in patients with mild to moderate Alzheimer's disease: ADAS-cog subscale results from the Alphase Study. JNHA-The Journal of Nutrition. Health and Aging 2009; 13(9): 808-12.

[91] Aisen PS, Gauthier S, Ferris SH, *et al.* Tramiprosate in mild-to-moderate Alzheimer's disease–a randomized, double-blind, placebo-controlled, multi-centre study (the Alphase Study). Archives of medical science. AMS 2011; 7(1): 102.

[92] Tanaka K, Takanaka S, Yoshida KI. A second-generation Bacillus cell factory for rare inositol production. Bioengineered 2014; 5(5): 331-4. [http://dx.doi.org/10.4161/bioe.29897]

[93] Ma K, Thomason LA, McLaurin J. Scyllo-inositol, preclinical, and clinical data for Alzheimer's disease. 2012.

[94] Salloway S, Sperling R, Keren R, *et al.* Scyllo-inositol, preclinical, and clinical data for Alzheimer's disease. In Advances in pharmacology 2012; 64: 177-212. Academic Press.

[95] Mandel SA, Amit T, Kalfon L, Reznichenko L, Weinreb O, Youdim MB. Cell signaling pathways and iron chelation in the neurorestorative activity of green tea polyphenols: special reference to epigallocatechin gallate (EGCG). J Alzheimers Dis 2008; 15(2): 211-22. [http://dx.doi.org/10.3233/JAD-2008-15207]

[96] Jelenković A, Jovanović MD, Stevanović I, *et al.* Influence of the green tea leaf extract on neurotoxicity of aluminium chloride in rats. Phytother Res 2014; 28(1): 82-7. [http://dx.doi.org/10.1002/ptr.4962]

[97] Sampson EL, Jenagaratnam L, McShane R. Metal protein attenuating compounds for the treatment of Alzheimer's dementia. Cochrane Database Syst Rev 2012; 5: CD005380.

[98] Adlard PA, Sedjahtera A, Gunawan L, *et al.* A novel approach to rapidly prevent age related cognitive decline. Aging Cell 2014; 13(2): 351-9. [http://dx.doi.org/10.1111/acel.12178]

[99] Adlard PA, Cherny RA, Finkelstein DI, *et al.* Rapid restoration of cognition in Alzheimer's transgenic mice with 8-hydroxy quinoline analogs is associated with decreased interstitial Aβ. Neuron 2008; 59(1): 43-55. [http://dx.doi.org/10.1016/j.neuron.2008.06.018]

[100] Galasko D, Bell J, Mancuso JY, *et al.* Clinical trial of an inhibitor of RAGE-Aβ interactions in Alzheimer disease. Neurology 2014; 82(17): 1536-42. [http://dx.doi.org/10.1212/WNL.0000000000000364]

[101] Habchi J, Arosio P, Perni M, *et al.* An anticancer drug suppresses the primary nucleation reaction that initiates the production of the toxic Aβ42 aggregates linked with Alzheimer's disease. Sci Adv 2016; 2(2): e1501244. [http://dx.doi.org/10.1126/sciadv.1501244]

[102] Matsuoka Y, Gray AJ, Hirata-Fukae C, *et al.* Intranasal NAP administration reduces accumulation of amyloid peptide and tau hyperphosphorylation in a transgenic mouse model of Alzheimer's disease at early pathological stage. J Mol Neurosci 2007; 31(2): 165-70.

[103] Kim D, Nguyen MD, Dobbin MM, *et al.* SIRT1 deacetylase protects against neurodegeneration in models for Alzheimer's disease and amyotrophic lateral sclerosis. EMBO J 2007; 26(13): 3169-79. [http://dx.doi.org/10.1038/sj.emboj.7601758]

[104] Kimura R, Ohno M. Impairments in remote memory stabilization precede hippocampal synaptic and cognitive failures in 5XFAD Alzheimer mouse model. Neurobiol Dis 2009; 33(2): 229-35.

[http://dx.doi.org/10.1016/j.nbd.2008.10.006]

[105] Paholikova K, Salingova B, Opattova A, *et al.* N-terminal truncation of microtubule associated protein tau dysregulates its cellular localization. J Alzheimers Dis 2015; 43(3): 915-26. [http://dx.doi.org/10.3233/JAD-140996]

[106] Theunis C, Crespo-Biel N, Gafner V, *et al.* Efficacy and safety of a liposome-based vaccine against protein Tau, assessed in tau. P301L mice that model tauopathy. PLoS One 2013; 8(8): e72301. [http://dx.doi.org/10.1371/journal.pone.0072301]

[107] Seripa D, Solfrizzi V, Imbimbo BP, *et al.* Tau-directed approaches for the treatment of Alzheimer's disease: focus on leuco-methylthioninium. Expert Rev Neurother 2016; 16(3): 259-77. [http://dx.doi.org/10.1586/14737175.2016.1140039]

[108] Wischik CM, Staff RT, Wischik DJ, *et al.* Tau aggregation inhibitor therapy: an exploratory phase 2 study in mild or moderate Alzheimer's disease. J Alzheimers Dis 2015; 44(2): 705-20. [http://dx.doi.org/10.3233/JAD-142874]

[109] Gauthier S, Feldman HH, Schneider LS, *et al.* Efficacy and safety of tau-aggregation inhibitor therapy in patients with mild or moderate Alzheimer's disease: a randomised, controlled, double-blind, parallel-arm, phase 3 trial. Lancet 2016; 388(10062): 2873-84. [http://dx.doi.org/10.1016/S0140-6736(16)31275-2]

[110] Rockenstein E, Torrance M, Adame A, *et al.* Neuroprotective effects of regulators of the glycogen synthase kinase-3β signaling pathway in a transgenic model of Alzheimer's disease are associated with reduced amyloid precursor protein phosphorylation. J Neurosci 2007; 27(8): 1981-91. [http://dx.doi.org/10.1523/JNEUROSCI.4321-06.2007]

[111] Domínguez JM, Fuertes A, Orozco L, del Monte-Millán M, Delgado E, Medina M. Evidence for the irreversible inhibition of glycogen synthase kinase-3β by tideglusib. Journal of Biological Chemistry. 2011; 18: jbc-M111.

[112] Lovestone S, Boada M, Dubois B, *et al.* A phase II trial of tideglusib in Alzheimer's disease. J Alzheimers Dis 2015; 45(1): 75-88. [http://dx.doi.org/10.3233/JAD-141959]

[113] Lad SP, Neet KE, Mufson EJ. Nerve growth factor: structure, function and therapeutic implications for Alzheimer's disease. Curr Drug Targets CNS Neurol Disord 2003; 2(5): 315-34. [http://dx.doi.org/10.2174/1568007033482724]

[114] Mandel RJ. CERE-110, an adeno-associated virus-based gene delivery vector expressing human nerve growth factor for the treatment of Alzheimer's disease. Curr Opin Mol Ther 2010; 12(2): 240-7.

[115] Rafii MS, Baumann TL, Bakay RA, *et al.* A phasel study of stereotactic gene delivery of AAV2-NGF for Alzheimer's disease. Alzheimers Dement 2014; 10(5): 571-81. [http://dx.doi.org/10.1016/j.jalz.2013.09.004]

[116] García-Escudero V, Martín-Maestro P, Perry G, Avila J. Deconstructing mitochondrial dysfunction in Alzheimer disease. Oxid Med Cell Longev 2013; 2013: 162152. [http://dx.doi.org/10.1155/2013/162152] [PMID: 23840916]

[117] Wang X, Wang W, Li L, Perry G, Lee HG, Zhu X. Oxidative stress and mitochondrial dysfunction in Alzheimer's disease. Biochimica et Biophysica Acta (BBA)-. Molecular Basis of Disease 2014; 1842(8): 1240-7. [http://dx.doi.org/10.1016/j.bbadis.2013.10.015]

[118] Eckert SH, Eckmann J, Renner K, Eckert GP, Leuner K, Muller WE. Dimebon ameliorates amyloid-β induced impairments of mitochondrial form and function. J Alzheimers Dis 2012; 31(1): 21-32. [http://dx.doi.org/10.3233/JAD-2012-120310]

[119] Perez SE, Nadeem M, Sadleir KR, *et al.* Dimebon alters hippocampal amyloid pathology in 3xTg-AD mice. Int J Physiol Pathophysiol Pharmacol 2012; 4(3): 115.

[120] Sabbagh MN, Shill HA. Latrepirdine, a potential novel treatment for Alzheimer's disease and Huntington's chorea. Curr Opin Investig Drugs 2010; 11(1): 80.

[121] Sleigh SH, Barton CL. Repurposing strategies for therapeutics. Pharmaceut Med 2010; 24(3): 151-9. [http://dx.doi.org/10.1007/BF03256811]

[122] Heneka MT, O'Banion MK. Inflammatory processes in Alzheimer's disease. J Neuroimmunol 2007; 184(1): 69-91. [http://dx.doi.org/10.1016/j.jneuroim.2006.11.017]

[123] Strachan MW, Reynolds RM, Marioni RE, Price JF. Cognitive function, dementia and type 2 diabetes mellitus in the elderly. Nat Rev Endocrinol 2011; 7(2): 108. [http://dx.doi.org/10.1038/nrendo.2010.228]

[124] Drochioiu G, Tudorachi L, Murariu M. NOSH aspirin may have a protective role in Alzheimer's disease. Med Hypotheses 2015; 84(3): 262-7. [http://dx.doi.org/10.1016/j.mehy.2015.01.008]

[125] Coma M, Sereno L, Da Rocha-Souto B, *et al.* Triflusal reduces dense-core plaque load, associated axonal alterations and inflammatory changes, and rescues cognition in a transgenic mouse model of Alzheimer's disease. Neurobiol Dis 2010; 38(3): 482-91. [http://dx.doi.org/10.1016/j.nbd.2010.01.019]

[126] Frautschy SA. Thinking outside the box about COX-1 in Alzheimer's disease. Neurobiol Dis 2010; 38(3): 492-4. [http://dx.doi.org/10.1016/j.nbd.2010.02.009]

[127] Valle M, Barbanoj MJ, Donner A, *et al.* Access of HTB, main metabolite of triflusal, to cerebrospinal fluid in healthy volunteers. Eur J Clin Pharmacol 2005; 61(2): 103-11. [http://dx.doi.org/10.1007/s00228-004-0887-0]

[128] Hirohata M, Ono K, Naiki H, Yamada M. Non-steroidal anti-inflammatory drugs have anti-amyloidogenic effects for Alzheimer's β-amyloid fibrils in vitro. Neuropharmacology 2005; 49(7): 1088-99. [http://dx.doi.org/10.1016/j.neuropharm.2005.07.004]

[129] Rich JB, Rasmusson DX, Folstein MF, Carson KA, Kawas C, Brandt J. Nonsteroidal anti-inflammatory drugs in Alzheimer's disease. Neurology 1995; 45(1): 51-5. [http://dx.doi.org/10.1212/WNL.45.1.51]

[130] Manev H, Chen H, Dzitoyeva S, Manev R. Cyclooxygenases and 5-lipoxygenase in Alzheimer's disease. Prog Neuropsychopharmacol Biol Psychiatry 2011; 35(2): 315-9. [http://dx.doi.org/10.1016/j.pnpbp.2010.07.032]

[131] Tabet N, Feldmand H. Ibuprofen for Alzheimer's disease. Cochrane Database Syst Rev 2003; 2.

[132] Mandal S, Mandal SD, Chuttani K, Sawant KK, Subudhi BB. Neuroprotective effect of ibuprofen by intranasal application of mucoadhesive nanoemulsion in MPTP induced Parkinson model. J Pharm Investig 2016; 46(1): 41-53. [http://dx.doi.org/10.1007/s40005-015-0212-1]

[133] Sahoo SP, Subudhi BB, Swain R. Synthesis and Evaluation of antioxidant and anti-inflammatory activity of Conjugates of Amino Acids with N-Aroyl-N, N′-Dicyclohexyl Urea. Asian J Res Chem 2011; 4(9): 1485-8.

[134] Abdullah R, Basak I, Patil KS, Alves G, Larsen JP, Moller SG. Parkinson's disease and age: the obvious but largely unexplored link. Exp Gerontol 2015; 68: 33-8. [http://dx.doi.org/10.1016/j.exger.2014.09.014]

[135] Kalra J, Kumar P, Majeed AB, Prakash A. Modulation of LOX and COX pathways via inhibition of amyloidogenesis contributes to mitoprotection against β-amyloid oligomer-induced toxicity in an animal model of Alzheimer's disease in rats. Pharmacol Biochem Behav 2016; 146: 1-2.

[http://dx.doi.org/10.1016/j.pbb.2016.04.002]

[136] Rozin SI. Case Series Using Montelukast in Patients with Memory Loss and Dementia. Open Neurol J 2017; 11: 7.
[http://dx.doi.org/10.2174/1874205X01711010007]

[137] Pernomian L, Pernomian L, Baraldi Araújo Restini C. Counter-regulatory effects played by the ACE-Ang II-AT1 and ACE2-Ang-(1-7)-Mas axes on the reactive oxygen species-mediated control of vascular function: perspectives to pharmacological approaches in controlling vascular complications. Vasa 2014; 43(6): 404-14.
[http://dx.doi.org/10.1024/0301-1526/a000387]

[138] Zhang F, Liu C, Wang L, Cao X, Wang YY, Yang JK. Antioxidant effect of angiotensin (1 7) in the protection of pancreatic β cell function. Mol Med Rep 2016; 14(3): 1963-9.
[http://dx.doi.org/10.3892/mmr.2016.5514]

[139] Singh N, Joshi S, Guo L, *et al.* ACE2/Ang-(1–7)/Mas axis stimulates vascular repair-relevant functions of CD34+ cells. Am J Physiol Heart Circ Physiol 2015; 309(10): H1697-707.
[http://dx.doi.org/10.1152/ajpheart.00854.2014]

[140] Brenner BM, Cooper ME, De Zeeuw D, *et al.* Effects of losartan on renal and cardiovascular outcomes in patients with type 2 diabetes and nephropathy. N Engl J Med 2001; 345(12): 861-9.
[http://dx.doi.org/10.1056/NEJMoa011161]

[141] Roncevic D. Does angiotensin II cross the blood–brain barrier? Hypertens Res 2012; 35(7): 775.
[http://dx.doi.org/10.1038/hr.2012.55]

[142] Biancardi VC, Son SJ, Ahmadi S, Filosa JA, Stern JE. Circulating angiotensin II gains access to the hypothalamus and brain stem during hypertension *via* breakdown of the blood–brain barrier. Hypertension. 2013; 1: hypertensionaha-113.

[143] Baltatu OC, Campos LA, Bader M. Local renin–angiotensin system and the brain—a continuous quest for knowledge. Peptides 2011; 32(5): 1083-6.
[http://dx.doi.org/10.1016/j.peptides.2011.02.008]

[144] Takeda S, Sato N, Ogihara T, Morishita R. The renin-angiotensin system, hypertension and cognitive dysfunction in Alzheimer's disease: new therapeutic potential. Front Biosci 2008; 13: 2253-65.
[http://dx.doi.org/10.2741/2839]

[145] Singh B, Sharma B, Jaggi AS, Singh N. Attenuating effect of lisinopril and telmisartan in intracerebroventricular streptozotocin induced experimental dementia of Alzheimer's disease type: possible involvement of PPAR-γ agonistic property. J Renin Angiotensin Aldosterone Syst 2013; 14(2): 124-36.
[http://dx.doi.org/10.1177/1470320312459977]

[146] Oliveira FFD, Bertolucci PH, Chen ES, Smith MC. Brain-penetrating angiotensin-converting enzyme inhibitors and cognitive change in patients with dementia due to Alzheimer's disease. J Alzheimers Dis 2014; 42(s3): S321-4.
[http://dx.doi.org/10.3233/JAD-132189]

[147] Solfrizzi V, Scafato E, Frisardi V, *et al.* Angiotensin-converting enzyme inhibitors and incidence of mild cognitive impairment. The Italian Longitudinal Study on Aging. Age (Dordr) 2013; 35(2): 441-53.
[http://dx.doi.org/10.1007/s11357-011-9360-z]

[148] O'Caoimh R, Healy L, Gao Y, *et al.* Effects of centrally acting angiotensin converting enzyme inhibitors on functional decline in patients with Alzheimer's disease. J Alzheimers Dis 2014; 40(3): 595-603.
[http://dx.doi.org/10.3233/JAD-131694]

[149] Wang J, Ho L, Chen L, *et al.* Valsartan lowers brain β-amyloid protein levels and improves spatial learning in a mouse model of Alzheimer disease. J Clin Invest 2007; 117(11): 3393-402.

[http://dx.doi.org/10.1172/JCI31547]

[150] Danielyan L, Klein R, Hanson LR, *et al.* Protective effects of intranasal losartan in the APP/PS1 transgenic mouse model of Alzheimer disease. Rejuvenation Res 2010; 13(2-3): 195-201. [http://dx.doi.org/10.1089/rej.2009.0944]

[151] Matzke A, Sargsyan V, Holtmann B, *et al.* Haploinsufficiency of c-Met in cd44−/− mice identifies a collaboration of CD44 and c-Met in vivo. Mol Cell Biol 2007; 27(24): 8797-806. [http://dx.doi.org/10.1128/MCB.01355-07]

[152] Mertens B, Vanderheyden P, Michotte Y, Sarre S. The role of the central renin-angiotensin system in Parkinson's disease. J Renin Angiotensin Aldosterone Syst 2010; 11(1): 49-56. [http://dx.doi.org/10.1177/1470320309347789]

[153] Wright JW, Harding JW. Brain renin-angiotensin—a new look at an old system. Prog Neurobiol 2011; 95(1): 49-67. [http://dx.doi.org/10.1016/j.pneurobio.2011.07.001]

[154] Wright JW, Harding JW. The brain renin–angiotensin system: a diversity of functions and implications for CNS diseases. Pflugers Arch 2013; 465(1): 133-51. [http://dx.doi.org/10.1007/s00424-012-1102-2]

[155] Gibson W, Gunter P. Eckert Urule Igbavboa and Walter E. Müller. Statins and neuroprotection: a prescription to move the field forward. Ann N Y Acad Sci 2010; 1199: 69-76. [http://dx.doi.org/10.1111/j.1749-6632.2009.05359.x]

[156] Pedrini S, Carter TL, Prendergast G, Petanceska S, Ehrlich ME, Gandy S. Modulation of statin-activated shedding of Alzheimer APP ectodomain by ROCK. PLoS Med 2005; 2(1): e18. [http://dx.doi.org/10.1371/journal.pmed.0020018]

[157] Koudinov AR, Berezov TT. Cholesterol, statins, and Alzheimer disease. PLoS Med 2005; 2(3): e81. [http://dx.doi.org/10.1371/journal.pmed.0020081]

[158] Geifman N, Brinton RD, Kennedy RE, Schneider LS, Butte AJ. Evidence for benefit of statins to modify cognitive decline and risk in Alzheimer's disease. Alzheimers Res Ther 2017; 9(1): 10. [http://dx.doi.org/10.1186/s13195-017-0237-y]

[159] Najem D, Bamji-Mirza M, Yang Z, Zhang W. Aβ-induced insulin resistance and the effects of insulin on the cholesterol synthesis pathway and Aβ secretion in neural cells. Neurosci Bull 2016; 32(3): 227-38. [http://dx.doi.org/10.1007/s12264-016-0034-9]

[160] Chen Y, Zhou K, Wang R, *et al.* Antidiabetic drug metformin (GlucophageR) increases biogenesis of Alzheimer's amyloid peptides via up-regulating BACE1 transcription. Proc Natl Acad Sci USA 2009; 106(10): 3907-12. [http://dx.doi.org/10.1073/pnas.0807991106]

[161] Chen S, Liu AR, An FM, Yao WB, Gao XD. Amelioration of neurodegenerative changes in cellular and rat models of diabetes-related Alzheimer's disease by exendin-4. Age (Dordr) 2012; 34(5): 1211-24. [http://dx.doi.org/10.1007/s11357-011-9303-8]

[162] Kim HS, Suh YH. Minocycline and neurodegenerative diseases. Behav Brain Res 2009; 196(2): 168-79. [http://dx.doi.org/10.1016/j.bbr.2008.09.040]

[163] Imfeld P, Bodmer M, Jick SS, Meier CR. Metformin, Other Antidiabetic Drugs, and Risk of Alzheimer's Disease: A Population based Case–Control Study. J Am Geriatr Soc 2012; 60(5): 916-21. [http://dx.doi.org/10.1111/j.1532-5415.2012.03916.x]

[164] Choi JS, Islam MN, Ali MY, Kim EJ, Kim YM, Jung HA. Effects of C-glycosylation on anti-diabetic, anti-Alzheimer's disease and anti-inflammatory potential of apigenin. Food Chem Toxicol 2014; 64: 27-33.

[http://dx.doi.org/10.1016/j.fct.2013.11.020]

[165] Kapogiannis D, Mattson MP. Disrupted energy metabolism and neuronal circuit dysfunction in cognitive impairment and Alzheimer's disease. Lancet Neurol 2011; 10(2): 187-98. [http://dx.doi.org/10.1016/S1474-4422(10)70277-5]

[166] Bomfim TR, Forny-Germano L, Sathler LB, *et al.* An anti-diabetes agent protects the mouse brain from defective insulin signaling caused by Alzheimer's disease–associated Aβ oligomers. J Clin Invest 2012; 122(4): 1339-53. [http://dx.doi.org/10.1172/JCI57256]

[167] Miller BW, Willett KC, Desilets AR. Rosiglitazone and pioglitazone for the treatment of Alzheimer's disease. Ann Pharmacother 2011; 45(11): 1416-24. [http://dx.doi.org/10.1345/aph.1Q238]

[168] Dysken MW, Sano M, Asthana S, *et al.* Effect of vitamin E and memantine on functional decline in Alzheimer disease: the TEAM-AD VA cooperative randomized trial. JAMA 2014; 311(1): 33-44. [http://dx.doi.org/10.1001/jama.2013.282834]

[169] Klatte ET, Scharre DW, Nagaraja HN, Davis RA, Beversdorf DQ. Combination therapy of donepezil and vitamin E in Alzheimer disease. Alzheimer Dis Assoc Disord 2003; 17(2): 113-6. [http://dx.doi.org/10.1097/00002093-200304000-00010]

[170] Littlejohns TJ, Henley WE, Lang IA, *et al.* Vitamin D and the risk of dementia and Alzheimer disease. Neurology 2014; 83(10): 920-8. [http://dx.doi.org/10.1212/WNL.0000000000000755]

[171] Schlogl M, Holick MF. Vitamin D and neurocognitive function. Clin Interv Aging 2014; 9: 559.

[172] Holick MF. Sunlight, Ultraviolet Radiation, Vitamin D and Skin Cancer.Sunlight, Vitamin D and Skin Cancer. New York, NY: Springer 2014; pp. 1-16. [http://dx.doi.org/10.1007/978-1-4939-0437-2_1]

[173] Annweiler C, Karras SN, Anagnostis P, Beauchet O. Vitamin D supplements: a novel therapeutic approach for Alzheimer patients. Front Pharmacol 2014; 5: 6. [http://dx.doi.org/10.3389/fphar.2014.00006]

[174] Shen L, Ji HF. Vitamin D deficiency is associated with increased risk of Alzheimer's disease and dementia: evidence from meta-analysis. Nutr J 2015; 14(1): 76. [http://dx.doi.org/10.1186/s12937-015-0063-7]

[175] Landel V, Millet P, Baranger K, Loriod B, Féron F. Vitamin D interacts with Esr1 and Igf1 to regulate molecular pathways relevant to Alzheimer's disease. Mol Neurodegener 2016; 11(1): 22. [http://dx.doi.org/10.1186/s13024-016-0087-2]

[176] Taylor CP, Traynelis SF, Siffert J, Pope LE, Matsumoto RR. Pharmacology of dextromethorphan: Relevance to dextromethorphan/quinidine (Nuedexta®) clinical use. Pharmacol Ther 2016; 164: 170-82. [http://dx.doi.org/10.1016/j.pharmthera.2016.04.010]

[177] http: //axsome.com/axs-05/agitation-in-patients-with-alzheimers-disease-ad/

[178] https: //www.alzforum.org/therapeutics/avp-786

[179] Athanasopoulos D, Karagiannis G, Tsolaki M. Recent findings in Alzheimer disease and nutrition focusing on epigenetics. Adv Nutr 2016; 7(5): 917-27. [http://dx.doi.org/10.3945/an.116.012229]

[180] Marcade M, Bourdin J, Loiseau N, *et al.* Etazolate, a neuroprotective drug linking GABAA receptor pharmacology to amyloid precursor protein processing. J Neurochem 2008; 106(1): 392-404. [http://dx.doi.org/10.1111/j.1471-4159.2008.05396.x]

[181] Wang Y, Lin SZ, Chiou AL, Williams LR, Hoffer BJ. Glial cell line-derived neurotrophic factor protects against ischemia-induced injury in the cerebral cortex. J Neurosci 1997; 17(11): 4341-8.

[http://dx.doi.org/10.1523/JNEUROSCI.17-11-04341.1997]

[182] Rodríguez JJ, Noristani HN, Verkhratsky A. The serotonergic system in ageing and Alzheimer's disease. Prog Neurobiol 2012; 99(1): 15-41. [http://dx.doi.org/10.1016/j.pneurobio.2012.06.010]

[183] Andrews M, Tousi B, Sabbagh MN. 5HT6 Antagonists in the Treatment of Alzheimer's Dementia: Current Progress. Neurol Ther 2018; 1: 1-8.

[184] Diana G, Malloni M, Pieri M. Effects of the synthetic cannabinoid nabilone on spatial learning and hippocampal neurotransmission. Pharmacol Biochem Behav 2003; 75(3): 585-91. [http://dx.doi.org/10.1016/S0091-3057(03)00127-8]

[185] Volicer L, Stelly M, Morris J. McLAUGHLIN JO, Volicer BJ. Effects of dronabinol on anorexia and disturbed behavior in patients with Alzheimer's disease. Int J Geriatr Psychiatry 1997; 12(9): 913-9. [http://dx.doi.org/10.1002/(SICI)1099-1166(199709)12:9<913::AID-GPS663>3.0.CO;2-D]

[186] Lakhan SE, Caro M, Hadzimichalis N. NMDA receptor activity in neuropsychiatric disorders. Front Psychiatry 2013; 4: 52. [http://dx.doi.org/10.3389/fpsyt.2013.00052]

[187] Moschetti V, Desch M, Goetz S, *et al.* Safety, tolerability and pharmacokinetics of oral BI 425809, a glycine transporter 1 inhibitor, in healthy male volunteers: a partially randomised, single-blind, placebo-controlled, first-in-human study. Eur J Drug Metab Pharmacokinet 2018; 43(2): 239-49. [http://dx.doi.org/10.1007/s13318-017-0440-z]

[188] Lipartiti M, Franceschini D, Zanoni R, *et al.* Neuroprotective effects of melatonin.Recent Advances in Tryptophan Research. Boston, MA: Springer 1996; pp. 315-21. [http://dx.doi.org/10.1007/978-1-4613-0381-7_49]

[189] Shukla M, Govitrapong P, Boontem P, Reiter RJ, Satayavivad J. Mechanisms of melatonin in alleviating Alzheimer's disease. Curr Neuropharmacol 2017; 15(7): 1010-31. [http://dx.doi.org/10.2174/1570159X15666170313123454]

[190] Diomede L, Cassata G, Fiordaliso F, *et al.* Tetracycline and its analogues protect Caenorhabditis elegans from β amyloid-induced toxicity by targeting oligomers. Neurobiol Dis 2010; 40(2): 424-31. [http://dx.doi.org/10.1016/j.nbd.2010.07.002]

[191] Choi Y, Kim HS, Shin KY, *et al.* Minocycline attenuates neuronal cell death and improves cognitive impairment in Alzheimer's disease models. Neuropsychopharmacology 2007; 32(11): 2393. [http://dx.doi.org/10.1038/sj.npp.1301377]

[192] Kim S, Moon M, Park S. Exendin-4 protects dopaminergic neurons by inhibition of microglial activation and matrix metalloproteinase-3 expression in an animal model of Parkinson's disease. J Endocrinol 2009; 202(3): 431-9. [http://dx.doi.org/10.1677/JOE-09-0132]

[193] Mehla J. Repurposing clinically used antibiotics for the treatment of Alzheimer's disease. J Pharmacol Rep 2017; 2: e102.

[194] Forloni G, Colombo L, Girola L, Tagliavini F, Salmona M. Anti□amyloidogenic activity of tetracyclines: studies in vitro. FEBS Lett 2001; 487(3): 404-7. [http://dx.doi.org/10.1016/S0014-5793(00)02380-2]

[195] Plane JM, Shen Y, Pleasure DE, Deng W. Prospects for minocycline neuroprotection. Arch Neurol 2010; 67(12): 1442-8. [http://dx.doi.org/10.1001/archneurol.2010.191]

[196] Budni JL, Garcez M, Medeiros JD, *et al.* The anti-inflammatory role of minocycline in Alzheimer s disease. Curr Alzheimer Res 2016; 13(12): 1319-29. [http://dx.doi.org/10.2174/1567205013666160819124206]

[197] Forlenza OV, Diniz BS, Radanovic M, Santos FS, Talib LL, Gattaz WF. Disease-modifying properties

of long-term lithium treatment for amnestic mild cognitive impairment: randomised controlled trial. Br J Psychiatry 2011; 198(5): 351-6.
[http://dx.doi.org/10.1192/bjp.bp.110.080044]

[198] Forlenza OV, de Paula VJ, Machado-Vieira R, Diniz BS, Gattaz WF. Does lithium prevent Alzheimer's disease? Drugs Aging 2012; 29(5): 335-42.
[http://dx.doi.org/10.2165/11599180-000000000-00000]

[199] Macdonald A, Briggs K, Poppe M, Higgins A, Velayudhan L, Lovestone S. A feasibility and tolerability study of lithium in Alzheimer's disease International Journal of Geriatric Psychiatry: A journal of the psychiatry of late life and allied sciences 2008; 23(7): 704-11.

[200] Qing H, He G, Ly PT, *et al.* Valproic acid inhibits Aβ production, neuritic plaque formation, and behavioral deficits in Alzheimer's disease mouse models. J Exp Med 2008; 205(12): 2781-9.
[http://dx.doi.org/10.1084/jem.20081588]

[201] Oz M, Lorke DE, Petroianu GA. Methylene blue and Alzheimer's disease. Biochem Pharmacol 2009; 78(8): 927-32.
[http://dx.doi.org/10.1016/j.bcp.2009.04.034]

[202] Graham AJ, Martin-Ruiz CM, Teaktong T, Ray MA. Human brain nicotinic receptors, their distribution and participation in neuropsychiatric disorders. Curr Drug Targets CNS Neurol Disord 2002; 1(4): 387-97.
[http://dx.doi.org/10.2174/1568007023339283]

[203] Wilson AL, Langley LK, Monley J, *et al.* Nicotine patches in Alzheimer's disease: pilot study on learning, memory, and safety. Pharmacol Biochem Behav 1995; 51(2-3): 509-14.
[http://dx.doi.org/10.1016/0091-3057(95)00043-V]

[204] Lopez Arrieta J, Sanz FJ. Nicotine for Alzheimer's disease. Cochrane Libr 2001.

[205] Rezvani AH, Levin ED. Cognitive effects of nicotine. Biol Psychiatry 2001; 49(3): 258-67.
[http://dx.doi.org/10.1016/S0006-3223(00)01094-5]

SUBJECT INDEX

A

B

C

D

E

F

M

N

O

P

Q

R

S

T

U

V

W

www.ingramcontent.com/pod-product-compliance
Lightning Source LLC
LaVergne TN
LVHW070948210926
848482LV00002B/143